# What Medical Professio...
## MOUTH M......

The sad news is that "real doctors" and medical students are likely to skip this book, sure they "already know" everything they need to ... and they would be WRONG! Our medical/illness system fails to teach – and almost always fails to treat – the root causes of many illnesses, even though they have been clearly identified in the scientific literature.

In this incredible book, noted author Carol Vander Stoep has done a masterful job of weaving together the concepts of "biological medicine" (going beyond using lab tests and complaints, to treat each person in all dimensions) and "biological dentistry" (dentistry practiced far beyond the "drill, fill, and bill" patchwork approach of past eras). As we learn more about the fields of pathophysiology, we will ever more appreciate the interconnections of hormones, immunity, infections, inflammation, metabolism, cell functions and division, and toxic chemicals and metals, as these all relate to failing health. This book charts an easy path for readers to more fully appreciate what we know now – and especially what actions we can take each day to help restore and preserve more robust health.

*Mouth Matters* is a "made simple" guide, one that should be read by every parent hoping to lead their children toward natural healing and away from an expectation of illness, medications, and surgery. While the sad news is that it is less likely to be on your doctor's bookshelf, the good news is it will be a treasured reference in many homes... and hopefully available in most dental offices.

Are you ready for a primer that makes modern medical and dental discoveries clearly within your reach, that shows you how small adjustments in your lifestyle can reap huge rewards? Then *Mouth Matters* is for you, right now! And strangely enough(?) this should be a gift you share with family and friends, to open for them the prospect of fewer pharmaceutical drugs, a lower likelihood of operations, only occasional doctor visits ... and the blessings of better health!

*John Parks Trowbridge M.D., FACAM*
*President, International Academy of Biological Dentistry and Medicine*
*Diplomate and Secretary to the Board of Directors of the American*
*    Board of Clinical Metal Toxicology*
*Co-author, The Yeast Syndrome*

Carol's book is eye opening for even the most conventional healthcare provider. Look at her information on nursing homes and reduction of pneumonia and flu. After reading her book I commented several times that every hospital and nursing home should employ a dental hygienist to assist patients in oral hygiene. Just imagine the impact if we could reduce secondary infections in coma patients, stroke patients etc. She is an inspiration!

*Dawn Ewing*
*Doctor of Integrative Medicine*

Carol comes from a unique position, in that she addresses very complex subject matter. She researches, understands, applies to clinical practice, and then writes about various topics. This allows her to present subjects in a way a layperson can comprehend and apply, greatly shortening their learning curve.

I strongly recommend this book as an easy path for any health professional who wants to become current in the fast evolving field of oral systemic health. The knowledge gained from her creation will also allow health professionals to better explain the connection and interactions between oral health and systemic health to the most important persons in our professional lives, our patients who are entrusting their health to our skills and knowledge.

*J Tim Rainey, DDS, MAGD*

Carol has that rare quality of coupling years of extensive hands-on experience with easy to understand scientific backing. This book brings years of important research to the forefront, allowing readers to understand the truth about dental health and the dangers of dental materials that are otherwise considered "everyday tools." The information in this book should not be taken lightly, but rather shared with others in the hope that change can happen when enough people make their voices heard.

*Griffin Cole, DDS, NMD, IBDM, FIAOMT*

You really amaze me. I can't believe your broad range of knowledge and comprehension. You have put together a masterpiece! Very few dentists could assemble the information with the clarity and cohesiveness that you have accomplished. If only all health care practitioners could read and absorb 1/4 of the information presented, health care would be forever altered for the better. Thank you for your excellence and dedication.

*John Laughlin III, D.D.S.*

Carol Vander Stoep has written 'the' definitive book, *Mouth Matters*, on oral-systemic connections and what the public can do to stay healthy. Yet this book is not for the public only, most health care professionals can learn from it too. Former Surgeon General C. Everett Koop, M.D., has often said, "You are not healthy without good oral health." Oral infections have systemic implications and systemic conditions have a reciprocal impact on oral health. Carol's wonderful book is a great textbook that is not meant to be read linearly, rather it truly becomes a 'go-to' resource to find answers on the oral connections with the heart, diabetes, sex hormones, osteoporosis and much more.

The real power of this work is Carol's book is its timely, accurate information written in a way readily accessible to most any reader. Carol is truly at the leading edge of this evolving field. This book takes philosophy into practical advice and is a must read for anyone looking to be healthy.

*Patti DiGangi, RDH, ADA Evidence-Based Champion, certified AGD presenter for Periodontal Disease*

Carol Vander Stoep's latest offering *Mouth Matters*, addresses oral and oral/systemic issues in a clear and comprehendible manner. The chapter on ozone therapy is very timely, as it addresses the most important paradigm shift to occur in dentistry in the last 60 years. This book is a must read for dentists, dental staff and patients.

*Robert E. Harris, Jr. DMD, NMD, IBDM*
*Co-founder American College of Integrative Medicine and Dentistry*

*Mouth Matters* belongs in the library of all dental professionals who want to be on the edge of the newly emerging science of the oral-systemic connection. Carol manages to explain things in accessible English so that this easily digested text can be shared with patients and staff alike.

*William C. Domb, DMD*
*Founding Board Member*
*American Academy for Oral Systemic Health*

*Mouth Matters* needs to be part of every dental school curriculum; it should be required reading for every mother... You have brought together some really great things I've never seen in print before.

*William Hang, DDS, MSD*
*American Association of Physiological Medicine and Dentistry*
*American Academy of Craniofacial Pain*
*North American Association of Facial Orthotropics®*
*International Association of Facial Growth Guidance*

## What Consumers are Saying About:
## *MOUTH MATTERS*

Thank you, Carol, for opening my eyes to the reasons why what we put in our bodies has such a direct impact on our health. For me specifically, gum disease has had wide ramifications. I am a 53 year old carpenter with a decent work ethic who unfortunately spent thirty years making some bad choices. Smoking one to two packs of cigarettes per day, consuming sugar, the wrong fats, and processed foods by the ton are examples. I have been battling gum disease for many years. I have spent thousands of dollars on gum treatments, extractions, and antibiotics with limited success. Until I met Carol and read her book I had no idea what exactly I was doing to myself, so much so that a few years prior I had a heart attack. My doctors attributed this solely to smoking. I learned otherwise as I became more educated about inflammation, plaque, consequences of poor dietary choices, etc. Carol's straightforward no-nonsense attention to my specific case has given me understandable guidance and positive results I am thankful for. I believe her unorthodox use of ozone has allowed me to keep my teeth. Needless to say my wife is happy, too. My hope is more dental professionals will adopt the procedures and practices that Carol has so well researched, studied and implemented. They are making a difference in people's lives... Thanks again to Carol. Sounds corny, but you are my hero. Keep it up, don't give up.

*C.K. Brazil*

I'm not done reading the whole book yet, however I do want to say I ended up putting my highlighter away since it seems to me that almost everything Carol writes needs to be highlighted, if you know what I mean. She gets right to the point with very useful information. I am enjoying this book because she reinforces what I already believe from lots of research, and then she adds even more information about each subject. So much I didn't know. So much I wanted to learn about! Very fortunate to learn about her through Dr. Mercola's site.

*Mari C.*

I'm not a doctor and I'm not a scientist, but I do have a brain and can discern Vander Stoep's approach makes sense! What we put into our body matters, and how we use our body matters. If we're using our mouths to do something another organ (our nose) was specifically designed for, (breathing), then yeah, we're gonna have problems! I so appreciate Carol's honest approach at sharing what she's learned.

*Jennifer R.*

*~ We inherit mechanisms, not outcomes.*
*~ All medicine should be about curing disease,*
*not just treating symptoms.*

# Mouth Matters
## Healthy Mouth
## Healthy Body

### How Your Mouth Ages Your Body and What You Can Do About It

*Revised Second Edition*

*I am a teacher; you are your own doctor.*

*To your best health!*
*Warm regards,*
*Carol Vander Stoep*

# Mouth Matters
## Healthy Mouth
## Healthy Body

**How Your Mouth Ages Your Body and What
You Can Do About It**

*Revised Second Edition*

## Carol Vander Stoep, RDH, BSDH

*"The most beautiful woman who's got my name written all over
her,
if she opens her mouth and smells like a truck driver ...
I'm out of there. Gone.*

*It always struck me (as) bizarre that women are willing to
paint their mouths beautifully with lipstick and
yet smoke and drink and make their breath smell like
a garbage heap."* [i]

**~ Gene Simmons of the rock band, KISS ~**

IANUA PUBLISHING
Austin, Texas

Mouth Matters: Healthy Mouth/Healthy Body by Carol Vander Stoep
Includes sources, glossary, appendices, and index
www.mouthmattersbook.com

ISBN: 978-0-9825869-0-7

Second Edition Copyright © 2011 by Ianua Publishing
Revised 2013

Address all inquiries to:
Ianua Publishing
P.O. Box 1403
Dripping Springs, TX  78620
www.mouthmattersbook.com

Printed in the United States of America at Lightning Source

Front cover design and graphics by Joe Peterson

All information herein is based on the author's extensive professional experience
and research. The author/publisher believes this information should be available.
It is designed to help you make informed decisions about your health and to help
you become a wise consumer. It is not intended as a substitute for any treatment
prescribed by your health care provider. There are a wide variety of individual
treatment options within all medical traditions. You should consult with a health
care provider for co-diagnosis and collaborative treatment. Neither the publisher
nor author is responsible for any adverse effects or consequences resulting from
the use of the suggestions or procedures discussed in this book.

Products, including vitamins, minerals and other dietary supplements, and any
claims made about those products throughout this book have not been evaluated
by the United States Food and Drug Administration and are not intended to diagnose, treat, cure or prevent disease.

For volume sales, consulting, or speaking engagements contact Carol Vander
Stoep: Carol@mouthmattersbook.com

*To my children, Tamara and Marina Zoch,
whose patience, support, and love, made this book possible,
and whose philosophical discussions concerning its content
made its production a pure joy.*

---

*Also to present and former clients. You helped
me realize how eager people are to receive this information.
You also generously shared your experiences
so I in turn, could share.*

# HONORING

This book was written in the hope future generations will be healthier – and more enlightened than my generation.

I am indebted to the many people whose stories grace the pages of this book. I hope they know their personal journeys inspire others. I am fortunate to live in Austin, a town of open minds, open hearts, and a vast interest in health.

I particularly honor my children, Marina and Tamara. Preparing this manuscript stole more precious family time from them than any of us would have liked, yet they remain supportive. I am grateful to have had the opportunity to discuss with them the ethics and values involved in developing the contents. I learned these amazing young women do not hesitate to make difficult philosophical decisions when security and economics vie for their perception of truth. I will always be proud of them.

I honor all practices that value prevention, early intervention, and an expansive view of health. This way of practicing requires courage and dedication. I appreciate the lifetime work of doctors such as Tim Rainey, Graeme Milicich, Brian Palmer, Chris Norton, John Mew, William Hang and so many others. Their professional passion shows in the development of their ideas and their willingness to share for the benefit of the public.

Casey Hein, a primary force behind the move to disseminate and implement what we know about oral-systemic medicine to practitioners throughout the United States and Canada, deserves special acknowledgement. She took the time from her diverse professional pursuits to review this manuscript and encourage its publication. Christine Nathe, Graduate Program Director at the University of New Mexico, provided the initial inspiration.

Joe Peterson offered invaluable personal support, technical assistance, graphic art abilities, and photographic skills for which I am appreciative.

I acknowledge those many visionaries in the professional dental world who strive to study, advocate for, and implement biological dentistry – those who understand that their work lies within the context of a larger framework – the entire human body.

I respect doctors Robert Harris, Phil Mollica, and Charles Reufenacht, who have a particularly good grasp on whole body wellness and who have developed novel modalities for restoring optimal health.

I particularly appreciate Dr. Griffin Cole, who first helped me feel comfortable with publicly expressing alternative viewpoints about mercury and fluoride toxicity. Dr. Hardy Limeback, Head of Preventive Dentistry at the University of Toronto, and Charles Brown, attorney for Consumers for Dental Choice also generously provided time and insight on these difficult subjects.

Meeting Tim Rainey was an excellent byproduct of having written the first edition of *Mouth Matters*. Being introduced to his life's work was mind altering. The offer to share his work, which dovetails beautifully with oral/systemic health, is a priceless gift to us all. When prevention fails, what Dr. Rainey observed and he, Dr. Alleman, Pascal Magne and others subsequently developed, must change how we treat the resulting damaged teeth. Rather than using 150-year-old techniques that doom teeth to expensive, uncomfortable, and repetitive failure, their methods preserve the structural strength of teeth. Lower lifetime costs and improved comfort, oral, and general health result. Chapter Thirteen, reviewing Minimally Invasive Dentistry, is worth your investment of time and resources in this book.

The same could be said for Chapter Twelve regarding respiration, pH, and "growing attractive faces" reflecting the work of Brian Palmer, John Mew, William Hang, Patrick McKeown, Joy Moeller and many others.

Last, I may not have completed this book without Ty Fain's encouragement, wise advice, and strong support. He always believed this work had enormous value and hoped, as I do, that it will not only bring health to those who can read and implement its simple suggestions, but that it will spur these people to work for the professional and political changes that can transform the health of those who can't.

# CONTENTS

# PREFACE

*"The information presented here could and should challenge the manner in which we think about the health of our mouths – personally, professionally, and politically."*

### ~ Ty Fain ~

Congratulations on your decision to educate yourself about how your mouth influences your vitality and longevity. Educating yourself means you welcome the opportunity to take control of your health and make decisions grounded in truth.

You are the most qualified person to do so. You hold the biggest stake in your treatment outcomes. Unlike your doctors, you only have to focus on your own health needs and those of your family. You understand that we each can learn how to naturally strengthen our own bodies so we can resist disease rather than create it.

Personal responsibility continues to gather importance as the world economy shifts. Contrary to common belief, the United States does not offer the highest quality medical care in the world. Americans spend a higher percent of their gross domestic product on healthcare than any other country, yet in 2000, the World Health Organization (WHO) ranked the United States healthcare system 37th out of 191 countries, after Dominica and Costa Rica.[1]

Several factors contribute to this dismal statistic. Some of these reflect pitfalls of our economic system. It begins as medical students become indoctrinated during training. Among other things, professors receive significant research money, which can influence their teaching.

Two-thirds of medical research is sponsored by pharmaceutical companies and unfavorable research does not always see the light of day. As the British medical journal *Lancet* reported, drug research, even from clinical trials sponsored by the U.S. federal government, is routinely suppressed. (January 3, 2012, "Missing Clinical Trial Data." BMJ 2012;344:d8158) The authors found only half of all NIH-funded clinical drug trials were published within 2.5 years, and one third were never published. An example the paper cited was the FDA-approved

---

1 *"The World Health Report 2000 – Health Systems: Improving Performance."* June 2000.

diabetes drug Avandia. In 2007, the FDA finally warned the public about Avandia risks – clinical studies showed the drug increases the risk of heart attack by 43 percent and can double heart failure risk after one year of treatment. The drug's maker, GlaxoSmithKline, had known of this risk before the drug was approved. Thirty-five out of forty-two studies of Avandia were never published. This information came to light only after a court required the pharmaceutical company to turn over data. This suppression harms patients while it increases healthcare costs, as patients succumb to serious side-effects.

Drug industry lobbying to the tune of one hundred million dollars a year is serious money for an industry that says it does not exert undue influence over government. Worse, a revolving door between positions of power within U.S. industry and government regulatory agencies also creates undue influence, as may the requirement of pharmaceutical companies to pay a portion of the FDA's operating costs.

Twenty-five percent of all ads on television are drug commercials. Does it influence you? Do you think it influences media news outlets? The drug industry nets about 300 billion dollars in North America. What would happen to sales if we had a health epidemic?

The food lobby may be more powerful than the pharmaceutical lobby, and likely influences our health more. As you will read, much is amiss with our food supply. In the 1960s the Department of Agriculture's motto became, "Get big or get OUT!" Industrial farming ramped up. Inflammatory disease rates skyrocketed after the move from sustainable agriculture to petroleum-based, non-sustainable agriculture.

Politicians may wring their hands over the obesity epidemic in this country, yet Congress subsidizes, that is, it delivers a price advantage to, foods we should avoid – including factory farmed meats, and GMO corn and soy in all their highly processed forms. Restaurants trying to stay competitive and cost-conscious consumers – whether shopping for their own pantries, or for schools and other institutions – often choose cheap products laden with high fructose corn syrup or corn or soybean oil. They also choose grain-fed animal protein, including beef, pork, eggs, milk, and many fish. These are well known contributors to obesity and chronic disease. In other words, Congress uses our tax dollars to help industrial farming operations grow more of the foods that make us sick on land that is degrading because of industrialized food production practices.[For more to chew on, go to: http://www.longevitywarehouse. com/Articles.asp?ID=622.] In 2009, that added up to roughly 79 billion dollars, or two-thirds of the USDA budget. Seventy-five percent of these taxpayer dollars went to the top-grossing ten percent of factory farms.

More and more people realize it is a bad idea to take drugs to fix old, malfunctioning cells. The body heals by making new ones. A body makes new healthy cells in the absence of toxins and when the proper nutrients are available. *Mouth Matters* explores some of these issues.

By now most Americans have heard that poor gum management leads to heart disease. This book clearly explains the connection – and in the process illustrates the model for the inflammatory processes that age all organs and tissues.

This book is for lay people who recognize the mouth is a part of the body and who realize that what goes on there reflects and influences inflammation, general health and aging in ways not imagined a few short years ago. *Mouth Matters* describes how the condition of your mouth and what enters it from infancy can affect your heart, blood vessels, lungs, bones, kidneys, artificial joints – and sexual responses.

It reviews how gum disease influences diabetes and pregnancy outcomes. *Mouth Matters* introduces oral cancer risks, critical reasons to breast feed infants, jaw-joint/clenching problems, and gluten intolerance. And of course it explains many people's biggest fear – how teeth are lost without pain or any other noticeable symptoms until the end stages of the disease that lead to their loss.

This book also tells you what you can do about it. If you want to live a long and vibrant life in our disease-ridden western society, you need to learn vital anti-aging strategies that control inflammation. The seeds for inflammation are sown decades before late-stage symptoms like heart attacks, erectile dysfunction (ED), Alzheimer's, osteoporosis, or diabetes appear. If you already suffer chronic inflammation, what you learn in these pages will help you douse these silent inflammatory fires.

For the reasons put forth in this book, it is ridiculous that ninety percent of dental hygiene procedures submitted to dental insurance companies are coded as "cleanings," a routine reserved for healthy mouths only. Translated, this means people are wrongly given a dental clearance for procedures like body part replacement, artificial insemination, and other procedures. The complications from an inappropriate clearance can be expensive and painful, if not life threatening. If a diabetic's endocrinologist were to ask, based on the procedures dental professionals are turning in to insurance companies, the dentist/hygienist would have to say their gums are healthy.

Yet roughly 80-85 percent of all adults have some level of gum disease. There is a disconnect from reality in dental health delivery and clients should fight it as though their lives depend on it. Because they do.

This book is designed to empower you to learn more and ask for more from your governing bodies and your health care professionals.

Case in point, a cardiology nurse/client mentioned that the cardiologists serving her hospital unit are aware of the connections between heart attacks and gum disease, yet their hospital exit protocol does not yet include a discussion about oral health or a suggestion to seek qualified dental services to clear the disease.

You may be disenchanted with our current health care system that undervalues preventive medicine and basic health education. You may not want to solve every health problem with medication. You do not want to become part of the statistics that Barbara Starfield of the Johns Hopkins School of Hygiene and Public Health reported in the *Journal of the American Medical Association* (Vol 284, July 26, 2000). Her review of statistics indicate that medically induced deaths are the third leading cause of death in the U.S. after heart disease and cancer – and that prescribed drugs play a major role.

You might not know this, but medical use of blood pressure and body temperature to measure health languished for almost 100 years before adoption. It is common knowledge that it takes at least 20 years to incorporate well-established research into widespread medical practice. We remain indifferent to experimentation or we are unable to grasp the implications of discoveries such as DNA in the 1800s. This indifference or inability to organize medicine caused one historian to call medicine the withered arm of science. The lag in what we know and what we do in almost all branches of medicine is notoriously long. "Perhaps as little as 8 percent of what dentists do is justified by peer-reviewed, published, and appropriately analyzed dental research."[2]

If you do not have the time or inclination to wait for oral-systemic medicine to percolate into the medical or dental practices you utilize, read this book. In its pages you will learn how to create – or seek wellbeing on levels you did not even know existed. I encourage you to pursue collaborative health care – to have open and amicable dialogues with your doctors about all aspects of your health, including the prescription drugs they suggest and alternative approaches you are practicing or considering. Since publication of the first edition, I have found most everyone, including traditional health care professionals, is more open to change than they were just a few short years ago. Let us all work together for optimal health at affordable costs!

---

2 Kao, R. "The Challenges of Transferring Evidence-based Dentistry Into Practice." *Journal of the California Dental Association.* 2006; Vol 34(6): 433-7.

# FOREWORD

Every once in a while, you come across a person you just know will make a difference in this world. Maybe it is their passion, creativity, or determination. For Carol Vander Stoep, I think it is fair to say, it's all the above. By virtue of my work, I have the privilege of meeting and dreaming with oral health care providers from around the world. Coming across Carol was one of the most memorable meetings I can remember, and I am deeply honored that she pulled me into her loop during the final stages of the development of *Mouth Matters*.

Several months before I spoke at the 2008 American Dental Association Annual Session in San Antonio, Carol e-mailed me to introduce herself and ask if I would get together with her at the meeting. It was then when she asked if I would be willing to review a manuscript in progress for what has become one of the most brilliant contributions in educating the consumer-public about the importance of oral health. I did review it, and I was awestruck with the depth and breadth of Carol's knowledge.

*Mouth Matters* is the quintessential road map for people who want to better understand the connection between oral and overall health. Carol has mastered the fine art of providing a thorough review of scientific evidence related to oral-systemic interrelationships and grounding this science by using terms everyone can understand. Indeed, this is a talent. No other author has been able to assimilate, synthesize, and craft the body of evidence that supports a role of infection and inflammation within the oral cavity in escalating risk for various chronic disease states with such clarity, and readability.

Many people have great ideas, but how many are so committed to a dream that they resolve to move it forward in spite of obstacles? Most of us just don't have that kind of heart. Carol does. Without her dogged determination in bringing this wonderful book to fruition, we would have lost a very valuable resource for consumer education. We are so lucky Carol saw this important work through. *Mouth Matters* is long overdue and a tribute to how one person's passion can be translated into helping others in such a meaningful way.

Congratulations Carol!

Casey Hein, BSDH, MBA
Assistant Professor; Division of Periodontics
Project Director, Interprofessional Oral-Systemic Curriculum
Development, Faculty of Dentistry
University of Manitoba

President, Casey Hein & Associates
www.caseyhein.com
Former editor-in-chief of the dental journal, Grand Rounds in Oral-Systemic Medicine

# INTRODUCTION

*"Inflammatory processes like atherosclerosis, Alzheimer's and
dementia may remain completely hidden for years.
They hold their secrets and when they confess,
the game may be just about over."* [i]

**~ Charles E. McCall, MD/
Inflammatory Disease Specialist ~**

## Connections: A Two-Way Street

You believe your life is precious. You expect health and dignity for a lifetime. You desire to stay forever young, keeping all mental and physical flags flying from the boardroom to the bedroom. Did you know if you overlook oral influences, you age faster? Your mouth reflects the lifetime care you have given yourself. Your mouth whispers secrets of current and future disease.

A tug-of-war between health and disease wages in your mouth because it teems with germs that can filter through and affect your entire body. If you do not know the tricks of winning that war, you can suffer complex diseases of your mouth and body as you age. Silent oral diseases influence and reflect the course of silent general diseases like diabetes, heart disease, Alzheimer's and osteoporosis.

A veterinarian's marquee reads, "Dental Screening Reveals Spleen in Trouble." Veterinarians often precede doctors in practicing integrated health. Though it is difficult to believe your pet has medical advantages, he does. His "health care system" is integrated. He automatically receives holistic medical care since veterinarians generally treat all organ systems like the unified whole they are.

When veterinarians speak to pet owners about oral care for animals, they emphasize that bacteria and other microbes from gum disease enter an animal's bloodstream where, as they stream through fragile organ tissues, constant low level infections begin in the heart, brain, kidney, liver, and stomach as well as within the highway of blood vessels that transport the microbes and their toxins. These infections cause permanent damage, threatening the animal's vitality and natural lifespan. It is no different for humans.

Most people are not aware a *Surgeon General's Report on Oral Health* exists. Released in 2000, the implications were at least as staggering as 1964's *Surgeon General's Report on Smoking and Health*, but it barely rippled the waters of public awareness.

No surprise. Smoking was sexy. It bestowed social cachet. In the 1930s and 1940s, pages of the *Journal of the American Medical Association (JAMA)* abounded with tobacco ads, claiming smoking conferred health benefits. One ad claimed Camel cigarettes aided digestion by stimulating digestive fluids. L&M cigarettes were "just what the doctor ordered." Philip Morris said its cigarettes were "recognized by eminent medical authorities." That a habit promoted by medical doctors could contribute to deadly diseases startled most Americans when it was made public in the 1950s. When they learned of it, thousands of people immediately quit, tossing their habit along with their cigarettes. At least today people *know* smoking harms them.

News flashes suggest consistent flossing adds years to life, but who has time to pay attention? It is a challenge to prioritize preventive oral care in our busy lives. Dated myths add more confusion, which leaves people uncertain about what works.

Ancient cultures understood oral health's influences on general health and designed fastidious oral care routines to prevent body contamination via this gateway. As they have for centuries, Eastern cultures use hundreds of essential oils that include oregano, cloves, cinnamon, rosemary, peppermint, and lavender. They also incorporate herbs and spices like turmeric, ginger, ginseng, curcumin, and myrrh as antibacterial/antiviral agents. Modern research confirms the powerful roles these ancient remedies play. Some not only fight germs, but also stimulate healing by either boosting immune responses or enhancing collagen[1] production.

---

1 Those who pursue beauty know collagen is an essential structural component of skin. As this protein degrades, our skin loses elasticity and structure, leading to wrinkles. Collagen is also the main building block of ligaments, tendons, bone, cartilage, and fascia.

Americans spend nine billion dollars on oral care products annually,[ii] but statistics reveal most people focus only on cosmetic care of this sensual and multifunctional gateway. Eyes glaze when I introduce clients to the shared pathways of oral/systemic health, yet incredulity and lively interaction rapidly replace boredom as they grasp the simple ways the body and mouth share disease – or health. As one client recently said, "That's the most logical thing I've ever heard about why I should invest some time on my mouth."

Hygienists would rather not just serve as "oral janitors". We do not want to repeatedly treat the symptoms of a bigger problem. We want to help you avoid a heart attack or stroke – or improve diseases such as diabetes, osteoporosis or other degenerative conditions. This book will guide you through simple steps to improved health that offers social, economic, and personal benefits.

## Inflammation: The Name of the Game

It is no secret many cultures fear aging, particularly aging poorly. But too many people are surprised when they learn inflammation is the primary villain of aging and deterioration. Beyond heart disease and diabetes – allergies, asthma, eczema, erectile dysfunction (ED), Alzheimer's disease, emphysema, irritable bowel disease, rheumatoid arthritis, lupus, Crohn's disease and psoriasis, all share common roots: inflammation and unbalanced body chemistry.

Do you remember your last injury? The trauma immediately activated your immune system. Blood vessels near the injury swelled so assorted cells could flood the area to heal it. Redness and warmth accompanied swelling and pain. Afterwards, scars may have remained as a testament to the battle waged at the site.

This inflammatory process is our body's primary system designed to heal us in crisis, but when it enters permanent, destructive overdrive as it often does in today's environment, our own defenses bombard us with friendly fire. We age prematurely and our quality of life deteriorates.

How does this protective immune system process work? Does lifestyle matter? Do you wonder if the seeds of inflammatory diseases are already sown deep within your own body?

Know that nearly every choice you make throughout life influences the answer. If you read this book, you will discover answers to important questions you never thought to ask. You will also know how the choices you make either flare or dampen your immune response and, thus, your propensity for disease.

Few Americans understand the synergy that exists between inadequate oral health and these diseases as damage and scarring override repair and healing. These connections were unimaginable a decade ago. Overlooked by most, gum disease – often registered as tender or bleeding gums – is a chronic inflammatory state. This book emphasizes oral health's role in promoting these diseases. And because these diseases also drive oral symptoms, these diseases are also explained from the viewpoint of their influences on oral health

Dr. Floyd Chilton, author of *Inflammation Nation*, asserts that more than half of American adults suffer from inflammatory disease. He outlines how numbers have soared over the past two decades. As most health professionals still do, this inflammation specialist overlooked gum disease, even though at least 80 percent of Americans suffer from it to some degree. If we can begin to accept integrative medicine – if we can agree the mouth is a body part and body systems influence each other – we must accept that most Americans suffer from inflammatory disease.

This book provides an introduction to oral/systemic disease for those 75 to 90 percent of Americans who suffer chronic inflammation. It is aimed at those who want to take charge of their health by learning easy ways to reduce their risk of shared diseases and support healthy aging.

Do you want to enjoy the full range of pleasures your mouth and body can experience for a lifetime? Do you demand and expect more from life than past generations have? If so, empower yourself. Learn how to modify the environmental factors that keep your immune system ramped up. Understand how and why your *Mouth Matters*.

## Collaboration

Recently, "a consensus paper on the relationship between heart disease and gum disease was published ... in ... the American Journal of Cardiology (AJC), a publication circulated to 30,000 cardiologists, and the Journal of Periodontology (JP), the official publication of the American Academy of Periodontology (AAP). Developed in concert by cardiologists, the physicians specialized in treating diseases of the heart, and periodontists, the dentists with advanced training in treatment and prevention of periodontal disease, the paper contains clinical recommendations for both medical and dental professionals to use in managing patients living with, or who are at risk for, either disease. As a result of the statement, cardiologists may now examine a patient's mouth, and periodontists may begin asking questions about heart health and family history of heart disease." [iii]

So, though currently about 46 percent of internists feel gum disease status is peripheral to their role, 69 percent are not comfortable with simple oral exams, 90 percent had no training about gum disease during medical school, and 82 percent never ask patients about gum disease, change is in the wind and you should expect collaboration by your health care providers.

**Author's Notes:** For some, the information in this book brings very little new. For others, the ideas presented are radically different from anything they have ever heard. With today's pace of research and rapid dissemination of findings, theories deeply believed today are sometimes debunked tomorrow. With all we know, there is far more we do not. It is likely some of what I offer here will not stand the test of time, just as some of the theories I debunk have not. What we must all do is to keep open minds as we continue to seek answers.

I mean no disrespect towards anyone in my writings. This is especially true of health care professionals who put their lives and energy on the line every day to raise the quality of people's lives. For instance, though I deplore practices such as the continued use of mercury/amalgam filling materials or their unsafe removal, I must conclude that doctors who use these materials and remove them following no special precautions, believe in their hearts they are doing the right thing and helping people. Otherwise they would not choose to put themselves at more risk of lifetime health problems than they do their clients.

I think too of orthodontists. A large fraction of our aging population is suffering all kinds of life threatening problems from orthodontic methods practiced years ago. Unfortunately, these methods persist. For those who have learned better ways and are horrified about what they may have done to so many, I empathize. There is much in the way I used to practice – and in the way I raised my precious children – that I would change if I could. But I can't. All we can acknowledge is that we now know better, and then move forward.

This book need not be read in depth or cover-to-cover. Scan the first three chapters for background information about how the mouth and body are connected. Then read chapters that most interest you. Because of the state of our food production and delivery system here in the United States, everyone should also read Chapter Five: Diabetes as an Accelerated Aging Model. When clients understand and use the anti-aging information in this chapter, diabetic or not, their health changes profoundly. Chapter Twelve also provides insight into oral influences on body chemistry/electrical imbalances. Keep in mind most people who suffer one inflammation-based disease, suffer others. Do not let this book's details impede you. They are there for professional credibility and for those who seek them. The "bottom line" is easy.

Visit: www.mouthmattersbook.com often for research updates about oral/systemic medicine, pertinent health-related articles, and blogs.

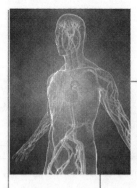

# HEALTH IS INTEGRATED BY DESIGN

*"The way the health care system functions, one might think the mouth isn't connected to the whole body. (It's) just as important as medical care, hospital care, and prescription drugs. It is inconsistent for society to recognize that oral health is important yet treat dental care as if it were discretionary.*

~ **William Maas, Director of the Division of Oral Health at the Centers for Disease Control (CDC)** ~

**Explore:**
1. What do the diseases we most fear have in common?
2. How can guarding your body's gateway save money and help you maintain a dynamic lifestyle?
3. How did we lose the notion that integrated body systems work well or suffer together?
4. How did the mouth lose its place in medical health models?
5. Can aspirated bacteria be deadly?

I am fortunate to work in Austin, Texas, a town dominated by people keenly interested in razor's edge thought and lifestyle. The town resonates with energy. Its enterprising population nourished the miraculous emergence of the Whole Foods empire, a thriving music and film industry, and some of the world's most recognizable high-tech companies.

Austinites are well informed, resourceful, and physically active. They passionately pursue health. A surprising exception is oral self-care. Most do not know oral health has life or death consequences until, to paraphrase inflammation specialist Dr. Charles McCall, the inflammatory process gives up its secrets and the game is just about over. Chronic inflammatory diseases silently steal health for years. It is no secret that an inflammatory system gone awry lies at the root of many mortal and painful diseases ravaging our health. Those who seek a robust, long life know this. Heart disease, diabetes, arthritis, allergies, asthma, and eczema, are but a few of the hundreds of diseases with unbridled, long-term inflammation as a root cause.

They also can share an intimate association with slimy biofilms, abundantly present in the mouth. Diet and obesity contribute to the inflammatory loads that aggravate these diseases. But gum disease, once considered a localized disease, shares the same pathways that create a web of damaging inflammation throughout the body. More than a decade after the *Surgeon General's Report on Oral Health* was released in 2000, gum disease may still be the most undiagnosed and under treated of all systemic diseases.

Politics and the unsophisticated science of the early 1900s may have marginalized oral health's place in overall health. This rift keeps many Americans uninformed and unable to fully care for their own wellbeing. It keeps us from forging public policy that could provide cost containment and improve lives.

## How Sexy Is It?

When news of the *Surgeon General's Report on Smoking and Health* captured headlines in 1964, smoking was sexy. Perceptions have since changed. Most smokers can list numerous reasons to quit and often try to. But Gene Simmons, of the rock band *KISS*, cuts through sound reasoning with a blunt assessment: Who wants to kiss a stinky, disease-ridden mouth?

Rising stars in any social or business strata know radiant smiles invite interaction; they project confidence, youth, vibrant health, intelligence, and success. To maximize your impact, you likely dash a brush over your teeth before social interactions to brighten and freshen your smile. From a vanity viewpoint, you know investing in your mouth enhances the likelihood of career and social advancement.

**Quote from a successful, handsome financial analyst after viewing enlarged images of his mouth:**
"Wow! After seeing my mouth 'up close and personal,' I feel really sorry for all those women I kiss! Ugh!"
**My Rejoinder:** "Don't feel so bad. Their mouths probably look about the same!"
**Look on his face:** Priceless!

Mouths are due some appreciation. They are the source of intense and varied pleasure from birth to death. They are a major visual and tactile trigger. We relish new pleasures, but may also use foods and oral habits to satisfy emotional needs. Nutrition and digestion start here. Mouths articulate verbal and nonverbal thoughts and emotions.

While a private place fraught with psychological associations, your mouth is also critical to your social face. You owe yourself the comfort, clear speech, and confidence a healthy mouth brings to your work and social interactions.

**My Smile Is My Image!**
Discussing smiles with the manager of a luxurious Tokyo hotel, a man enthusiastically described the importance of his. "Oh, yes! Of course! I tell people all the time I wouldn't be where I am professionally, nor could I operate effectively without my trademark smile. My smile is my image and my image must be impeccable. I depend on it...."

But to keep your confident smile as part of a fully functioning body, think beyond cosmetics. How seriously can you take vague news stories linking increased vitality and lifespan to flossing? What does that mean? How does this information affect you or your family? Shouldn't news stories explain more? I applaud the media as they tell us oral diseases and other inflammatory diseases are intertwined. But they should also indicate that poor oral conditions don't just drive other diseases; they also reflect poor overall health. Offering simple answers like brushing, flossing, and visiting a dental professional twice yearly plays into the Western tradition of treating disease symptoms, not their root causes. Cavities and gum disease are symptoms of imbalances within the body.

We will never cure disease until we change our Western mind set and think of healing from the inside out. What prematurely ages us is not bad germs, bad genes, or bad luck. It is not taking care of ourselves – not eating right, not moving enough, and perhaps cloudy thinking.

Biochemistry researchers believe microorganisms drive most diseases, but there is much more to the story. While high concentrations of germs reside in the mouth, there is a balance between beneficial and disease-causing bacteria. If you know how to balance your body chemistry and pay attention to oral health, you will make your body inhospitable to both oral and systemic diseases.

The following chapters will help you learn to ward off or minimize inflammatory diseases, even those to which you are genetically inclined, through balancing oral and whole body chemistry. This story of general health is told through via the lens of oral health.

## Will You Be Healthier in Five Years Than You Are Now?

You can be if you choose to. You replace about one hundred million cells a day. If you know how to shape your environment, the new cells can be healthier than the cells you are replacing and your biological age decreases. Further, you are born with an innate capacity to fight disease – to keep your body humming. Your immune system works full-time to keep a complex interplay of inflammatory diseases at bay. By adjusting your lifestyle, you can encourage your body to increase cellular repair and slow the destructive scarring caused by exaggerated immune responses.

A small, painless, chronic oral infection that afflicts – and is ignored by – most people influences inflammatory diseases. Initially it is hard to grasp the far-reaching effects of even minor gum inflammation. Can an overlooked cranny, the size of half a Popsicle stick (5cm²) exponentially ramp up your body's inflammatory response? Can germs teeming there invade arterial blood vessel walls and inflame this tennis court-sized area? Can they damage your heart, joints, or even harm an unborn child? What does that mean? Read on.

You probably think your gums provide as protective a barrier against germ invasion as the rest of your skin does. But often, the fragile oral barriers are breached. The gates are thrown open. Worse, there is no more hospitable place on your body for germs to breed – a warm, dark, moist nook blessed with a constant food source. No wonder gum disease is so prevalent. Acute symptoms of gum disease become obvious only as teeth become sore, loosen, drift, or abscess. Mild, early signs like bleeding or tenderness while flossing or brushing are often ignored. Would you tolerate consistent bleeding and tenderness anywhere else in your body?

Most of us don't choose to believe our mouths sport an "open oral wound", but at least three-fourths[ii] of Americans' mouths do. Denial plays a major role in the development of most chronic, hidden diseases.

**Denial**
Another observation, stumblingly delivered with a derisive smile after seeing his mouth magnified on a video screen: "I can't imagine what I was ever thinking.... I ... I obviously haven't been thinking at all I guess.... I can't run and hide from the reality of what I just saw... How can I change what I see?"

In your mouth, virulent germs can breed unhindered within a concealed reservoir. The skin lining the walls of this reservoir is unique. Unlike other skin, it is missing its top protective layer – its shield. Thus, like a skinned knee, it invites bacterial invasion. When the delicate balance between body defenses and microbes shifts here, it affects organs such as your brain, heart, lungs, stomach, and kidneys.

Absence of pain does not mean absence of injury. The complex chemistry that underlies gum disease is overlooked because the structures it affects and the microscopic germs that alter complex chemistry are hidden.

There are other ways for poor oral conditions to poison us. Sometimes news stories focus attention on tragic examples, but stories like these quickly fade:

- "A young, nonverbal autistic California woman began to act out and hit other residents of her community residential care facility. She was admitted to a locked psychiatric facility at a cost of $150,000 per year to the State of California. Fortunately, caregivers eventually discovered she had dental problems. Once her dental problems were treated, her acting out behaviors ceased and she was able to return to her community." [iii]

- "In Louisiana, a $70 tooth extraction would have saved an elderly patient fifteen days in the hospital, including two days in an intensive care unit, and a $35,000 medical bill." [iv]
- In February of 2007, *The New York Times* reported the death of 12-year-old Deamonte Driver who died of a toothache. "By the time Deamonte's… aching tooth got any attention, the bacteria from the abscess had spread to his brain, doctors said. After two operations and more than six weeks of hospital care, the Prince George's County boy died… A routine, $80 tooth extraction might have saved him." [v]

It is amazing such stories still bring so little attention, reflection, or calls for change. How tragic that the roughly quarter of a million dollar bill to Maryland Medicaid for Deamonte's two-week hospital stay, could neither save his life nor go toward preventing similar catastrophes.

Most stories do not make the news. While conducting research for this book, people told me personal tales related to the mouth's potential influence on overall health. One friend mentioned how an aunt's knee replacement failed after oral bacteria entered her bloodstream and colonized her artificial joint. Another missed a kayaking trip due to an emergency hospital stay. The heart infection that almost killed him was traced to his gum disease. A client told me her mother uses rubber bands to stabilize her few remaining teeth. When I suggested researchers use something similar to induce gum disease in study rats, she shook her head and explained that without the rubber bands, her mother's teeth would immediately fall out. Compromised nutrition was just one part of general health affected by her mouth infection. Another acquaintance told me a pathological cyst found on a relative's spinal cord was traced to an oral infection.

Think for a moment. You may know someone whose health was dramatically affected by poorly managed oral care.

While these stories are common, they are not common knowledge. General public awareness about the integration of body systems is cursory at best. Many people admit they feel comfortable about having mild or moderate gum disease because they do not notice immediate problems and they say so. I help them see the future through their oral health; it commands their attention.

## Gum Disease: Another Source of Lung Pollution?

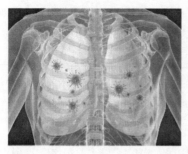

Recently, NPR radio aired a story called, "Think Music Heals? Trombone Player Begs to Differ."[vi] A music professor developed something now being called "trombone player's lung."

After fifteen years of suffering with a constant sore throat, low-grade fever, and bouts of serious weight loss, a Professor Bean traveled without his horn – and felt better. A doctor, checking his horn, explained what made him sick. Organisms like mycobacterium, a TB-like organism, accompanied the air he blew into his trombone. Inside the closed, dark horn these microscopic organisms flourished. They also broke off and entered his lungs each time he inhaled.

Similarly, our lungs pick up and culture microorganisms from our mouths, delivered by tiny aerosolized saliva droplets. When one has gum disease, saliva enzyme activity increases. These enzymes induce disease-causing microorganisms to become extra sticky. They easily colonize in the throat and lungs where they continue their inflammatory destruction. We succumb to respiratory diseases when our resistance is weak. This is particularly true for the elderly, who often die as the result of respiratory infections.

Evidence of links between poor oral care and respiratory diseases like pneumonia, chronic bronchitis, and chronic obstructive pulmonary disease (COPD) continue to grow. Those with gum disease suffer respiratory diseases from infectious germs far more often than those with healthy mouths. If they mouth breathe, they face additional risk. Those with COPD cannot easily eliminate these sticky organisms from their lungs. They suffer frequent infections that cause irreversible damage, so it is particularly important for them to follow thorough oral self-care and schedule routine, competent professional oral care.

Researchers surmise enzymes from gum disease encourage the growth of respiratory disease organisms around teeth. The inflammation generated by this infection may alter lung cells so they are more susceptible to disease as patients aspirate the bacteria common to respiratory and gum disease. The general inflammatory response cascades to further increase a person's susceptibility to respiratory infection.[vii]

Studies show improved personal and professional oral care reduces the progression or occurrence of respiratory diseases, especially among high-risk elderly adults living in nursing homes. A stronger correlation holds for those in intensive care units. Those who depend on others for oral care are at significantly higher risk for pneumonia.[viii] In one study, there were from 34 to 83 percent less cases of pneumonia and other respiratory infections for people with good personal and professional oral care compared to those who did not.[ix]

Research should illuminate improved strategies for avoiding the serious complications of pneumonia and influenza in hospital and nursing home settings.

A related Japanese experiment indicates a potent reason to relax current tight state regulatory control over preventive dental professionals (hygienists) in most states. The researchers proved that the presence of two destructive anaerobic oral bacteria[1] commonly found in gum disease induced inflammatory messengers in the body, which then resulted in pneumonia.

Then they studied the impact of improved oral care on the number of deaths from pneumonia. They instituted a 24-month program of weekly oral cleansing care to elderly patients in nursing homes requiring help with basic daily living skills. Dental hygienists administered the weekly oral care, which resulted in significant reduction of yeast, staphylococcus, and other anaerobic organisms as well as a decline in fatal aspiration pneumonia cases. Why aren't these professional activities allowed more widely?

In another Japanese program, dental hygienists administered frequent oral care to elderly persons in nursing homes for the six months of flu season. This effort resulted in fewer influenza cases, also known for higher mortality rates among older populations.[x][xi]

Research links between respiratory diseases and gum disease are well established. We must work to change how we care for immuno-compromised patients and those in hospital settings on respirators and in intensive care units.

In a dental setting, if you or someone you love has COPD and gum disease, be sure your dental professional encourages a pre-procedural rinse. Ozonated water, water infused with an essential oil such as

---

1 *Porphyromonas gingivalis* and *Treponema denticola*

Thieves, or in the traditional vein, the non-alcohol version of Listerine or chlorhexidine will do. This temporarily lowers oral bacterial counts. They must also use high-speed suction, especially if they use ultrasonic instruments. The separate water supply should also be ozonated water or contain a biocide like chlorhexidine, since studies show plain tap water moving through dental lines carry water with 10 – 100 times more bacterial colonies than the FDA allows[2] for safe drinking water. This is in addition to methods dentists use for purging and disinfecting. I prefer ozonated water because of its biocompatibility and it does not interfere with resin bond strength. The air supply must also be designed to be contaminant free (see Resources section).

## Medicine's Stepchild: Dentistry

How, one might wonder, did oral health, prevention, and general dentistry become discretionary? The origins of dentistry's isolation from medicine may have begun in the early 1900s. At the time, many dentists believed abscessing teeth and infected gums were so septic they created widespread health damage. Advertising themselves as "one hundred percenters" these practitioners proposed that pulling 100 percent of a person's teeth would cure many diseases.

The practice of full mouth extractions continued for years until a study concluded the radical solution conferred no measurable health benefits. Did the solution overreach its premise? These dentists addressed whole body wellness far ahead of their time. Perhaps they were not as far off the mark as it initially sounds. Of course their evaluation tools were too crude to measure health improvements. It is possible these diseases they studied were too established to reverse by the time they initiated "treatment."

Other factors may have contributed. Cavitations likely occurred at many of these extraction sites. When a practitioner does not thoroughly remove a tooth's surrounding ligament and nearby infected bone during an extraction, cavitations can occur in the jaw

---

2 Boil water notices go out when Colony Forming Units (CFUs) go above 500. The ADA recommends waterlines should contain no more than 200 CFUs. In a study by Ketterig J, Munoz C, Stephens J, et al (Comparison of methods for reducing dental unit waterline bacteria and biofilm.) presented in 1997, dental units with chlorhexidine solution demonstrated no bacterial growth for the duration of the study while the units containing tap water regardless of additional methods for purging and disinfecting, continuously had CFUs in the range of 500,000 to 5,000,000.

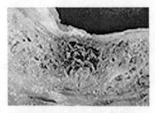

**Cavitation in the jaw bone.**

bone. Bone may fill in over the site, but bacteria may be trapped in an oxygen-free environment and incubate potent toxins. More colorfully stated, cavitations are areas of rotted, dead bone embedded within live bone. (Dr. Hal Huggins notes that in surgical intervention of over 1000 extraction sites, 99% show partial or totally unhealed bone.) As with gum disease, the trapped toxic waste products do not stay local, but circulate and weaken the whole body. Many medical professionals and most veterinarians recognize and treat cavitations within skeletal bone, yet dental professionals are slow to recognize their existence, much less their impact on human health. When present, they are a constant source of whole body infection long after teeth are removed. In cavitated bone, anaerobic bacteria are trapped within the site. They feed into the circulatory system and spark low-grade chronic inflammation that constantly challenges the immune system. Cavitations are thought to be a particular risk in sites where extracted teeth had prior root canal treatment, were severely compromised at the time of the extraction, or when the ligament surrounding the root was incompletely removed during a crude extraction.

Dentistry continues to recover from the tremendous loss of respect it suffered. Only the last decade has brought an understanding of inflammation's crucial role in the diseases of aging, thus more insight to some dentists.

This book will illuminate the dark gateway most people dismiss. It is a personal wake up call for those with sizeable, untended "oral wounds" and for those responsible for the public policy keeping this awareness muted. This book provides information for people whose doctors are not paying attention to the significant and growing body of research about oral health's impact on wellbeing. It also offers proactive suggestions designed to empower those without access to care, as well as a minimal but targeted oral care routine that, if used, will enhance the lives of many. If we are all lucky, it can help forge progressive public policy. This book is for:

- Everyone suffering from an inflammatory disease like heart disease, allergies, asthma, eczema, erectile dysfunction (ED), Alzheimer's disease, emphysema, irritable bowel disease, rheumatoid arthritis, lupus, Crohn's disease or psoriasis – or has a loved one whose health is impaired by inflammation.

- Children under age 12 who have not yet completed their orofacial development. These children have a chance to optimize their genes and influence facial growth using correct oral posture. This includes nasal breathing, proper tongue rest position and swallowing, and when necessary, "face forward" orthodontic intervention.
- The 850,000 Americans admitted to hospital emergency rooms annually due to life threatening abscesses from gum disease.
- A client from Ten Sleep, Wyoming who must drive to Montana for dental care or wait until she visits relatives who live in towns that offer dental services.
- A friend who mistrusts dentists; he believes their goals to be solely pecuniary. He rarely seeks care and has no knowledge of the link between oral and general health.
- The friend who routinely seeks dental care for her children because she wants the best for them. She knows "twice a year" visits are recommended. She lacks dental insurance, sees an attractive smile reflected in her mirror, and thus does not perceive the need to budget wellness visits for herself. As a result, she is left in the dark about the far ranging effects her mouth can have on her general health.
- The many Americans who pursue "dental tourism." These people combine dentistry with trips to foreign countries as a way of reducing costs – and sometimes to receive care unavailable in the U.S. Not having a close relationship with a trusted dentist could limit ongoing preventive monitoring and advice.
- Younger versions of the woman I heard about on a morning radio program. She was poor and lived a hard day's journey from dental care. As years progressed, she began to suffer severe oral pain and carefully saved money until she could travel to a dentist who would extract all her teeth. She wanted pain relief and to eat and feel better than she had for many years. Only in her later years, as she began to suffer, did she recognize the significance of oral health.

- The woman so hesitant to schedule her first dental visit she attempted to use her camera phone to visualize and solve her own oral problems.
- The patient referred to a hospital by a dermatologist friend of mine whose eyeball was very nearly expulsed. The dermatologist correctly guessed an oral infection was the underlying cause and immediately referred the patient to a hospital.
- Any child who contributes to the statistic of 51 million school hours lost annually to dental related illness or adult who contributes to the statistic of 164 million work hours lost annually to dental disease or emergency dental visits.
- Those with asthma, apnea, erectile dysfunction, jaw joint problems, ADHD, a clouded memory, unexplained weight gain, thyroid problems, or perhaps even Tourette's syndrome.
- Those who shape restrictive public policy denying access to dental care in multiple ways.

*How many diseases are there?* *

*Raymond Francis, M. Sc. describes a simple, elegant disease theory:
One disease: malfunctioning cells
Two causes: deficiency and toxicity
Six pathways between health and disease: nutrition, toxin, psychology, physical, genetic and medical.
Choose health!

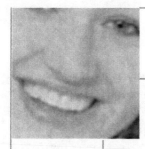

# GUARDING THE GATES

*Where will you live if you don't take care of your body?*

**Explore:**
1. The unique mouth/body interface.
2. What is a professional "cleaning"? Why are the necessary?
3. What is plaque?
4. Why can't antibiotics and chemicals control gum disease?
5. How do simple carbohydrates challenge your immune system?
6. Can plaque destroy the jawbone that anchors your teeth?

Airline pilots obsess over the purity of their airplane's jet fuel and the cleanliness of its fuel lines. If they fail to detect contaminants, a cascade of failures in the intricate engine/fuel line/computer complex can trigger a cataclysmic event. A seemingly small failure can crash a jet.

Our fuel and fuel lines are just as critical to our survival. As with any complex system, we jeopardize our own vitality when we ignore essential health components. Inflammatory diseases like those of the heart and gums are essentially diseases of blood vessel walls. How we fuel ourselves determines how well we keep our own fuel lines open.

A whole is greater than the sum of its parts. Insurance companies may soon trump individuals and medical systems as they implement this philosophy. They know guarding the body's gateway optimizes whole body health and their bottom line.

Some insurance companies offer 100 percent coverage for initial gum disease treatment (periodontal scaling) and maintenance (quarterly wellness visits) for those at risk for stroke or those diagnosed with diabetes and cardiovascular disease. For instance, Aetna found increasing access to oral health care for patients with chronic degenerative diseases reduced their overall medical care costs by as much as 16 percent.

Costs for diabetes care declined 9 percent, cardiovascular disease 16 percent and stroke treatment costs declined 11 percent. [11]

Remarkably, these are not specified benefits in dental plans but in medical insurance plans. This is a radical departure from typical medical benefit schedules. Additionally, medical and dental policies are both beginning to cover orofacial myofunctional therapy because of the cascade of positive health benefits resulting from proper orofacial posture.

Some medical policies offer participants financial incentives to encourage the use of dental benefits. Though cost is just one barrier to dental care, insurance companies think financial encouragement might overcome other obstacles. Insurance companies offer these because they expect to reduce the cost of treating diabetes and heart disease by controlling gum disease.

Wise employers may offer these integrated insurance plans as a way to diminish the staggering statistic of 160+ million lost work hours each year due directly to dental disease.[ii] What if your insurance plan does not offer these benefits? Should you let that dictate the level of health you desire and deserve?

Claire is a client who recently decided to take charge of her health. She came to me with a limited awareness of how oral and general health influence each other. She had few cavities, so she felt immune to dental problems. As many do, she forgot teeth are just one part of a healthy mouth. In fact, there are many others.

## CLAIRE

Claire's early adult life was turbulent. She contended with a difficult marriage, emotional volatility, and young children. She struggled to keep regular preventive appointments, but eventually disappeared from our practice while she reorganized her life and health. During her absence, she was diagnosed with the bipolar disorder she had self-medicated with alcohol during her marriage. After diagnosis, she took conventional medications but soon decided she did not like the side effects. She believed they exacerbated her rheumatoid arthritis, an inflammatory derangement of the immune system, so she turned to alternative medical therapies.

She believes conventional Western medicine best treats infectious diseases, and symptoms of acute end-stage disease. She feels treating symptoms rather than their root causes is reductionist science. She knows

---

1 A similar study in Japan looked at more than 4,000 middle-aged patients and found cumulative health care costs were 21 percent higher in patients with severe gum disease than those with no gum disease.

alternative therapies indirectly combat her diseases by strengthening the natural function of her organs and immune system, thus treating underlying causes. Therefore Claire chooses a collaborative approach to health. She meditates and practices yoga and positive thinking. She goes to bed at 10PM, sleeps eight hours nightly, exercises regularly, eats fresh, nutrient-dense foods correct for her body type, takes enzymes to support digestion, her immune system and adrenal glands[2] and takes pre- and probiotics to keep gut bacteria healthy. She is fortunate to live in a town with proximity to complementary health care options.

Claire enjoys her redesigned life and radiates a joie de vivre. She knows she needs a healthy mouth to have a healthy body. She flosses twice a week and uses an electric toothbrush daily. This exceeds most people's oral care efforts, so our conversations focus on other health matters. One day, she told me her gums felt tender and bled lightly when she flossed. This frustrated her. She wanted a healthier mouth, but didn't know how to improve. She was ready to move forward.

Magnified video observation is often disturbing, but it always stimulates conversation about the surprising and unimaginable chemical signaling unhealthy gums activate throughout the body. Using the camera increased Claire's accountability to herself and helped us design solutions for treating her tender, bleeding gums. Understanding what she saw strengthened her motivation and reorganized her priorities.

A back tooth's inside surface is the best place to illustrate an overlooked breeding ground where potent bacteria often colonize. These bacteria can form a pool of inflammation encircling each tooth. The inflammation is responsible for far-ranging health consequences.

---

2 The adrenal and pituitary glands, and the brain's hypothalamus comprise the neuro-endocrine system. Interactions between the nervous system and the body's hormone systems regulate the immune system, sexuality, digestion, mood, and stress. This hormone system is theorized to be partially regulated by gut microbiota![iii] People develop one of three distinct microbial ecosystems in their gut that exert discreet health effects and influence brain function. For example: one of these ecosystems produces more enzymes for making the B vitamin biotin, another, more enzymes for the B vitamin thiamine. Another example: in a study, mice lacking certain gut bacteria had neurochemical differences in their brain and behaved differently from mice whose gut hosted these gut bacteria. These mice engaged more frequently in "high-risk behavior."[iv]

It would seem prudent to establish what kinds of foods work best for your personal body type, partially determined by your gut microbiota. Try playing with Dr. Mercola's free nutritional typing test online, found at: http://nutritionaltyping.mercola.com/Pre-Test.aspx. Taking this test years ago, I was so out of tune with my body I had no idea how to answer the questions. Researching this book led to a few small changes that have made huge differences in my energy levels and feelings of wellbeing. I breezed through the test years later and knew the results before I started.

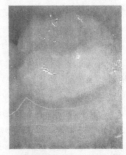

**Tooth pooled in biofilm. Deep supporting tissues remain intact, but the darkened gums encircling the tooth are mildly infected. Healthy gums are a uniform light pink and exhibit no swelling.**

## Intricate Dental Design

CAROL: "Claire, I know magnification is unsettling, but it can help define your challenges.

"Let's think differently about your teeth. We say teeth erupt. Erupt is a violent word we usually reserve for volcanoes and anger. Think about it. Your most durable internal body tissue partially erupts through your gums. No other living body part protrudes through enveloping protective skin to function externally while anchored within your body. Teeth balance precariously between the two worlds. Unfortunately the seal around each tooth is an imperfect, vulnerable interface.

"The curved shape of your teeth from chewing surface to gum line deflects food away from your gums so chewing doesn't constantly nick and expose them to oral bacteria. Now that we live longer, this shape can be a liability because it forms a mild undercut. Germs collect at the base of teeth and, to complicate things, the gums through which your teeth erupted don't seal at the top edge. They seal a few millimeters down from the gum's margin so a loose collar forms around the neck of every tooth. In dentistry, we call the collar a pocket. Dead cells, bacteria, fungi, and their toxic by-products mature within the pocket when left undisturbed. They and their systemic influences are concealed from your awareness.

CLAIRE: "Wow! That's a wild way to think of it. So obviously I'm missing something critical?"

CAROL: "You can see by the way your teeth gleam that you work at it. But if you look at your gums beside the thin line of visible plaque, you can see a dark, thick red line across the top edge. Your gum margins are inflamed. Plaque extends from the neck of the tooth into this shallow pocket where some complicated chemistry happens. This is partially why your gums are tender and sometimes bleed when you floss. You can't avoid inflammation without the skills to sweep debris out of the pocket.

"You probably brush as most do, aiming the bristles ninety degrees to the sides of your teeth. These two images illustrate why that fails:

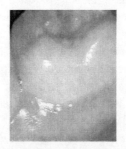 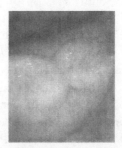

**Typically, bulging tissues surrounding curved teeth form an undercut below the gum margin, hindering effective cleaning in the "pocket."**

"When you brush, the bristle tips take a sweeping leap over bulging gum surfaces, only to touch down onto the tooth a small distance from the gum's edge. The bulk of the tooth is sparkling! But you didn't know there was a pocket at the base of an undercut. You did not know to scoop the debris out of it. It's unfortunate, but this tricky pocket around each tooth can have enormous health repercussions." (Refer to Chapter Sixteen for a more effective brushing technique.)

"Bill Domb, DDS, colorfully describes typical oral conditions this way: 'Pull off some forearm skin, then go rub some toilet water over what's left 24/7... That gives your body less exposure to germs than the exposure you get daily from what is going on in your mouth.' He continues, 'And what about those that let abscesses go untreated in an upper back tooth? I tell them just don't turn any somersaults. Those bad boy germs will migrate right into the Circle of Willis.'" The Circle of Willis is a ring of blood vessels that supply blood to the brain. This pathway may well be what led to Deamonte Driver's death, whose story was told in the last chapter.

"Thirty years ago we practiced under many primitive assumptions, which are still dogma for many today. One misconception was that the crusty, mineralized deposits called tartar (or calculus) were the source of gum problems. People often schedule dental "cleanings" based on what they see accumulating on the inside of their lower front teeth. But mineralized deposits are a symptom of deeper health problems, not the cause.

"Still, crusty deposit accumulations are a valid reason to seek professional services, though they often lie ignored within the pocket. Years ago, we were certain this tartar damaged gums. It 'obviously' acted like a long-embedded splinter that irritated the gums. When eased out from under gum margins, the gums it displaced were raw and bled profusely. If given proper care, these damaged gums healed soon after its removal. But our observations did not hold up to scientific scrutiny.

"We now know tartar requires removal, but mainly because it is porous. The crusty build-up hosts the real destructive culprit – the soft masses of microscopic bacterial colonies and their toxic by-products (endotoxins), which can trigger a vast and destructive response from your immune system. These bacterial toxins penetrate the hard deposit's porous surface and invade the tissues that touch it. Hygienists remove the mineralized plaques to eradicate the toxins and their bacterial nesting sites. Doing so gives you somewhat of a clean slate so you can effectively fight the bacterial masses. But soft deposits reform daily, so you are really the one in control of your oral health status."

## Laser Therapy

Hygienists are gaining the right in some states to use lasers for nonsurgical gum disease therapy.[3] Properly used, lasers seal off blood vessels to speed healing time and increase postoperative comfort. They also reduce germ populations, selectively vaporize bacterially invaded diseased tissue, and alkalize pocket pH by oxygenating the tissues. Alkaline tissues promote "good" bacteria. Lasers require anesthetic, which hygienists have safely administered for years in 44 states without incident. Ozone therapy delivers similar, perhaps better results without anesthetic. Ozone gas clears microscopic tooth tubules of bacteria.

## Know Your Enemy

Van Leeuwenhoek provided the first recorded microscopic observations of living bacteria after examining the soft, white masses harvested from his own teeth. In 1683, he wrote, "… in the said matter there were many

3 See one in action at: http://www.youtube.com/watch?v=U8S_NM-s6oU&feature=related)

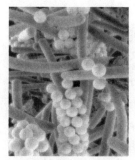

**Dental Plaque**

very little living animalcules, very prettily moving. The biggest sort... had a very strong and swift motion, and shot through the water (or spittle) like a pike does through the water. The second sort... spun round like a top... and these were far more in number."ᵛ You probably call these masses "plaque," but this does not describe much.

Children think plaque is black. They engage when I explain germs are smart; they employ stealth technology and camouflage to remain undetected so they can live and breed undisturbed.

## Biofilms are Like Adolescent Female Cliques: Complex, Socially Sophisticated, and Protective

Plaque is a biofilm (think "pond scum"). Initially, isolated bacteria called planktonic bacteria drift solo in liquids, but under favorable conditions they form biofilms: the bacteria multiply rapidly, coalesce, and begin to adhere to solid surfaces using the slimy adhesives they produce. In your mouth, biofilms attach to teeth. Eventually, the bacteria produce so much protective slime that the slime outweighs the bacteria!

As the colony matures, the germs begin to communicate. Electrical and chemical signals elicit gene changes in the bacteria. In other words, bacteria morph as biofilms mature. They behave differently than their suspended individual forms. Like teenage girls learning social rules, they morph and form groups. Their behavior changes radically as they take on new roles. They become social, learn to work together, protect each other, and act in ways never imagined in the name of group survival.

The colony grows as the bacteria clone and recruit. More potent and complex bacteria taxi to the comfortable environment created by the slimy matrix. At this point, the mass expands rapidly. Like cliques, the highly structured, communicative colony begins to act as a single, complex organism. Just as the whole of our bodies is greater than the sum of its parts, this biofilm colony is much more than the sum of its parts. The bacteria share nutrients and defenses to protect and feed the community's interior. At this stage, they are impenetrable and therefore resistant to detergents, antibiotics, and the body's defenses.

Biofilms protect themselves in other ways, too. Bacteria are powerful survivors that can lie dormant for decades, possibly centuries.

For instance, during starvation or under a siege of antibiotics, they will tightly pack their DNA, shrink, and slow metabolic activity to a virtual standstill. In this way they elude starvation and are immune to antibiotics. As food or liquids again become available, or when antibiotic levels drop, certain genes switch back on and bacteria multiply furiously to repopulate the biofilm.

This is one reason antibiotics cannot control biofilms. Another reason is because current antibiotics target only planktonic bacteria. Since bacteria in biofilms have morphed, current antibiotics do not work. Occasionally, depending on an individual's biofilm bacterial profile *and* if used in conjunction with professional therapy that breaks up the biofilm, antibiotics may be helpful.

However, bacteria are not the only oral pathogens contributing to disease. Fungi, parasites and viruses play a role. If one focuses only on eradicating bacteria, these other pathogens easily gain a stronger foothold, fungi in particular. Additionally, some bacteria consume viruses, so after die-off, they release the viral remains as toxins.

It is my belief antibiotics often turn acute infections into chronic infections – or worse, turn them into superinfections. The best approach is to create an optimal, balanced environment. Stay tuned to learn more about that and about ozone's superiority over antibiotics. **Hint:** Ozone kills most pathogens and their endotoxins; it oxygenates and alkalizes sluggish tissues, while also making white blood cells more effective at killing the "bad guys".

CAROL: "Estimates of the total bacterial load in one person's mouth range from 6 billion to somewhere in the in the trillions. No matter how you look at it, these are substantial numbers! Species counts continually revise upward. So far, around nineteen thousand genotypes of bacteria have been identified."

## Immune System Challenges

CLAIRE: "You mean I might have thousands of kinds of bacteria in my mouth right now?"

CAROL: "Certainly not. You realistically host about two hundred. Besides, not all bacteria are virulent; some are beneficial. And your body has amazing defenses to keep bad species in check. As you know from your struggles with your immune system and arthritis, you have to play an active role in keeping those systems strong. Since arthritis and diseases of the gums[3] share immune system dysfunction, you already have a supportive lifestyle. An important remaining key is refining how you mechanically remove your biofilm.

"So far, we've only talked about the germs that cause oral inflammation. How your body reacts to them is more important. Follow my thoughts, but don't sweat the details. You may recognize common themes from exploring arthritis control.

## Infection at This Interface is Not Casual

"The majority of your body's skin provides a protective barrier. Though skin absorbs more than half of what we slather on it, it shields you from most bacteria, viruses, and fungi because of the thin, tough outer layer we strive to keep intact. But say you skin your knee; it is a minor wound, a break in your protective armor. What do you do? You probably wash it, apply antibiotic ointment to keep bacteria from festering, and then cover it with a bandage until it heals.

"Unfortunately the unique tissue lining each tooth is missing this protective layer. Your dark, warm, moist mouth provides a hospitable environment for germs. The crevice between your teeth and gums is a breeding ground where biofilms develop undisturbed because you are unaware of them. No wonder oral infections are the most common human infections! Yet infections at the interface between your mouth and body are far from casual. They fire up inflammation throughout your body and profoundly change its chemistry.

"In health, this potential breeding ground measures about 5 square centimeters – roughly the size of half a popsicle stick. If microbial destruction erodes a tooth's surrounding gums and bone, the "wound" often ranges from 8 to 20 square centimeters. Severe cases can provoke a 44 square centimeter interface, about the size of the palm of your hand. Most anyone with a visibly infected wound of that size anywhere else on his or her body would speed to a doctor in alarm! But because gum disease is neither painful nor readily visible, most people don't seek treatment until teeth begin to abscess. As with other silent diseases, like heart disease, nothing appears unusual until its end stages.

3 Other conditions in which a compromised immune system can lead to oral and systemic disease interactions include: Sjogren's syndrome, systemic lupus, HIV/AIDS, diabetes, Hashimoto's thyroiditis, cancer therapy, organ transplantation, high stress levels, inadequate nutrition, or a lifestyle generally understood to be unsupportive of health.

"Let's take a closer look at this vulnerable site: Do you see the swollen red tissue in these pictures? It is a result of biofilm accumulation in the 'pocket.' Look at the tissue between your teeth. Can you see how it scallops into a peak?

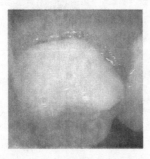 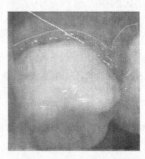

**The plaque has been removed from this tooth to better visualize the inflamed, swollen gums surrounding this tooth. Right image: note the gum attachment level (white scalloped line) and the floss path (straight white line).**

"Thankfully, your gums fill the space so broccoli and meat don't have to, but that means there is more interface area to clean compared to the interface where the brush reaches. In health, the gums between the teeth connect at the base of the scallop. The wall of the pocket is about 3 millimeters deep. This is critical because the deepest you can slide your floss is the level you have in health – 3 millimeters! Can you see where the tissue you clean with the brush blocks the floss from sliding deeper?

"When you don't clean between your teeth, chronic inflammation activates a process that destroys the gum's attachment to them and the underlying bone that anchors them. The bacteria invade deeper into these protected niches and continue their destruction. Unfortunately, there is more surface area in the "unshielded oral wound" cleaned by floss than the area cleaned by your toothbrush. Because of its relative surface area, it is more important to clean between teeth than to brush visible tooth surfaces. (See appendices or www.mouthmattersbook for brushing and flossing tips.)

"Over time, random oral bacteria morph into complex biofilms. For ideal wound management, you should disrupt these biofilms at least every 24 hours to keep them from affecting wound surfaces. As time lengthens between disruptions, your biofilm colonies mature; they become more sticky, dense and complex. Over time, your body's defense system intensifies its fight against the resulting infection in increasingly sophisticated ways. The results have surprising consequences."

CLAIRE: "So I guess flossing twice a week isn't enough?"

CAROL: "Flossing twice a week as you do is good, but no, it doesn't rid you of the constant, low grade inflammation you notice as slight bleeding and mild aching when you floss. If you floss daily, biofilms do not establish, inflammation ceases and tenderness disappears. Flossing twice a week keeps your body's most active defense systems at bay but it doesn't rid you of the chronic, mild inflammation called gingivitis. "When you have gingivitis, the damage is reversible. Underlying bone remains intact in this early stage of gum disease. You can acquire or heal gingivitis in about three days. Some clients forget about flossing for six months, then floss the morning of a dental appointment. They wonder how I know it isn't a regular habit!

"But back to you. If your gums continue to bleed after flossing daily for a while, you'll know the balance between healing and destruction has shifted towards destruction because of an underlying systemic condition. Or you might be enjoying a food trigger. You know your genes dealt you an easily compromised immune system. While sugar intake, stress, and poor nutrition challenge everyone, it compromises you more than most."

At this point, Claire mentioned her new husband loves eating dessert after dinner. Feeling deprived while watching him, she recently joined him, despite knowing the many ways sugars degrade her health. Claire should be especially cautious about ingesting sugar since it is an inflammatory trigger for arthritis, it stresses her adrenals, and the sugar highs and lows accentuate the roller coaster ride of her bipolar disorder. She also knows these simple carbohydrates negate the unpasteurized fermented foods she eats such as kefir and sauerkraut, and other probiotics she takes to maintain the proper "friendly bacteria" human digestive systems require.

Sugar wipes out beneficial bacteria in the digestive tract, leaving a niche in which harmful bacteria thrive. She knows a crucial part of her immune system depends on these beneficial bacteria. They help her body distinguish between disease-causing germs and non-harmful antigens. When the beneficial ratio of good/bad bacteria is imbalanced, the immune system can overreact to non-harmful antigens, which creates allergies. Friendly bacteria also help produce the antibodies required to fight pathogens entering her body.

After our discussion, Claire was ready to address her sugar intake. I suggested, "For now, let's see if daily wound management brings about the results you want. One last thing: developing sound hygiene practices boosts your immune system and may help keep your rheumatoid arthritis in check!" [vi vii viii ix]

**Immune System Sings the Sugar Blues:**
**How sugar and other simple carbohydrates destroy the**
**circulatory and immune system.**

Overdoing refined carbohydrates like sugars and white flour products crank up two of our most powerful aging inflammatory processes, oxidation and glycation. Combining these with poor oral care creates a disastrous recipe for aging. I will return to these processes throughout the book as they relate to specific diseases, but they must be introduced early because they influence many biological functions.

We should manage free radicals in our bodies because these reduced, unstable molecules are missing an electron. They aggressively search for molecules from which to steal one. Once they do, the victimized donor molecule destabilizes and becomes a free radical. We call the resulting chain reaction "oxidation." As oxidative damage to cells accumulates, the cells lose function and eventually die. We quench oxidative fires when we eat a steady supply of foods rich in antioxidants like beta-carotene, vitamins A, C, and E, and complexes like CoQ10 (in the reduced form, ubiquinol) that recycle important antioxidants. Ideally, distribute antioxidant intake throughout the day so they are continuously available as oxidative fires start. Many antioxidants are water-soluble. Our bodies eliminate them if not immediately needed. (See Chapters Five and Twelve for a more thorough discussion of oxidation and how to control it.)

Strangely enough, the oxidation story begins with a surprising twist. Our bodies convert natural sugars into the blood sugar, glucose. Glucose is a precursor of vitamin C so the chemical structure of sugar and vitamin C is similar. This is where problems begin. This similarity didn't matter much when simple carbohydrates were scarce, but it has assumed paramount importance with today's high carbohydrate diets.

You see, vitamin C and sugar compete with each other for insulin use. Our cells need compounds that often require a transport molecule to help them cross a cell's membrane barrier. This is one of insulin's powerful roles, to either ferry sugar out of the bloodstream and into target cells or to enable vitamin C to cross cell membranes for its multiple positive uses, particularly to extinguish fiery oxidative chain reactions. Since sugars are so massively damaging, as you will see in a moment and explore more thoroughly in Chapters Five and Fourteen, insulin is biologically programmed to remove sugars from the bloodstream preferentially. When taken at the same time as sugar, vitamin C, being water-soluble, is excreted long before it can be absorbed. Believe it or not, this has been common knowledge in scientific circles since the 1970s.

So when vitamin C and sugar are ingested at the same time, general health suffers because they compete for insulin uptake. Think about the common temptation to get vitamin C through orange juice. Whole fruits and vegetables contain a mixture of simple and complex carbohydrates. Juice manufacturers remove the complex carbohydrates that slow down absorption of the simple carbohydrates. This leaves high calorie juices that are concentrated forms of fruit sugars, called fructose. Sugars unable to swiftly enter fat or muscle cells for storage or energy use remain in the bloodstream too long. With delayed absorption, these sticky, circulating molecules have more time to irrevocably combine, or glycate, with red blood cells, proteins, and fats in the blood.

This leads to a second major inflammatory aging process. These enlarged, sharp, and sticky molecules play a key role in aging many cells of the human body. Pointedly, they are called advanced glycation end products, or AGEs. They cause terrible damage throughout the body. This is partly because they are powerful oxidizers, so they intensify the first major aging process. Vitamin C, probably the best known antioxidant, could help contain the damage, but delays in vitamin C uptake mean most of this crucial vitamin passes out of the body before it is absorbed for use.

The following points explain how a diet high in simple carbohydrates allows oxidation to damage tissues and organs as it competes with vitamin C for absorption:

- Neutrophils make up 65 percent of the immune system's white blood cells. Like PacMen, neutrophils engulf and destroy bacteria and other foreign invaders. But these cells need about 50 times more vitamin C in their interiors than most cells to function properly. Their performance suffers in direct correlation to their lack of appropriate vitamin C levels.

  The phagocytic index is the scorecard that shows the number of virus, bacteria, or cancer cells a white blood cell can gobble over a limited amount of time. A study showed that 100 grams of any simple sugar like glucose, sucrose, honey, or even fruit sugar like that found in a small glass of orange juice are enough to reduce neutrophil function within 30 minutes of ingestion. Within two hours, neutrophils operate at 50 percent capacity and the effects last for at least five hours.[x] A blood sugar value of 120 reduces the phagocytic index by 75 percent so the immune system is slowed to a crawl.

  This led Linus Pauling to believe high doses of vitamin C helped combat cold viruses and many other illnesses. This is the same reason excessive carbohydrate ingestion leaves you unable to fight oral inflammation from bacterial tissue invasion.

- Free radicals, like AGE products, increase cancer risks, compromise cell wall function, make bones brittle, and promote wrinkles, kidney failure, and eye damage such as cataracts and macular degeneration. To fight free radicals, infection-fighting proteins and white blood cells flood, then irreversibly damage blood vessels. This leads to a rise in stroke and heart attack risks.

  **Note:** When you take vitamin C as a supplement, it acts as an antioxidant, but it can also have opposite the desired effect. It can start a chain reaction of free radicals, especially when taken in high doses. Its reputation as a powerful antioxidant is mainly deserved when taken as part of a whole food. In whole foods, antioxidants are biochemically balanced. Supplements lack this balance. For instance researchers once thought uncontrolled diabetics would benefit from high-dose antioxidant supplementation since, through poor blood sugar management, they often experience low vitamin C levels as well as excessive oxidative damage.

Researchers believed increasing antioxidants would lower diabetics' risks of stroke and heart attacks. Instead, fortifying with 300 milligrams of vitamin C per day more than doubled their risk of death from both diseases. When antioxidants interact with free radicals, they become pro-oxidants, which must be detoxified by other antioxidants that may not be available in the balance needed when taken as a supplement.[xi] Vitamin C supplements cause similar difficulties for smokers. Because smoking generates massive amounts of free radicals, vitamin C reacts with these free radicals and in the process, become pro-oxidants. These two groups of people in particular would do better eating whole foods rich in antioxidants compared to taking the fractionated nutrients in vitamins.

- With circulating high sugar levels, low vitamin C levels in blood vessel walls contribute to atherosclerosis development and other blood vessel abnormalities.[xii] Surprisingly this is partly because sharp, sticky AGEs damage blood vessel walls. They scratch or embed themselves in the walls and create serious oxidative damage that may be poorly repaired due to low vitamin C levels. Damage is even more serious when these AGEs try to squeeze single file through capillaries, our tiniest blood vessels. Because they are too large to flow through easily, they cause particular damage to the delicate vessels of the eyes and kidneys.

- There is another reason diabetics suffer vision loss from low vitamin C levels. Vitamin C concentrates in the retina about 100 times more than in normal tissue. This is to combat the massive numbers of free radicals formed when the eye lens focuses UV sunlight on the retina. When blood sugar is poorly controlled, vitamin C levels in the retina are too low to prevent oxidative damage.

- Vitamin C helps build collagen, a critical protein building block of cells. Adequate vitamin C absorption thus supports healthy blood vessels, scar tissue, cartilage and bone. Vitamin C also enables cells to generate energy and enhances tissue repair.

Refer to Chapters Five and Fourteen to learn about other effects of high blood sugar loads.

## More Than Tooth Support

Claire had latent concerns.

CLAIRE: "Please explain how oral bacteria cause this inflammatory chain of events. I have heard news stories linking flossing to heart health. I would like to understand that better. My dad has heart disease, gum disease, and diabetes. I want to explain some of this to him. I wonder, too, if I could have inherited some of his genes for these diseases?"

CAROL: "Most of the diseases of aging, like those from which your dad suffers, are related to the destructive inflammatory process. Inflammation creates a web of interconnecting pathways throughout the body. It is possible your genes may be coded for an enhanced susceptibility to these diseases, but an emerging field of study called epigenetics explores how environmental factors like nutrition chemically modifies how those genes are activated. As the environmental influences that you control accumulate over time, your gene expression changes and diseases of aging surface. Supporting your immune system in distinct ways profoundly affects health outcomes. Excellent self care matters.

"Any time you host an infection your body mounts an inflammatory response to promote healing, right? As biofilms mature, that response escalates. If you don't remove the biofilm under your gums for a week, advanced biochemical reactions can take place as these bacteria and their toxic by-products, or endotoxins, enter your infection-fighting lymph system and your bloodstream.

"If this were to happen, your immune system would launch a series of messengers, or inflammatory mediators, to help fight your oral infection, mild as it seems to you. Two of these, Interleukin-I and C-Reactive protein (CRP), trigger other molecules like osteoclasts, which destroy bone, and collagenases, which destroy cartilage and other tissues, to multiply within your oral pocket tissue. This would signal the beginning of the destruction of your jawbone.

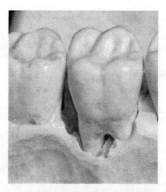 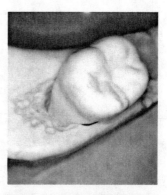

**Models show bone destruction due to chronic inflammation around a tooth's support structure.**

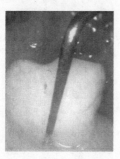 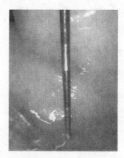

**Gum tissue can mask bone loss so it is not visibly apparent. The left picture shows a slim probe inserted into a defect. It measures the extent of bone loss in millimeters. The right picture shows the same probe lying to the outside of the gum on the same tooth to the same depth. The extensive bone loss measures 7 millimeters on a 12 millimeter-long root). Each colored band on this probe measures 3 millimeters.**

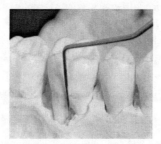

**This model illustrates the approximate bone loss experienced by this client.**

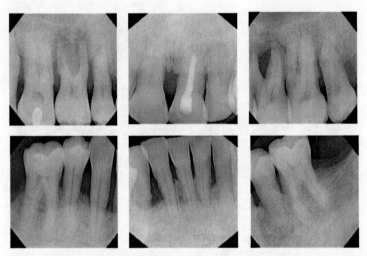

**X-rays are the most illustrative. The jawbone on this client is seriously eroded, yet overlying gums still mask the loss.**

## Little Systemic Terrorists

"Once bone loss occurs, only a skilled dental professional can remove the complex biofilm and calcified deposits that form deep in the crevice.[4] Because it is such a tight, closed area, devoid of oxygen, the predominant germs are anaerobic. In other words, these potent germs[5] thrive without oxygen. Because of the immune system's response to these bacteria and their toxic by-products, I call these little systemic terrorists, the bad boys of gum disease."

"Claire, you correctly grouped the three chronic degenerative diseases your father has: gum disease, heart disease, and diabetes. Genetics influence most diseases, so you may have inherited a tendency to develop all three. But these are primarily lifestyle diseases. Constant immune system bombardment can trigger the genetic expression of any of these diseases. Our immune systems and liver struggle to contend with synthesized chemicals that run rampant in our environment. A few toxins include heavy metals, pesticides and herbicides, product

---

4 Note: advanced cases are referred to a periodontist or specialist in treating gums.
5 Some of the most prolific and destructive are: *Porphyromonas gingivalis, Actinomyces actinomycetemcomitans, Treponema denticola* (a spirochete), *Tannerella forsythia, Prevotella intermedia, Fusobacterium nucleatum,* and *Campylobacter rectus.* In a terrorist class all their own: oral spirochetes. These will be discussed separately.

additives, and byproducts of viruses and bacteria. In today's world, to maintain a long, vibrant life, it is critical to try to control as many negative influences as possible. It is not surprising a rising number of people suffer from diseases and cancers given how often we voluntarily compromise our health with smoking, excessive alcohol intake, drugs, chemical exposure, and high carbohydrate consumption. I know you are concerned about your father's three diseases, but let's just talk about heart disease for now."

**Note 1:** Claire suffered from acute rheumatoid arthritis, "a common, systemic autoimmune disease, which leads to destruction of the joint architecture and consequent disability."[xiii]

In the years since I treated her, science continues to illuminate the connections between gum disease and rheumatoid arthritis. *P. gingivalis* is one of the most prevalent of all oral pathogens and a strong driving agent of gum disease. A recent Chinese study looked at this particular link between the two. It describes how *P. gingivalis* causes pain and disability. *P. gingivalis* continuously produces a particular enzyme (considered an endotoxin or bacterial waste product for our purposes) that targets joints. Within the joint space, this enzyme rapidly converts an amino acid arginine and other proteins into citrulline, in a process called citrullination. In susceptible people, this P gingivalis-mediated citrullination of bacterial and other host proteins in joints is likely a key way the body generates antigens that drive the rheumatoid arthritis autoimmune response. The earlier the intervention, the less irritating the build-up of waste products in joints. Good oral care is a must.

Ozone therapy can destroy *P. gingivalis*. Wouldn't it be interesting to study the effects of ozone within joints? Is it possible ozone could generate healing stem cells within them?

**Note 2.** Processed foods can create havoc with our bodies in unimagined ways. Who would dream something as lowly as refined table salt could be a problem? Yet a steady released by Harvard and Yale researchers suggest refined salt may play a role in creating autoimmune diseases wherein the immune system begins to attack healthy tissues.

Some autoimmune diseases are associated with an overproduction of the immune system cell called a T-cell, specifically the Th17 cell. Rheumatoid arthritis, multiple sclerosis, psoriasis, and ankylosing spondylities have been associated with Th17. Refined salts make these Th17 cells more aggressive, so more likely to assault the host.

Mice fed a diet high in refined salts saw a dramatic increase in the number of Th17 cells in their nervous systems that promoted inflammation. Laboratory tests revealed refined salt exposure caused Th17 cells to release levels of the inflammatory messengers at ten times the usual level. They were also more likely to develop a severe form of a disease associated with multiple sclerosis in humans.

Particularly interested in multiple sclerosis, one of the study's co-authors, Professor David Hafler, from Yale University,  said, "Nature had clearly not intended for the immune system to attack its host body, so I expected an external factor was playing a part. These are not diseases of bad genes alone or diseases caused by the environment, but diseases of a bad interaction between genes and the environment.

"Humans were genetically selected for conditions in sub-Saharan Africa, where there was no salt. It's one of the reasons that having a particular gene may make African Americans much more sensitive to salt. Today, Western diets all have high salt content and that has led to increase in hypertension and perhaps autoimmune disease as well."

On the other hand, unrefined salts are important to our diets. When a salt is filled with dozens of minerals such as the rose-colored Himalayan rock salt crystals or grey Celtic salt crystals, our bodies benefit tremendously for their incorporation into our diet. Too few minerals, rather than too much salt, may be to blame for health problems.[xiv]

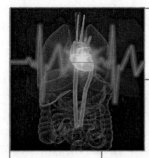

# 3

# WHAT'S THE HEART GOT TO DO, GOT TO DO WITH IT?

*"Illness enters via the mouth; ills exit it."*

**~ Chinese proverb ~**

**Explore:**
1. What is heart disease?
2. What numbers matter more than cholesterol numbers?
3. How do blood vessel walls stiffen and cause high blood pressure?
4. What are LDL "cholesterols"?
5. How does gum inflammation promote heart disease and high blood pressure?
6. How do oral microbes invade your body and exponentially accelerate inappropriate inflammation to create disease?
7. Genetics and inflammatory diseases. Genetic susceptibility test.
8. What is a bacterial shower? Who should be concerned and how can you protect yourself?
9. As we learn more about how mouth germs affect our bodies, does it make sense to reduce antibiotic coverage for those at risk?
10. If not antibiotics, then what?
11. How do bacterial showers from gum disease into the bloodstream affect me if I have an implanted medical device or have had orthopedic surgery?

## Cardiovascular Disease

In only fifty percent of heart attacks are cholesterol numbers high. High cholesterol numbers are merely a symptom of inflammation, characterized by damage to blood vessel walls. The term cardiovascular disease, or CVD, encompasses several related diseases of the heart and circulatory system. Atherosclerosis is common and occurs when mineralized plaques build in artery walls. Arteries are the highways that carry oxygenated blood to our tissues. These plaques constrict and stiffen these highways. Because the heart is our hardest working organ, its oxygen demands are enormous. As plaques build, the amount of oxygen delivered to the heart muscle declines, which causes a rise in heart attack risk. Atherosclerosis occurring in the heart and nearby neck and chest arteries can also cause ischemic strokes if they obstruct oxygenated blood flow to the brain. Risks increase with poor oral health.

Plaques arise in blood vessel walls as a response to injury. The damage can come from high homocysteine blood levels from genetic influences or from environmental influences. The following list illustrates how lifestyle choices bombard blood vessel walls to cause damage:

- high meat intake, which raises homocystine levels
- inadequate B complex vitamins or their poor absorption. B vitamins mitigate homocysteine damage.
- constant high insulin levels found most commonly in people with pre-diabetes or uncontrolled diabetes
- glycation (AGE) damage from eating sugar and other simple carbohydrates
- high blood pressure
- nicotine irritation from smoking
- constant release of the stress hormone cortisol
- apnea
- microbes such as those of gum disease or other infections
- trans fat and other poor fat ingestion
- heavy metal (like mercury) toxicity

Gum disease can also accelerate blood vessel damage because it is one of many infections that increase blood levels of C-reactive protein, or CRP. CRPs are addressed more thoroughly below.

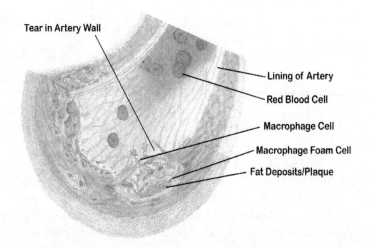

Tear in Artery Wall

Lining of Artery

Red Blood Cell

Macrophage Cell

Macrophage Foam Cell

Fat Deposits/Plaque

**Section of Plaque-filled Artery:** Plaques do not form in the open channels of blood vessels. They form just beneath the interior arterial walls. To repair damage, low-density lipoprotein cholesterol carriers, or LDLs, bring cholesterol to the site where they aggregate with blood platelets to repair the damage. LDLs tend to oxidize as they flow through oxygen-rich arterial blood, so as this complex infiltrates the single cell lining of the artery, or endothelium, white blood cells called macrophages (shown as blue star shapes on website) engulf them. Unfortunately, these macrophages cannot process oxidized LDLs. Together, they form "foam cells" (rust-colored on website), an important component of the damaging plaques found within the walls of our arteries. These foam cells grow, rupture, and signal the need for more cholesterol repair, which is brought by more oxidized LDLs in an endless damaging cycle.

Smooth muscle cells and a protective fibrous cap line and thicken the artery wall to keep blood flowing smoothly, but foam cells secrete a substance capable of breeching this protective layer. Debris from the plaques escapes into the bloodstream if the wall ruptures. Clotting occurs quickly. A clot, escaped debris, or both can narrow or block blood vessels. This occurs at the injury site or in smaller downstream vessels.

## Active Oral Infections Pour Oil on Inflammatory Fires

CAROL: "Claire, a study released to periodontists, or gum surgeons, in 2004 flatly stated, 'The periodontal (gum) health of patients admitted to the Coronary[1] Care unit due to acute coronary syndrome is unacceptable.'[i] In fact, those with chronic gum disease develop heart disease one and a half times more often than those with healthy mouths.

"As I said, long-term active oral infections initiate a cascade of biological responses. The immune system functions by flooding the body with chemical messenger molecules designed to help your body heal.[2] These healing molecules help most when they fight acute infections. They are problematic and destructive when they attempt to manage chronic, prolonged infections like gum and heart diseases, the chronic diseases that can begin in childhood, but surface as we age.

"These messenger molecules stimulate the liver to make C-reactive proteins or CRPs. The media most frequently link high levels of CRPs to heart disease. A test for circulating CRPs can give you an indication of your cumulative inflammatory risk from all sources. CRP levels are consistently higher in people with gum disease compared to those with healthy gums.[ii] Knowing your CRP numbers is more important than knowing your cholesterol numbers.

"Some of these infection messengers do more than communicate; they initiate atherosclerosis. These messengers[3] stimulate foam cell formation within blood vessel walls. Foam cells are a major component of the plaques that narrow and stiffen arteries. These foam cells don't just narrow the arteries; they also secrete the chemicals responsible for weakening and rupturing blood vessel walls. When a wall ruptures, plaque and other debris escapes, a clot forms and blood flow is blocked. When it occurs in the heart, it's a heart attack. When it occurs in the brain or nearby artery and the clot moves into the brain, it is a stroke.

---

1 The term coronary pertains to the heart, particularly when discussing health.
2 When gums are infected, tumor necrosis factor alpha (TNF-alpha), Interleukin-1, Interleukin-6, lipopolysaccaharides (LPS), and prostaglandins are just some of the released messenger molecules.
3 TNF and IL-6

### High Sensitivity C-Reactive Protein, or hs-CRP Test

A high sensitivity CRP test, or hs-CRP test, measures CRPs in number of milligrams per liter of blood. Elevated CRP levels may be a strong predictor for heart attack risk, especially in conjunction with high triglyceride levels and low HDL levels. According to the American Heart Association, "High levels of hs-CRP consistently predict recurrent coronary events in patients with unstable angina and ... heart attack. Higher hs-CRP levels also are associated with lower survival rates in these patients... After adjusting for other prognostic factors, hs-CRP is useful as a risk predictor. [iii]

These inflammatory markers produced in the liver reflect cumulative risks from many sources. Inflammation can multiply levels 1,000 times. The following guide indicates risk levels:

- CRP less than 1 mg per liter represents a low risk.
- CRPs between 1 and 3 milligrams per liter represents an average   risk.
- CRPs greater than 3 milligrams per liter represent a high risk. [iv] [v]

Other conditions that prompt a rise in CRP blood levels: trauma, surgery, burns, cancers, smoking, stress, other inflammatory diseases, alcohol abuse, and certainly dietary habits. For example, in a study of 700 nurses, 20 percent of nurses with the highest intake of trans fats had blood levels of C-reactive protein 73 percent higher than those in the lowest 20 percent.[vi] Gum disease can be a chronic or acute stimulus of CRPs and increase the risks of heart diseases and other inflammatory diseases.[vii]

Some suggest that only 20 to 40 percent of gum disease cases have a genetic basis for high levels of hsCRP.[viii]

Cholesterol and hs-CRP tests are inexpensive and can be run on the same blood sample. Self-test kits are available. Go to www.mouthmattersbook.com for links.

## LDLs (the "Bad Cholesterols")

"If you have high levels of low-density lipoproteins (LDLs) and high triglyceride levels, it's an indication arterial plaque formation is likely in full swing. LDLs are markers for cholesterol and the body's need for them. They are fat/protein molecules found in the blood that transport cholesterols made in the liver to places in the body where they are needed for cell repair.

"How you eat determines the size of LDL proteins. The very small LDLs (VLDLs) are the most destructive. It is the VLDLs, produced in the liver largely as a byproduct of fructose metabolism, that tend to migrate into the tiny crevices of blood vessel walls where they oxidize and promote inflammation and scarring. This is how LDLs earned their reputation as "bad" cholesterols. Cholesterols are called upon to repair blood vessel wall damage.

"The presence of oxidized LDLs together with inflammatory messengers, triggers foam cell formation within the blood vessel walls. Surprisingly, ruptures in vessels with newer, less stable, and non-calcified plaques more often cause heart attacks and strokes. These typically occur where blood vessel openings are only constricted about 20 percent. But blood vessels with more significantly reduced flows carry a two-fold danger. First, they are easier to block by debris or a clot. Second, the heart must work much harder to pump the blood through narrower, less elastic channels. This effort alone can seriously tax the heart and lead to a full-blown heart attack.

"Atherosclerosis is associated with high blood pressure. High blood pressure means blood vessel walls lack elasticity. Arteries are muscular and elastic when healthy. They stretch when the heart pumps blood through them. The amount they stretch depends on the amount of force exerted by the blood. A recent study revealed patients with inflammatory diseases such as high blood pressure, diabetes, early kidney disease, and rheumatoid arthritis had stiff blood vessels with low elasticity. Notably, it also showed that when periodontal (gum) disease was treated, not only did CRP levels decrease, but also small artery elasticity increased.[x]

"So gum disease is an important way atherosclerosis begins and advances in blood vessels. [xi] [xii] Treating gum disease and keeping it under tight control helps reverse damage.

# Gum Disease and
# Heart Disease

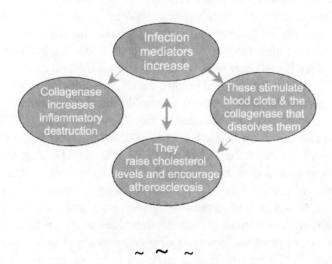

~ ~ ~

# Aetna Study

**Treating gum disease decreases costs for treating other degenerative diseases.**

Cost savings after therapy

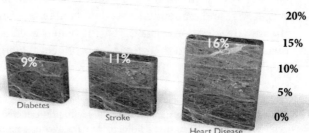

Albert DA, Sadowsky D, Papapanou P, et al. "An Examination of periodontal treatment and per member per month (OMOM) medical costs in an insured population." *BMC Health Serv Res.* 2006; 6: 103.

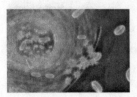

## Huge Playground for Germs

"There is another way gum disease damages the entire circulatory system. As anaerobic bacteria embed themselves in inaccessible gum tissue, the local inflammatory response causes blood vessel walls there to become porous and leaky. Bacteria and their toxins easily seep into the blood stream, and begin to circulate. The bacteria invade arterial walls and other sites far removed from the oral cavity.

"An estimate of the total surface area of an adult's blood vessel walls is at least $1,000^2$ meters, which is roughly the size of a tennis court.[xiii] Habitation of this huge area has tremendous consequences. There is a whole alphabet soup of bad bacteria we could call "systemic terrorists". Some of the ones that inoculate your arteries are: *Fusobacterium nucleatum,*[4] found in 80 percent; *Tannerella forsythia,* just under 50 percent; *C. pneumoniae,* significantly associated with coronary artery plaques,[xvi] and a major cause of pneumonia and possibly asthma, Alzheimer's and interstitial cystitis,[5] embedded in just under 30 percent. *Heliobacter pylori,* the germ responsible for many stomach ulcers and cancers, and *Haemophilus influenzae* are found in approximately four percent of artery walls.[xvii] Researchers think an oral reservoir of *H. pylori* makes it difficult to eradicate these bacteria from the gut, complicating stomach ulcer treatment. (H. pylori is a spirochete; see next section.)

"*Porphyromonas gingivalis* (*pG*), is usually the most common germ hiding under gums. *PG* is also found in atherosclerotic plaques, numerous cancers, and within brain abscesses. The mouth is always its source. This germ initiates and enhances atherosclerosis[xiv] and directly causes bone loss around teeth. [xv] One of its fatty by-products can inappropriately rev up the immune system to cause autoimmune disease. *PG* has been found embedded in 100 percent of arterial walls.

"Your inflammatory response stays roaring when a consistently large load of bad organisms and their toxic by-products are embedded in your circulatory system. This condition exacerbates many inflammatory conditions."

---

4 Facilitates colonization of other bacteria. It is associated with pre-term and still-births. It has been isolated from the amniotic fluid, placenta, and chorioamnionic membranes of women delivering prematurely. Mouse injection resulted in premature delivery, stillbirths, and non-sustained live births.

5 Interstitial cystitis is a syndrome characterized by urinary frequency, urgency, nocturia, and pain with bladder filling.

## Spirochetes

What has the Center for Disease Control (CDC) most concerned right now? Mycobacterium, the class of germs the trombone player from Chapter One fought. MRSA belongs to it. So does tuberculosis.

Many bacteria in this class have a characteristic receiving renewed attention – they have several life phases, an adaptation that gives them powerful survival strategies.

As described in the last chapter, current antibiotics target individual bacteria not protected by germs organized into biofilms. Antibiotics and the ultrasonics used in dentistry, kill by disrupting a bacteria's cell walls. What if a microorganism has no cell wall?

Many bacterial species have life phases during which they do not. They shrink from their typically large size to form a spores or cysts about the size of a virus – so small our immune systems cannot detect them. In these dormant forms, they do not cause symptoms; yet similar to bacteria in biofilms, most survive starvation, pH changes, temperature variations, and attempts at oxidation with hydrogen peroxide.[xv]

Spirochetes are a primary concern. Lyme Disease and Syphilis are familiar diseases caused by spirochetes. There are fifty-three known strains of oral spirochetes. Their corkscrew-shaped active forms easily drill into cell walls of dense tissues like bone that other organisms can't enter. They arrive and infect via the circulatory system. Their active forms regularly release neurotoxins. Brains and blood of Alzheimer's patients often contain a too-common spirochete of oral origin called *Treponema denticola*.[xvi] The outer membrane of *Treponema* strains contribute to their ability to penetrate blood vessel walls and cause virulence.

Remember when I suggested inflammatory diseases are essentially diseases of blood vessel walls? Blood vessel walls in diseased gum pockets match blood vessel walls described in atherosclerotic plaques. In other words, blood vessels throughout the body including the heart are affected as well as those in infected gum tissues.

There is an intimate and direct relationship between the function of capillaries throughout the body and seriousness of gum disease. Microscopically, advanced gum disease lesions show considerably remodeled blood vessels – the deeper the lesion, the more vessels are increased in diameter and number and the more leaky they will be.

Blood vessel wall function and localized blood congestion improves following successful gum disease therapy.

One of the ways bacteria resist our control efforts is their ability to exchange genes asexually between species. Species thriving close together, such as those in oral biofilms, have ample opportunity to gain diversity and resistance within plaques. *Treponema* organisms are particularly good at asexual gene swapping.

Active spirochetes go dormant when threatened or when the immune system is strong. When conditions become more favorable for them, they convert back to their active drill bit form. When spirochetes are cultured in a lab, carefully matched antibiotics create a kill zone in their immediate vicinity, but off to the edge of the medium, dormant cystic forms proliferate. This is consistent with retrospective research by Dr. Nordquist, a leading dentist and researcher. Over many years he took electronic recordings of the microscopic sessions he had with his clients. When he realized spirochetes have a dormant phase, he reviewed his archived data and saw spirochetal spores everywhere, particularly prevalent in those just finishing antibiotic therapy.[xvii] It could be said antibiotics encourage the non-motile dormant phase/proliferation of these bacteria.

*H. pylori,* an oral organism previously mentioned as being associated with ulcers and stomach cancers, is difficult to eradicate without treating gum disease at the same time. *H. pylori* is a spirochete. Could it be that treating gum disease concurrently is not enough for long-term success?

Dr. Nordquist surmises oral spirochetes may be the "smoking gun" connecting gum and heart disease. He believes the dormant forms reactivate in the lining of the blood vessels of the heart in particular, "causing a final inflammatory response that results in a heart attack". He believes spore activation in blood vessels results in blood clots and that these events affect people in their later, more vulnerable years.[xviii] Spores can also activate when the immune system is challenged by extreme stress.

There are a few high-level dentists interested in eradicating oral spirochetes. They are evaluating treatments developed for Lyme disease. While laser, chemical curettage, or ozone therapy may work well within the mouth and are important adjuncts, remember they are localized, temporary therapy. Keeping the body chemically balanced is part of keeping your whole body strong and resistant.

To kill off the spore forms, alternative therapies with promise utilize various ozone gas treatment modalities or complicated multi-year courses of pulsed very low dose antibiotics in conjunction with Olmesartan (the Marshall Protocol) and glutathione. (See Resources section.)

**Fun Facts: Those Incredible Survivors!***

- Live bacteria survive in the petrified gut of a forty million year old bee.
- The most amazing thing ever brought back from the moon was a live bacterial colony. It survived a space launch, the vacuum of space, continual radiation exposure, frigid space temperatures, and a lack of food, energy, or water for three years.
- *D. Radiodurans* (What humorists scientists can be!) can survive almost 10,000 times the dose of radiation lethal to humans.
- Bacteria are the oldest life form on earth – more than 3.5 billion years old.
- Your body has ten times more bacterial cells than human cells.
- Scientists have trained *E. coli* bugs, the most numerous bacteria found in the colon, to assemble into glowing bull's eye shapes on command.
- *R. metallidurans* can turn dissolved gold into solid particles.
- Hydrothermal vent bacteria, never considered to be able to survive in humans, has been found on prosthetic hip joints.

*Thank you Betsy Reynolds, RDH, MS, oral biologist, for these insights into an unseen world.

What will you do with all this information?

Pause here and remember: I did not write this book to scare you. Fear has nothing to recommend it. "Living with fear" is an oxymoron.

Bacteria are clearly survivalists. And they are fascinating. I hope you gain a sense of wonder – wonder at the intricacies of the biology and wonder that we live as well as we do. We humans are quite ingenious and resilient ourselves. If we pay attention – if we keep our minds and hearts open – we experience a far richer and likely longer life.

Learn about the fascinating connections, then enjoy learning about how to implement solutions. We are all just beginning to appreciate the miraculous world of the unseen.

## Genetics Is Not Destiny

CLAIRE: "Do you think I'm genetically coded for this? Must I be more meticulous than my friends because my father has heart disease and high blood pressure?"

CAROL: "Genes influence everything. A simple PST test, a one-time screening tool based on a genetic variation of the inflammatory messenger Interleukin-1, measures how strong a person's immune system will respond to disease microbes. I test smokers because studies show heavy smoking and this genetic variance work aggressively together to cause early tooth loss.[xviii] Both contribute to an exaggerated immune response, partially through elevated IL-1 levels. Smokers are seven times more likely to suffer severe gum disease anyway.[xix] Because your family and personal health history is riddled with inflammatory diseases, it may help us determine how aggressive we need to be to keep you healthy. Keep in mind however, quite frequently, people without a genetic predisposition have advanced gum disease largely due to lifestyle.

"We should consult with your rheumatologist, because arthritis also raises Interleukin levels. Researchers have long guessed these two diseases are closely related through common underlying dysfunction of inflammatory mechanisms.[xx] I know you don't take a prescription to control your arthritis so if Interleukin levels were low it could be because you already boost your immune system to keep symptoms bearable. You walk daily and chase your kids for exercise. You minimize stress through yoga, meditation, and positive thinking. You don't smoke, your diet is excellent except for your recent sugar indulgences, and you don't carry excess abdominal fat.

"Between now and your next visit, why don't you try to limit your desserts and develop sound hygiene practices, what I call 'daily wound management.' Your gums will likely improve, and you might have fewer arthritis flare-ups! It's a win-win deal. Try to floss in front of your children. They don't listen to us; they mimic us!

"If your gums don't improve, we can order a PST test, a pathogen test, and consider diabetes screening, because the disease runs in your family. You may want to relay this information to your father. I sense he has a casual attitude about his gum disease, which he ignores it at his peril. If he treated his gum disease, he will likely reduce his cardiovascular risk and gain better control of his diabetes. We'll discuss that next time, because gum disease plays a role in blood sugar control.

"To summarize, your mouth is your body's gateway. Poor dental health and heart disease are strongly linked and the odds of having a heart attack increase in proportion to the severity of the gum disease.

While this is clear, remember smoking, obesity, diabetes, arthritis, and stress, are shared risk factors. But isn't it wonderful to know you can control a significant risk factor for many diseases with a few attentive minutes every day?"

## Interleukin-1 (IL-1) Genetic Test (PST)

Interleukin-1s recruit so many other inflammatory messengers they are considered the "master mediator" of the inflammatory response. IL-1s stimulate bone loss throughout the body. The jawbone supporting the teeth, is not spared. The PST test measures a genetic variation on the IL-1 genes that indicate an amplified immune response to gum disease microbes. This trait is but one of the contributing factors to gum disease. Even in the absence of obvious infection, a positive genotype can indicate a predisposition to aggressive gum disease.[xxi] The theory is that some people with periodontal disease show an Interleukin-1 level two to six times higher than others with similar disease levels because of a genetic susceptibility. The enhanced inflammatory response for genetically susceptible individuals would initiate more body damage compared to those with a muted response.

There are other reasons for elevated IL-1 levels beyond bacterial stimulus, genetic predisposition and smoking. For example, some diabetics show an IL-1 level thirty times that of a healthy person.[xxii] See Chapter Five to learn why diabetics have serious immune system challenges.

Though we should always treat gum disease aggressively, some want to determine risk. Oral DNA Labs (Quest Labs subsidiary: 877-577-9055) offers the "MyPeriodID PST" test, which looks at the IL-1 DNA to help determine genetic risk for accelerated bone loss. A non-invasive test, a saliva sample is sent to a lab for molecular analysis. If someone is at genetic risk and has other complicating factors like smoking, diabetes, High VLDL cholesterol readings, or heart disease, appropriate therapy might include assessing some of the disease-causing bacteria present. Some dentists target them with matched high dose antibiotics during *active* periodontal therapy. This is because ultrasonic instrumentation breaks up biofilm, therefore some bacteria become susceptible to antibiotics. Because gum disease should always be treated aggressively for reasons that will become clear, I avoid antibiotics and use more certain therapies you will read about later.

Consider this and the following test before placing implants for maximum success.

**Note:** A person must fast for 12 hours prior to testing.

### My PerioPath Test

Oral DNA Labs has another interesting test. Knowing risk factors and what germs live in the reservoir is important. From a saliva sample, MyPerioPath shows the DNA signature of about 13 organisms.

I resisted this test because it was presented to me as a way to design antibiotic therapy. Learning about spirochetes, knowing most researchers think antibiotics will become a thing of the past for many reasons, and knowing there are far more pathogens than this test looks for, it may be obvious why I did not use it. Nonetheless, knowing the identity of some of the bad players* and their characteristics helps profile risk – and powerfully motivates people. Not only does it help me measure the success or failure of therapy based on the presence or absence of these indicator bugs, it helps clients work harder to change their terrain, the substrate** they make of their bodies through lifestyle choices.

Alternatively, clinicians skilled at using Darkfield microscopes can use them to identify spores or spirochete cysts.

*This tests includes one spirochetal organism, *Treponema denticola*.
**Substrate**: the base on which an organism lives.

## Bacterial Showers/Damaged Heart Valves

Did you ever neglect a sore throat only to have it develop into a massive strep throat case? Many of us have done so without knowing it can devolve into rheumatic fever. Rheumatic fever is dangerous because it can permanently damage heart valves. It can result in immediate heart failure or put you at risk of heart failure for a lifetime. Damaged heart valves can also result from open-heart surgery or congestive heart failure. Sometimes one is born with faulty valves.

Bacterial showers, like those that gum disease induces, become an every day risk for those with faulty heart valves.

The list on the following page is not an enviable list. These are well-known people who have died suddenly because of endocarditis, an uncommon, but serious infection occurring on heart valves or the lining of the heart's blood vessels:

- Gustav Mahler, composer, 1860–1911
- Robert Burns, poet, 1759–1796
- Alois Alzheimer, physician, 1864–1915
- Orville Gibson, guitar manufacturer, 1856–1918
- Rudolph Valentino, actor, 1895–1926;
- Jack Glascock, bass player for Jethro Tull, 1951–1997

When a surge of adherent bacteria like oral biofilms shower the circulatory system, these bacteria can attach to and colonize damaged heart structures. Endocarditis from bacterial showers can result from any infection. Oral infections are a frequent culprit, but past wisdom suggested this occurred only during certain dental procedures. Research has changed what we know of this phenomenon; infective endocarditis can be a serious complication of daily dental neglect.

Imagine a waterfall. Downstream from its churning base, leaves and other debris swirl in tranquil side eddies. Metaphorically, this is a quiet location downstream from an ineffective heart valve. Faulty valves disrupt normally smooth blood flow. These eddies are the hospitable locations where adherent biofilms grow to become potentially life threatening infections.

Where do these bacterial showers originate? Certainly any infection in the body can flood the bloodstream with bacterial culprits known to trigger endocarditis. Urinary tract infections, pneumonia, and cellulitis are examples.

Surgical and dental procedures involving contaminated tissues have been especially blamed in the past. This has kept the American Heart Association and dentists struggling for decades to manage these risks.

The American Heart Association continually evaluates and revises guidelines for antibiotic coverage during dental procedures. Thirty years ago, they recommended at-risk clients to take antibiotics for four days. Since then, the recommended antibiotic dosage and frequency has downgraded several times. By the late 1990s, the recommendation was for one sizeable antibiotic dose an hour prior to dental procedures.

This sounds sensible and reduces the risk of already rare cases of endocarditis. Consider what you now know about the health implications of raw oral tissues teeming with morphed bacteria in biofilms, which are specialized to adhere to blood vessel walls. This unhealthy state is common in many adults. It is easy to understand how toxins from a pocket can shower the bloodstream when highly inflamed and fragile tissues are manipulated to remove biofilm and mineralized deposits. For this reason, I believe it is critical for dental professionals to begin immune system support therapy for clients prior to therapy.[5]

Finally, in 2007, the American Heart Association released new dental antibiotic coverage guidelines. These guidelines strictly curtail antibiotic coverage, reflecting a subtle, yet important reality.

## Infected Gums are Not a Casual Concern

A casual attitude towards infected gums is a dangerous attitude for everyone. For those at high risk, it is more dangerous. As oral-systemic infection links become clearer, it seems odd to curtail antibiotic coverage, yet these guidelines implicate an interesting reality. Dental procedures are a transient event. An average extraction subjects patients to a six-minute intense bacterial shower. A "cleaning" is a more serious and lengthy procedure, yet still low risk, all things considered.

Bacteremia, the presence of a high bacterial load in the bloodstream, of oral cause is an everyday risk. Daily chewing represents the biggest risk. Blood levels of endotoxins (toxic bacterial end products) and inflammatory messengers quadrupled in circulating blood after subjects gently chewed gum lightly for 50 times on each side of the mouth.[xxiii] Informed estimates suggest eating rough foods like corn chips, tooth brushing (especially with a hard or rough, natural brush), flossing (particularly incorrectly), and other oral habits subject a person to bacteremias for over ninety hours a month![xiv] That is roughly three hours every day. So there is a chronic release of bacteria, their endotoxins, and the mediators that combat them into the bloodstream.

Both the incidence and the magnitude of bacteremias of oral origin are proportional to the degree of oral inflammation and infection.[xxv] [xxvi] Active inflammation matters more than the surface area of the "oral wound." People with healthy mouths are at far less daily risk of life threatening bacteremias.

The implications are enormous and are compounded when one learns the risk of infective endocarditis[6] and chronic inflammatory diseases are on the rise.

---

5 I use ozone gel in pockets before therapy to avoid precipitating bacterial showers. In the meantime, clients boost their immune systems. (Chapter Fifteen and Appendices IX and X) Doctors can fabricate PerioProtect trays and have the client use them with 1.7% hydrogen peroxide daily for two weeks. Note: spirochetes are resistant to hydrogen peroxide, but not ozone. Smokers should avoid hydrogen peroxide, as use multiplies cancer risks.

6 Currently reported at 3.3 cases/100,000 population/year in the U.S. and the U.K.

This knowledge is critical, especially to clients with heart concerns. Most people surrender their health to dental hygienists, thinking "twice a year" dental "cleanings" protect their oral health. Some schedule wellness visits quarterly, but often with the same objective: to hand their health over to professionals. This is not true primary prevention. Detoxifying teeth with a cleaning simply removes evidence of disease to give you a new chance to heal yourself. If you and your hygienist work together toward optimal health, your preventive visits will help you monitor your general health.

The risks from oral complications are no different than they ever were. These guidelines simply acknowledge the reality that dental manipulations are insignificant compared to the daily oral risks people choose to manage or not manage.

The new guidelines suggest covering only those with the highest risk of death as a complication of infective endocarditis.[7] It turns out allergic reactions caused by antibiotic coverage lead to more deaths than deaths from complications of non-antibiotic-covered dental treatment. Be accountable.

## Bacterial Showers and Orthopedic Surgery/Implanted Medical Devices

Biofilms also colonize medical devices such as joint replacements or ports. Though rare, the consequences of medical device failure are catastrophic. Again, because bacteria in biofilms have genetically morphed, they have an enhanced ability to adhere to joint replacements and other implanted medical devices. Worse, these biofilms are resistant to antibiotics and human immune responses. (See Chapter Two for a biofilm review.)

Previously, at-risk orthopedic surgery patients were also pre-medicated with antibiotics prior to dental treatment. These guidelines have been modified for the same reasons. The risks are small, though serious. Risks for antibiotic reactions are higher than the risk of developing a biofilm on a joint replacement. You *must* collaborate with your dental team and your doctors to devise an appropriate regimen that reflects your risks.

7 People with organ transplants *must* always be premedicated. Consider it or therapies indicated in the previous footnote if you have: body piercings, use intravenous drugs or drink excessive amounts of alcohol, which suppresses the immune system. HIV/ AIDS also increases susceptibility to bacterial showers.

Think of what you have learned about inflammation and gum disease. Then consider the age group that usually receives joint replacements is people over age 50. Seniors have had more time to develop inflammatory diseases. They likely have unmet dental needs. Many seniors are missing teeth. Missing teeth leads to malnutrition because of ineffective chewing. Other possible dental challenges include untreated or uncontrolled gum disease, numerous root canals, and unfilled or abscessing teeth. Remember, people visit dentists when they are well and physicians when they are sick. Seniors often spend limited health care time and resources on medical care outside of dentistry.

Everyone must be evaluated and treated by a dental professional prior to elective medical implant surgery. This elective surgery is absolutely contraindicated whenever there is an infection elsewhere in the body. These infections must be treated and controlled. Commit to a successful surgery.

**Note:** Many orthopedic surgeons request dental clearance prior to joint replacement surgery, but advance notice is essential. It takes time to complete extensive dental plans. Unfortunately, many people postpone joint replacement until the joint completely fails. This is a poor time to begin a comprehensive project designed to regain oral health. Pre-surgical clearance from health specialists like cardiologists, internists, and endocrinologists are still obtained more often than from dental teams.

Symptoms of joint replacement infection include fatigue and weakness, sore throat, weight loss, fever, chills, night sweats, aches and pains, painful nodes in the pads of fingers and toes, red spots on the skin of palms and soles, swelling of feet, legs, and abdomen, shortness of breath with activity, and blood in the urine. Complications other than serious illness and death can be blood clots, stroke, heart rhythm problems, abscesses, and other infections.

Many dental offices offer genetic tests and hs-C-Reactive Protein tests as an adjunct to treating gum disease and its risks. These are administered in-office or in the privacy of one's home. See the Resources Section for more information.

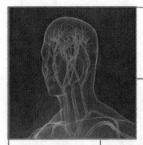

# 4

# STROKE/CAROTID ARTERY DISEASE

**Explore:**
1. What is a stroke?
2. How do gum disease, atherosclerosis, and other diseases of the blood vessels influence one another?
3. How does gum disease increase stroke risk?

Carotid artery disease is a specific form of the heart disease discussed in the last chapter. The risks and inflammatory pathways are the same, but this form deserves special attention, since oral organisms target carotid neck arteries. System-wide damage occurs jointly, but strokes are a frequent result of this specific area of plaque accumulation.

Postmenopausal women disproportionately account for more than 60 percent of the deaths in the U.S. attributed to stroke. Panoramic x-rays, taken in some dental offices, can show calcification of carotid arteries. Though not the preferred diagnostic path for stroke risk, if your dentist takes these, you might ask if he or she sees anything.[i]

## JAMES

James is a local rancher who has survived 72 hard years. After a 12-year hiatus from dental offices, he recently strolled into ours. The following pictures show he did not enthusiastically participate in his oral health, but intimate views of his teeth made him less indifferent.[1]

---

1 The following photographs are courtesy of Dr. David Yu, Austin, TX.

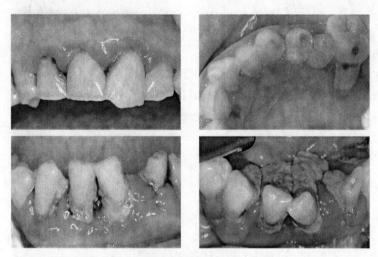

**James: "I just want to maintain what I have."**

He was as interested as he was surprised. While carefully explaining our observations, I mentioned how bad oral bacteria enter the circulatory system and often target the carotid arteries of the neck. James's face lit up in recognition because he had just had a CIMT scan[2] of his carotid artery and it had shown serious atherosclerosis. Since his doctor mentioned the link between stroke and gum disease, James wanted to know more.

CAROL: "James, as your doctor probably explained, an ischemic stroke causes damage to the brain. If a blood clot or a portion of artery clogging plaque itself is expelled into the arteries of the brain or arteries downstream from the breakaway site, it obstructs blood flow. This means oxygen and necessary nutrients can't reach your brain to nourish it. Subsequently starved areas lose function.

"Your two carotid arteries are major upstream arteries. They run up each side of your neck to connect the large blood vessel carrying oxygenated blood from your heart to the blood vessels of your brain. Many clots originate in the carotid arteries.

"Stroke risk factors are diabetes, heart disease, high blood pressure, smoking, and gum disease. The processes active in promoting heart disease also lead to strokes.

---

2 A CIMT (Carotid Intima-Media Thickness) test reveals the amount of plaque build-up in carotid arteries. See image at end of this chapter.

"Mouth infections are the most common of all human infections. The oral reservoir of bacteria and their toxic wastes initiate damaging biochemical pathways." (Here I explained the principals I discussed in the last chapter.)

"The inflammatory markers, atherosclerosis, and loss of blood vessel elasticity exist for both heart disease and stroke risk. With stroke risk, there is an increased chance of blood clot formation in the carotid artery because that blood vessel is targeted for heavy plaque formation.

"Three more things:

1. As two inflammatory markers increase,[3] so does the possibility of blood clot formation because these markers turn blood thick, sticky, sluggish and stimulate blood clots. A stroke occurs when a blood clot forms in the carotid artery and travels to the brain. A heart attack happens when a clot blocks a heart artery. Those with high levels of hs-CRPs have two to three times greater risk for stroke.

2. Another inflammatory messenger, TNF-alpha, raises blood triglyceride levels associated with the plaques and stiffened blood vessels of atherosclerosis.

3. Some of the same inflammatory messengers[4] released as a result of gum disease or other infections that contribute to atherosclerosis also generate collagenase, the protein-destroying enzyme that attacks the tissue foundation of the teeth. But collagenase also dissolves and releases arterial plaques into the blood stream. It is the biochemical response dental professionals battle.

"Many alternative care providers view blood with Dark Field Microscopes to check for a condition called rouleau, an indication of sticky red blood cells and a non-specific disease indicator. They know sticky red blood cells are prone to clotting and may result from inflammation and increased levels of CRP in their blood, diet imbalances, anemia, and emotional stress. When two weeks of eating properly do not resolve the condition, they begin to consider a network of inflammatory disease possibilities. Rouleau favors the growth of unhealthy organisms, which tolerate oxygen-poor environments.

---

3 Hs-CRPs and fibrinogen. For every fibrinogen increase of 100 mg/dl, risk for stroke increases 82%.

4 Example: prostaglandins.

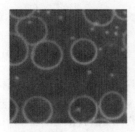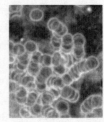

Left: Dark Field microscopic images of normal, free-flowing red blood cells. Right: "stacked" red blood cells of rouleau (referrs to how red blood cells look like a roll of coins). It indicates sticky, thick blood prone to clotting. Stacked blood cells do not carry or exchange oxygen and carbon dioxide well.

"Inflammatory markers elicited by gum disease both encourage arterial plaque formation and provoke the collagenase production that breaks down the protective cap that walls off atherosclerotic damage. Dissolving this cap can lead to clots. To complete the cycle, collagenase worsens gum disease. The process feeds on itself."

"Several major studies show that the heavier the load of bacteria derived from gum disease found in the carotid neck artery, the thicker and more constricted the carotid artery walls, which increases the risk for heart attack and stroke.[ii] [5] In fact, had you not asked about this, we would have referred you for a CMIT scan of your carotid arteries because of the influences each one has on the other. Many studies recommend carotid scans if you have significant gum disease.[iii]

"Another study's conclusion was short and succinct: dental health condition, oral hygiene, and particularly tooth loss (most teeth are lost due to gum disease) are associated with the degree of carotid artery narrowing and predict future progression of the disease.[iv] The assumption: spiraling inflammatory responses draw upon the huge and constant septic bacterial 'sink' the mouth often is.  Consider your situation. It makes sense with what we know; people with long-standing and serious periodontal disease carry the highest risk.

---

5 The finding that bacterial components of carotid artery plaque are similar to plaque around a person's teeth is consistent with a study that concluded, "Overall periodontal bacteria burden (defined by the score of *Actinobacillus actinomycetemcomitans, Porphyromonas gingivalis, Tannerella forsythensis,* and *Treponima denticola*) was significantly related to carotid intimal thickness (and) have been associated with increased risk of myocardial infarction [heart attack] and stroke, particularly in adults 65 years of age or older." (Intimal thickness is the thickness of the innermost lining of the blood vessel, indicating various degrees of atherosclerosis in this area.)

One study analyzing bacterial burden risks found subjects with severe gum disease had a 4.3-fold increase of cerebral ischemia (stroke) over those with mild or no periodontitis. Soder PO, Soder B, Nowak J, et al. **Early Carotid Atherosclerosis in Subjects With Periodontal Diseases**. *Stroke,* June 1, 2005; 36(6): 1195 - 1200. http://stroke.ahajournals.org/cgi/reprint/36/6/1195. Accessed 2/14/2009.

"I know you understand this, but you'll enjoy this study because of your ranching background. A research group took 36 pigs and fed half of them low fat chow and half of them high fat chow. Then they injected half of each of these two groups with one of the most prevalent bacteria found in gum disease[6] three times a week for five months. When they euthanized the pigs and looked at their coronary arteries – the arteries that supply the heart – and aortas – the major blood vessels that lead from the heart – they found the bacteria began atherosclerotic lesions even in pigs eating low-fat pig chow. It increased lesions for the pigs on high-fat chow." [v]

JAMES: "It looks like I should lose the high-fat chow and reduce my bacterial load!"

CAROL: "Yes. We need to improve your odds. Today we'll talk about your diet, how to boost your immune system, and how we'll begin to spiff up your mouth and work to change your chemistry both orally and throughout your body. Phase two will likely be referral to a specialist."

James became an interested, active partner in his oral health. He intently observed his treatment in a mirror. He was cooperative and worked hard on self-care. He was referred to a periodontist (a specialist in treatment of the supportive tissues around the teeth) for further assessment and surgery. He lost several teeth because considerable bone loss had rendered them hopeless. Still, he was thrilled with his treatment results. Anecdotally, he said what I often hear from clients, which is that he was far more energetic after treatment. Psychologically and physiologically, we both knew he had done something good for himself, something he deserved.

---

6 *P. gingivalis*. More recent studies also show this germ significantly accelerates atherosclerotic plaques. The lipopolysaccharide outer membrane of these anaerobic, gram negative bacteria are a part of their toxicity. Human enzymes cannot digest them, so our bodies try to wall them off with proteins. When these bacteria contact a blood vessel wall, they attract immune system cells. These cells (monocytes) produce enzymes which dissolve the elastic layer of the wall, leading to their rupture. The LP-PLA$_2$ Index measures lipoprotein levels in blood. Gum disease raises these levels. Stroke risks elevate when readings are >200. Treating gum disease improves LP-PLA$_2$ levels. (Lösche W, Marshal GJ, Krause S, et al. "Lipoprotein-associated phospholipase A2 and plasma lipids in patients with destructive periodontal disease ." *Journal of Clin Perio 2005*. 32(6);640–644. ) So far, The PLAC Test which measures LP-PLA$_2$ levels, is the only blood test cleared by the FDA to aid in assessing risk for both coronary heart disease (CHD) and ischemic stroke associated with atherosclerosis.

**Note:** James provides a dramatic example of gum disease. Most clients, even with severe disease, show few symptoms and would look "normal" during self-observation. Nonetheless, they likely have many measurable markers for disease. For example, I also arranged for James to be checked for insulin resistance. When a person is insulin resistant, he likely has reduced brain function, reduced blood flow to the heart, and is three times more likely to have a stroke than someone with normal sugar metabolism. Insulin resistance damages arteries regardless of blood sugar levels. Eighty percent of those with insulin resistance die from heart attack or stroke. Not surprising, James bordered on being diabetic.

Initially, I tested James's salivary pH, which was exceptionally low (acidic). While not a great test, it opened the discussion about how dependent he was on simple carbohydrates – his sugary snacks and love of potatoes – and how they affected his body. Discussed later, most white foods are acutely inflammatory. Simple carbohydrates require significant buffering capacity. One of the body's buffering systems mobilizes needed minerals out of skeletal bone including the jawbone; dental professionals should be concerned. These minerals then precipitate in the most inappropriate places such as cancers (calcium precipitation into tumors makes cancers visible on x-rays), atherosclerotic plaques and kidneys. Just as these minerals deposit into plaques in blood vessel walls, they deposit into oral biofilms.

We also asked James to complete a sleep study; it was determined he had sleep apnea, which affected his oral and general health.

Examining James's story, it is obvious oral conditions are not localized. If we had just "cleaned" his teeth, we would have only treated his symptoms – and actually may have triggered a stroke. Symptom-driven treatment does not deliver health.

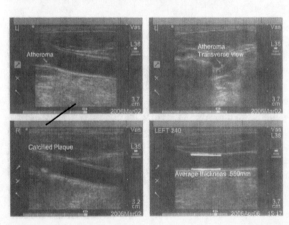

CMIT Scan courtesy of Vasolabs, Inc. (www.vasolabs.com). These carotid artery scans provide your physician a visualized plaque and atherosclerotic burden assessment along with a written report describing risk with 95% confidence.

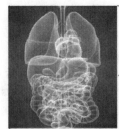

# 5

# DIABETES AS AN ACCELERATED AGING MODEL

*"The cost of a thing is the amount of ... life which is required to be exchanged for it, immediately or in the long run."*

**~Henry David Thoreau ~**

This chapter is for you if you are diabetic, pre-diabetic, or simply at risk of developing diabetes. That covers most of us. Diabetes is another way of saying you are at risk for blindness, heart attack and other cardiovascular disease, sexual dysfunction, kidney failure, extremity amputation, nerve disorders, gum disease and other oral infections, tooth loss, dry mouth, cavities, difficulty with wound healing, and premature death. Is that blunt enough? This extensive list makes it clear that healthy aging depends on how well you and your body manage insulin, sugar, and energy.

**Explore:**
1. What oral clues alert dental professionals to suggest a client test for diabetes or pre-diabetes?
2. What are the benefits of early diagnosis?
3. What are "end organs" and how does diabetes affect them?
4. How does one acquire insulin resistance or diabetes?
5. What do marijuana and abdominal fat have in common?
6. What is leptin?
7. How does insulin influence aging?
8. How are diabetes and gum disease linked?
9. Do AGE products affect everyone? Why do they matter?
10. How can you boost energy metabolism?
11. What is a food's glycemic index?
12. What are symptoms of insulin resistance and diabetes?

A hygienist's potential influence is probably greatest on clients with diabetes. People tend to visit doctors when they believe they are sick. They visit dentists when they believe they are healthy. This means dental professionals regularly treat people with symptoms of disease that are so subtle the client is usually unaware of any illness.

## The First Clinical Sign of Diabetes is Gum Disease

Gum disease is the first symptom to emerge in those with diabetes, often showing itself in childhood before all other complications. [i][ii][iii] Organs with rich capillary beds are called end organs. Diabetes is an "end-organ" disease; the gums surrounding the teeth are a highly visible and accessible end organ. A hygienist's unique medical niche is as first-line "oral tissue" caregiver. An observant, knowledgeable clinician can detect clues signaling an inability to correctly process energy, taken into the body as simple carbohydrates. These carbohydrates are found in refined sugars and grains not associated with fiber. Hygienists are well positioned to suggest referrals when classic oral symptoms appear, thus providing earlier life-giving intervention.

Most of us know diabetes rates are spiraling. The Center for Disease Control (CDC) estimates 23.6 million Americans have diabetes, though a *third of them are undiagnosed*. Probably twice that many are pre-diabetic. That is a fourth of our population! The CDC projects a third of the population born after 2000 will be diagnosed with the disease in their lifetime.

Undiagnosed diabetics have type 2 diabetes. They can and usually do live for years with unidentified symptoms while the disease ages them at accelerated rates. It destroys their eyes, nerves, circulatory system, kidneys, and extremities, especially the feet. Skin infections appear more frequently and heal slowly. The earlier a diabetic diagnoses and addresses their metabolic problem, the less damage occurs. Diabetics are twice as likely to develop gum disease, partly because they are susceptible to infections in the first place. Type 2 diabetes is a lifestyle disease.

Only five percent of diabetics have type 1 diabetes. They suffer so acutely at the onset of the disease, it is impossible to dismiss their symptoms. They must rapidly seek treatment or risk death. (See Appendix III.)

The influence hygienists can have on individuals through preventive counseling, early-stage referral, and meticulous gum disease management, could improve lives and reduce treatment costs. Currently most hygienists do not have the knowledge or freedom to accomplish counseling or referrals. I want people to envision the possibility of a larger role for hygienists in disease screening, counseling and accelerated referrals for early diagnosis and treatment. In 2007, diabetes care accounted for $132 billion, or one in ten health care dollars spent. Indirect costs accounted for another $58 billion. This is unsustainable. Diabetics on average spend $11,744.00 per year on care.

## Diabetes as an End Organ Disease

If left undiagnosed and untreated, diabetes can devastate one's life. The disease accounts for more than eight percent of all deaths in the US.[iv] When you take into consideration that more than half of deaths attributed to strokes and heart attacks have diabetes as the underlying cause, you realize this is an understated statistic.

Organs with rich capillary beds are called end organs. Diabetes affects all end organs. Nutrient exchange between tissues and the blood occurs in the capillaries, which are the smallest part of the circulatory system and are the point of the whole heart/lung/blood vessel circulatory system.

Think of capillaries as being like a soaker hose with zillions of pinpoint punctures. Capillary walls normally allow only the smallest nutrients and tiny oxygen molecules to exit through their small pores to nurture surrounding cells. These small pores also allow molecular movement in the other direction. Carbon dioxide and waste products diffuse into the blood to be carried away. Unfortunately, diabetes makes the walls of these tiny capillaries thick and leaky, allowing larger molecules like proteins to escape through the larger pores. The following two examples focus on end organs particularly damaged by diabetes: the eyes and kidneys.

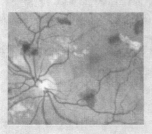

### Eyes and Kidneys as End Organs

Proteins such as albumin leak out of porous blood vessels throughout the body, including those of the eye. The albumen then forms little plugs. This prompts the formation of more blood vessels to circumvent the plugs so the eye can continue to function. But the new blood vessels tend to be even more fragile than the old ones. They also leak, form plugs, additional blood vessels form to circumvent these plugs, and so on. This circular process continues, eroding one's vision.

Further eye damage occurs because diabetics are troubled by sugar control, thus vitamin C absorption. Because UV rays from the sun focus on the retina to facilitate vision, the area is prone to extremely high oxidative stresses. Glycation of sugars with red blood cells (see Chapter One) create large, sharp molecules. These scratch and oxidize fragile retinal capillaries. To combat the enormous amount of free radicals caused by oxidative stress, retinal levels of vitamin C are 100 times that of most other body tissues. Because diabetics frequently have low vitamin C levels, free radical damage accumulates rapidly. Further, since vitamin C is crucial for collagen building, blood vessels in the retina and elsewhere are more fragile in diabetics than in non-diabetics.

Blood vessel leakiness occurs on a larger scale in the kidneys. These end organs filter the body's waste products from the blood and pass them into the urine to be excreted. When we are healthy, critical large molecules in the blood including proteins and red blood cells cannot pass through capillary walls and are retained in the blood. But as blood vessel walls become leaky and damaged from the same process that destroys the diabetic retina, albumin proteins also leak into the kidneys. This is why doctors look for albumin levels in urine to screen for kidney damage.

As kidneys fail, waste products build up in the blood. These wastes become so life threatening, they require either a kidney transplant or regular dialysis treatments to artificially cleanse the blood. A protein-rich diet increases the strain on already struggling kidneys, so a diabetic should discuss the wisdom of following a high protein weight loss diet with their doctors.

Understanding how diabetes affects the eye and kidney end organs is easy. Less well known and appreciated is how diabetes and the oral end organ influence each other.

The following stories reveal how my professional life brought me into contact with three people struggling with energy management and gum disease control. Each needed something different.

## MARK
## Needed: Diabetes Screening, Guidance, and Encouragement

Mark followed me to the door of my treatment room, but did not immediately sit. Instead, he stood at the door, met my eyes with an unwavering gaze, and threw down a stack of clipped papers. I needed a moment to remember the details of our last appointment.

He saw the tumblers click and assisted me, "This is a list of my new medications and information from my physician's office."

Oh yes. Mark's case was unusual. I promptly recalled that he had suffered a few job reversals, which kept him from seeing a dentist for five years. During his first visit with me, a standard gum disease evaluation showed several classic signs of gum disease: tissue swelling, easy bleeding, and significant bone and tissue loss around his teeth.

During therapy, I found few mineralized deposits under the tissue collar around his teeth. Even the biofilm was minimal. Moderate bone loss and easy bleeding without the usual complement of deposits suggests a systemic complication. So as I worked, I considered his health history.

When I noticed Mark had not had a physical in years, I suggested he should. I reevaluated his heavy 6'6" frame and his elevated blood pressure reading while considering the fact that obesity fuels inflammation. To be obese is to be chronically inflamed. Most know obesity is linked to high blood pressure, diabetes, heart disease, and stroke, but I was also concerned about his heightened risk of developing osteoarthritis, gout, and some cancers. I discussed with Mark my primary suspicion that he suffered a common trio of degenerative diseases: heart disease, diabetes, and gum disease.

"Mark, this is good news/bad news. The good news is today's visit was much simpler for both of us than I'd expected. But I will lean on you to schedule a physical. You have no obvious localized cause for the degree of bone loss and gum inflammation you show. You likely have a systemic health complication. Diabetes or pre-diabetes is possible. Diabetes signals a failure in two major hormones that regulate energy metabolism: insulin and leptin. Insulin tells individual cells whether they should burn or store sugars and fats and directs energy use. Leptin, secreted by fat cells, regulates appetite, activity levels, and energy storage on a larger scale through the brain via the hypothalamus.[1] Disturbances in both of these pathways are probably necessary to trigger diabetes. Diabetes is an important disease to diagnose because of the silent damage it causes in its early stages."

"Please return in two months so we can see how you responded to today's visit and to clear out the biofilm from those inaccessible areas. I would also like you to have had a complete physical by then."

And so he had. I snapped to the present. "Oh wonderful! You had a physical but I sense you're frustrated. What happened?"

## Diagnosis

MARK: "You wouldn't believe how high my blood sugar reading was; somewhere in the 300s. Scary. And I have developed high blood pressure as well. The doctor is trying to establish effective drugs and doses for me. Here's the list of what I am currently trying. I'd like to know how you guessed my condition and where do we go from here?"

I appraised him respectfully. In the years of guiding clients toward diabetes screening, I have learned to query them carefully on subsequent visits. Denial is frequent. Many people are not ready to face the lifestyle changes required to regain control over their body's metabolic function, thus the quality of their lives. It is more difficult to "own" diabetes than gum disease. When clients follow through on referrals and receive a positive diagnosis for this chronic degenerative disease, they often erupt in frustration. I was impressed by Mark's initiative. He followed my recommendation and was ready to regain his health through educated management.

CAROL: "Mark, as you've learned from the diabetes management training I hope you received, diabetes is an end organ disease. I am sure you learned how leaky blood vessels affect many of your organs, but I wonder if oral health was stressed at all? Remember when I discussed "wound management" during your last appointment? The wound area contains a rich network of capillaries, as do other end organs like your eyes and kidneys. Gums should be light pink, have a firm texture, and

1 The hypothalamus controls many passive/automatic body functions such as hunger, fat storage and burning, heart rate, temperature, reproductive urges, stress response, and bone growth.

should wrap tightly around the teeth. Your gums were red, spongy, and slightly swollen. They bled profusely without provocation and without an obvious inflammatory source.[v] These symptoms led me to believe your physical would indicate a metabolic disorder. Diabetics are easily infected, yet slow to heal.

"Your high blood pressure reading also suggested a loss of elasticity in your blood vessel walls. Before we talk about diabetes and its connection to oral health, know the news is not all negative. If you can regain control over leptin signaling and insulin levels, tissue damage will be limited. I know it's a challenge and can be overwhelming, but you should know control is possible. You can live a long, energetic life if you choose." (Note: Mark's case was almost a decade ago. I would no longer treat him first and ask questions later. I would be sure he was stabilized before beginning gum disease therapy.)

## Acquiring Insulin Resistance, Leptin Resistance, and Diabetes

Diabetes is the symptom of a fouled energy metabolism. A diabetic's body no longer uses or stores energy properly. Insulin, a potent healing factor at micro levels, turns deadly at constant high levels, as you will see in a moment. Currently, most people recognize insulin as the hormone that regulates carbohydrate energy metabolism, its least important role up until the last two centuries when refined sugar consumption began to soar.

Produced in the pancreas, insulin helps store energy and nutrients. The liver always stores small amounts of sugar as glycogen, which provides instant energy when required. All other sugars are converted and stored as fat for future energy needs.

Normal metabolism requires muscle, fat, and liver cells to increase their sensitivity to insulin after meals. Insulin is the key that unlocks these cells' doors so large sugar molecules (glucose) can enter. This is crucial because sugar molecules should exit the bloodstream before they activate many destructive conditions related to heart disease. Sugars and their glycated products known as AGEs (see "Immune System Sings the Sugar Blues" in Chapter Two) damage blood vessel walls and require the cholesterol repair discussed at the opening of Chapter Three. Incoming sugars our bodies do not immediately need for energy, short-term liver storage, or that are not glycated, are converted into fats including "bad" LDLs and triglycerides. Contrary to popular belief, triglycerides are primarily derived from excess sugars that have not been used for energy, not from excess dietary fat.

HDLs and LDLs are not cholesterols at all, but cholesterol carriers. They indicate the direction of cholesterol movement. LDLs carry cholesterol from the liver to blood vessel walls to plug damage, so elevated levels mark disease. HDLs move cholesterol away from atherosclerotic lesions back to the liver for recycling or eventual excretion. Components of HDL also help limit inflammation and oxidation unless inflammatory diseases have made them dysfunctional.

LDL complexes oxidize easily as they carry cholesterol to repair damaged blood vessel walls. These complexes also react with homocysteine molecules that may have damaged blood vessel walls in the first place. Immune cells gobble up these oxidized LDLs as they enter the pitted crevices of blood vessel walls and turn them into foam cells, the most damaging component of atherosclerotic arterial plaques.[2] High LDL levels, then, are the symptom of a problem. They indicate damaged arteries need help. Cholesterol is the bandage our bodies use to heal arterial damage. Most cholesterol is produced in the liver and is influenced by insulin levels. If you can control insulin, you can usually control cholesterol.

To summarize, sugars indirectly lower good HDL cholesterols, and raise bad LDL cholesterols. Stroke, heart attack risk and stiffened blood vessels result.[3] If blood vessels cannot expand when the heart pumps,

---

2 Statin drugs like Crestor and Lipitor – and red rice yeast, if you prefer a non-pharmaceutical, are common treatments for high cholesterol. These substances shut down an enzyme necessary for cholesterol production. In other words these drugs lower levels of LDL carrier molecules because there is little cholesterol available to ferry to the damage. They also block production of a powerful antioxidant, Coenzyme Q10 (CoQ10), that helps slow glycation/oxidation damage because the same enzyme that helps the body produce cholesterol also helps the body make CoQ10. CoQ10 functions far beyond its role as an antioxidant. It helps generate energy in every cell in the form of ATP. Almost all energy in the human body is generated this way. Heart cells beat relentlessly, so they are the cells with the highest energy requirements and the highest CoQ10 concentrations. Low CoQ10 levels threaten heart health, often causing an enlarged heart. CoQ10 therapy can reverse this. The liver also has high energy requirements and benefits from CoQ10 therapy when natural levels are deficient.
3 Very low density lipoproteins (VLDLs) are far more harmful than LDLs. The more insulin resistant a person is, the more VLDLs that person will have compared to LDLs. HDLs diminish in size and number. These trends both drive and indicate major cardiovascular damage. It is important to know that conventional lipid panels underestimate cardiovascular disease risk because they do not sub-classify all the particle sizes. (Garvey WT, Kwon S, Zheng D, et al. "Effects of Insulin Resistance and Type 2 Diabetes on

the temporary increase in blood volume exerts excessive pressure on the non-elastic vessel walls, resulting in high blood pressure readings and further blood vessel damage.

A person has insulin resistance when desensitized liver, muscle and fat cells cannot respond to normal insulin levels, so sugar molecules are locked out of these cells. The pancreas must produce copious amounts of insulin to try to trigger these cells' sensitivity. This can work for a while, but when cellular insulin resistance increases or when the overworked pancreas can no longer churn out enough insulin to remove over-abundant blood glucose, the person progresses into type 2 diabetes. If not diagnosed and managed, damaging high blood sugar levels *and* high insulin levels continue.

Various conditions lead to insulin resistance. Genes are influential, however population studies suggest lifestyle matters more.[vi] Genetic expression for diabetes occurs when too many lifestyle triggers overwhelm the immune system. Inflammation increases insulin resistance.[vii] High levels of circulating inflammatory messengers are implicated, so gum disease is part of the inflammatory load. For instance, TNF-alpha strongly increases insulin resistance.

Fat stores within muscle and liver cells also create insulin resistance. They impair the function of the mitochondria, the energy producing furnaces, in these cells. Poor mitochondrial function makes it hard for muscles to burn off these internal fat stores, even in lean people. They also impair muscle and liver cell function in general. The more oxidative damage your cell's mitochondria face, the quicker these cells die and the faster you age.

Obesity-associated inflammation is a major driver of insulin resistance. Abdominal fat is considered an endocrine gland because abdominal fat cells are a primary source of many kinds of hormonal messengers. For instance, as one carries more and more abdominal fat, each fat cell enlarges and secretes far more hormones and inflammatory messengers than normal. These include many I've mentioned: IL1-betas, CRPs, and TNF-alpha for instance. These messengers, in turn, increase insulin resistance in a continuous cycle.

Abdominal fat cells also manufacture cannabinoid receptors. Simply stated, cannabinoids trigger hunger. They were named after marijuana (cannabis) because the hormone shares the same molecule found in cannabis well known to cause "the munchies." Cannabinoids are hormones we manufacture from the omega-6 fatty acids so prevalent in typical American diets because our diets are largely corn-based. Corn, and everything fattened on corn, is abundant in pro-inflammatory omega-6 fatty acids. This includes all meat, dairy, and egg products from animals that are not pasture-raised including farm-raised fish.

A hungry brain is always looking for a quick jolt. From our ancestral beginnings, the human brain was designed to swim in the feel good chemicals fatty foods and sugars generate. This survival mechanism encouraged our ancestors to search for energy dense foods to sustain them during famines. However in modern times, eating the subsidized and thus, abundant and highly processed foods supplied by current agribusiness, this mechanism often proves lethal.

Today, those who consume a typical diet rich in sugars and omega-6 fatty acids crave the junk foods that only accelerate fat storage and its ensuing problems. Worse, cannabinoids impede insulin's ability to move blood sugar into cells, the very definition of insulin resistance. If your brain does not receive the feedback it needs that it has been fed, you eat more, gain weight, and increase insulin resistance. This results in the manufacture of more cannabinoids, which prompts you to eat more, which leads to more weight gain, in a self-perpetuating cycle. All the while, the foods you crave are usually high in the bad fats and sugars that cause cellular and arterial damage through oxidation and glycation (introduced in Chapter Two and explained more thoroughly in a moment).

Other contributors to insulin resistance can be:

- **A sedentary lifestyle.** Resistance exercise (putting load on muscles) immediately increases muscle cell sensitivity to insulin; aerobic exercise generates more mitochondria per cell. Mitochondria are the energy generators of each cell. Lance Armstrong's muscle fibers are jam-packed with mitochondria (23,000/cell). Since diabetics have trouble in all ways with energy use and storage, they should not overlook the importance of multiplying their mitochondria with exercise. It is a powerful key to blood sugar control.
- **Taking anti-inflammatory and immunosuppressive drugs called glucocorticoids.** These are prescribed to treat autoimmune diseases and cancer. Examples include Hydrocortisone, Prednisone, Prednisolone, Aldosterone, and Lupron. Lupron is used for treating prostate cancer.

- **Conditions contributing to acidosis, or increased blood acidity.** This occurs in several ways. Examples are infrequent or irregular eating as in anorexia and mouth breathing.

## Leptin Resistance

Leptin is a neurotransmitter produced in response to eating. Abdominal fat cells produce leptin that, along with cannabinoids, regulate appetite. For people with normal metabolism, low leptin levels signal them to eat and store fat while high leptin levels reduce appetite and encourage fat burning. As with insulin resistance, brain cells can lose sensitivity and become leptin resistant. Specialized brain neurons in the hypothalamus become insensitive to leptin-signaling. In this case, normal signaling breaks down. The body increases leptin production in order to trigger sensitivity. In turn the brain's hunger center becomes more leptin resistant, does not turn off, signals the body to eat more and then stores what it can as fat. This fat in turn makes more leptin.

Leptin also works with the liver and insulin to maintain stable low glucose levels. It tells the liver what to do with glucose – burn it, store it, or signal that more is needed. When a person is leptin resistant, they build fat stores. This increase in fat stores contributes to both leptin and insulin resistance.

Leptin also:

- **Regulates activity levels.** Most people with type 2 diabetes are obese and have difficulty losing weight because they have low energy. Restoring leptin sensitivity in the brain doubles activity levels.[viii]
- **Raises blood fat levels.**
- **Inhibits insulin production.** [ix]
- **Is pro-inflammatory.** It triggers fat cells to manufacture the potent pro-inflammatory molecules discussed in this book.[x]

Leptin works through the hypothalamus of the brain, therefore leptin influences other functions too. Some of these are stress response through the adrenal glands, bone growth, thyroid function, the sympathetic nervous system, and reproductive behavior. Leptin is considered a biomarker for fat. Its role is often overlooked.

A person with leptin resistance always thinks they are hungry. Leptin resistance can come from excessive fructose or sucrose consumption – think processed foods and beverages – or from carrying excess body fat.

## Constant High Insulin Levels and the Aging Process

Most people who live into very old age do so largely because they have maintained consistently low triglyceride, sugar, and insulin levels for years. Insulin is a complicated molecule that positively influences healing and longevity. Found in the earliest single-celled organisms, many human metabolic processes are built upon it, yet in high doses, such as those that occur in pre-diabetes, it is troublesome. Insulin regulates far more than blood sugar levels. It also contributes to the following:

- High blood pressure. High insulin levels exert a host of influences on blood pressure. A sharp rise in insulin triggers the part of the nervous system that causes blood vessels to constrict, which leads to a spike in blood pressure.[4] Insulin helps the body retain sodium, leading to excessive blood volume. The excess blood creates pressure against blood vessel walls that cannot relax. Magnesium could help these blood vessel walls to relax, but diabetics and those with insulin resistance are often low in this mineral because of diet, accelerated magnesium excretion and an altered ability to properly use it.[5][6] Finally, high insulin levels keep blood vessel walls from producing adequate nitric oxide. Nitric oxide also helps blood vessel walls relax.

---

4 Heart attacks happen more than twice as often after high-carbohydrate meals than after high-fat meals.

5 Magnesium is necessary for insulin production and action. If you have insufficient magnesium (highly likely if you eat a lot of processed foods), you become more insulin resistant. High sugar intake as well as excessive calcium, phosphates, and vitamin D intake reduces magnesium levels.

6 Magnesium influences a critical enzyme that converts certain omega-3 and -6 fatty acids into forms that could positively impact their disease course. GLA cannot be made when one is deficient in magnesium, zinc, and the nicotinic acid portion of the B$_3$ vitamin (as say, many asthmatics are), or diets include too many poor quality saturated fats, trans fatty acids, or alcohol. GLA, DGLA, EPA and DHA are fatty acids that change the course of inflammation.

- Insulin elevates homocysteine levels.[xi] Homocysteine pits blood vessel walls and inhibits their structural repair. More indirectly, B vitamins keep homocysteine under control. Anything that depletes B vitamins like excess sugars, alcohol, certain fats, animal proteins, or smoking enhances homocysteine damage to blood vessel walls. This in turn requires LDLs to carry cholesterol to the area for repair.
- Insulin promotes inflammation and blood clotting.[xii]
- The sex hormones estrogen, progesterone and testosterone are derived from cholesterol.[7] Among other things, these hormones promote bone health.[8] Insulin tells these hormones where to deposit calcium. When that signaling goes awry, one can get osteoporosis while liberated calcium makes its way to undesirable locations such as blood vessel walls, kidneys, or tumors. Often free calcium ends up in the mouth as tartar or stones within tooth pulps. Remember, osteoporosis affects the jawbone that anchors teeth, too.
- High levels of insulin also cause calcium excretion, which contributes to osteoporosis.
- As we age, or *as insulin resistance rises*, we produce less of an adrenal steroid called DHEA. Low DHEA levels increase abdominal fat. Low DHEA levels also encourage diabetes through several pathways, including increased inflammation, decreased insulin sensitivity, and control of fat to muscle ratios. Several forms of dementia are increasingly associated with diabetes and low DHEA levels.
- Some cells are not as insulin resistant as others. Insulin accelerates proliferation of these cells, so constant high levels of insulin are associated with tumor growth, particularly in the breast and colon.
- As unchecked insulin levels make the liver insulin resistant, the liver cannot convert thyroid hormone T4 to a usable state, T3. This is important because doctors often check T4 levels to ascertain thyroid function. T4 levels may be normal, while usable T3 is inadequate. This is troublesome for diabetics and those with insulin resistance because it is T3 that turns on the ATP energy-making machinery inside each cell.

---

7 Insulin also influences sex hormone carriers, thus the availability of sex hormones. Derangements of these sex hormone carriers may also play a role in insulin resistance.

8 So do the insulin-like growth factors (IGFs) that are almost bio-identical to insulin.

- High insulin levels in pre-diabetics suppress the action of the glucagon hormone.[xiii] Glucagon burns fats and sugars. Persistent low levels of glucagon promote muscle wasting.[xiv] Said another way, high insulin levels make it difficult to gain muscle or lose fat.

The U.S. Department of Health and Human Services estimated that in 2002, over half the U.S. population between the ages of 40 and 74 (54 million adults) is pre-diabetic. Most people with pre-diabetes develop type 2 diabetes within ten years unless they lose five to seven percent of their body weight.

Pre-diabetics with gum disease are more likely to become diabetic.[xv]

**BOTTOM LINE: Avoid blood sugar spikes and emphasize quality fats to improve leptin and insulin sensitivity. Refer to Chapter Fourteen to learn about good fats.**

## Diabetes and Gum Disease are Synergistic Inflammatory Events

CAROL: "Mark, diabetes and gum disease are bidirectional. Perhaps your physician explored how diabetes develops, but it sounds as though you want to know how uncontrolled diabetes affects your mouth. I can answer that for you.

"First of all, diabetics tend to have exaggerated immune responses. Generally, a person with poorly regulated sugar levels[9] has nearly double the circulating levels of inflammatory messengers like IL-1s compared to someone with better control.[xvi] Diabetics can actually have 30 times as many IL-1s as a non-diabetic with a similar bacterial load![xv] You are certain to have elevated levels of these infection messengers throughout your body, especially in the fluids that continuously bathe your gum pockets.[xvii xviii]

"Do you remember when I said these inflammatory mediators kicked off tissue breakdown around your teeth because they recruit the destructive collagenase enzyme? This is also how these molecules enhance osteoporosis throughout your body, including the bone supporting your teeth. This breakdown marks the beginning of an active destructive cycle. As the collagenase silently destroyed the

---

9 A1c higher than eight

gums and the jawbone around your teeth, it allowed the bacteria to multiply. They burrowed ever deeper into and under your gums and created a larger germ reservoir. The anaerobic germs found the warm, wet, nutritive, and now acidic environment next to your wound a hospitable place to live and breed unhindered. With an immune system compromised by constant high levels of blood sugar, these bacteria faced little disruption from an active immune system. Remember, wound healing in diabetics is slow because sugar sharply reduces the germ-gobbling capacity of white blood cells.

"Another mediator recruited during inflammation is TNF-alpha. It unbalances the normal bone remodeling that constantly occurs in your body. Normally, one kind of cell (an osteoclast) breaks down bone so another kind of cell (osteoblast) can lay down fresh bone to keep your skeleton strong. It is an important way your skeleton deals with all the stresses and minor injuries you accumulate during an active life. But TNF-alpha decouples that process, so bone destruction outweighs bone rebuilding. This is just as true for your jaw bones as it is for the rest of your skeleton.

"To review your case, high levels of circulating blood sugar overwhelmed your immune system. When your body sent out the white blood cells [10] whose job it is to destroy and engulf invading bacteria, they were unable to do so as effectively as they should. The abilities of these cells to chemically move to, attach to, and destroy their targets, were all impaired.[xix xx] If just two teaspoons of sugar impair the immune response for hours in a person with normal metabolism, imagine an immune system under siege with constant high blood sugar levels! In the latter case the delicate balance between the healing and destruction normally present at the wound site severely tilts towards destruction.

"As this complex biofilm matured and grew, some of these bacteria and their toxins caused your blood vessels to become inflamed. Do you remember when I alluded to the tennis court-sized lining of your blood vessels? Inhabiting a territory of that size, in addition to your enlarging oral pockets, caused levels of inflammatory messengers to accelerate in a destructive spiral.

"You can be sure glucose was also building in the pockets around your teeth.[xxi] Anaerobic germs thrive in a sugar-rich, acidic environment. Also, high glucose levels in the pockets incapacitate the fibroblasts that help heal you. Remember my analogy to Velcro?

---

10 The phagocytes called neutrophils and monocytes

The fibroblast's hooks are necessary for tissue reconnection to the tooth. If the fibroblasts do not get the chemical direction to move to the right place, they do not attach well.[xxii] In this case, little healing or reattachment occurs.[11] Last, because bone-building cells (osteoblasts) have a shortened life cycle, the balance tips towards bone loss.[xxiii xxiv]

## Glycation Aging Theory

"Glycation plays a powerful role in the inflammatory aging process diabetics struggle to control. In medical terms, we call it glycation, but cooks call it caramelization. It happens when meats or vegetables brown, or when sugar turns to caramel.

"As you know, your body converts simple carbohydrates into glucose, which like all sugars, is sticky. If you consume more carbohydrates than your body's store of insulin can move into cells, its extended circulation time allows it to clump irreversibly with proteins, fats, and red blood cells in your bloodstream. These bonded cells are called advanced glycation end products or AGEs. Glycation damages proteins beyond use so they cannot be recycled. White blood cells gobble some of these ruined proteins, but many of them accumulate over a lifetime, which causes widespread damage. AGEs complicate diabetes. Serious damage accumulates in tissues with a slow turnover rate, such as nerves, bone, cartilage, and collagen.

"AGEs are highly pro-inflammatory. First, they recruit destructive inflammatory mediators. Second, cross-linked proteins generate many times more free radicals than non-cross-linked proteins. Oxidation leads to degenerative aging. This means the two aging theories of glycation and oxidation are linked.

"While a person with properly functioning kidneys excretes at least a third of preformed dietary AGEs, there is more uncertainty about the longevity of AGEs formed when we indulge in excessive simple carbohydrates. Degradation and clearance of AGEs is very slow. In fact, as we accumulate AGEs over time, they damage our kidneys. When this happens, the kidney structures that filter blood become less and less efficient.

"Glycated red blood cells are large and jagged. AGEs are almost too large to pass through delicate capillaries. They are certainly too rough, but nevertheless, our hearts must pump these complexes through them

---

11 Elevated sugar levels in the fluid at the wound site also promote cavities.

single file. AGEs cause damage to all blood vessel walls as they pass, but the most narrow and fragile of them, the capillaries, are most injured. Particularly vulnerable are the capillaries of the eyes and kidneys, two organ systems already easily damaged by diabetes.

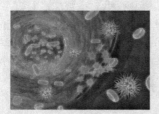

## AGEs

As described by a paper published in the journal, *Clinical Diabetes*, "AGEs form at a constant but slow rate in the normal body, starting in early embryonic development, and accumulate with time. Their formation is markedly accelerated in diabetes because of increased of glucose availability." [xxiv]

You can see a similar chemical combination occurring between proteins, fats, and sugars as you cook foods at high temperatures. AGEs are the browned parts of grilled, browned, broiled or fried meats and cheeses. Roasted, pasteurized, and sterilized foods also contain them. Because we enjoy their unique flavor, food chemists create synthetic AGEs to add to many of the processed food products we buy. Smokers introduce particularly potent AGEs into their bodies that are directly reflected in their arteries and the lenses of their eyes.

AGEs are a key reason why diabetics are at high risk for nerve, artery, and kidney damage. AGEs accelerate atherosclerosis by several routes, damage the most basic structure of a diabetic's kidneys (the glomeruli), cause retinal problems, modify LDL cholesterols so they easily oxidize and embed themselves within arterial walls, perpetuate and enhance oxidation and inflammation, accelerate the programmed death of cells, and stiffen blood vessel walls by promoting calcium accumulation. Throughout the body, their presence leads to cellular degradation.

From the *Clinical Diabetes Journal:* "Current evidence points to glucose not only as the body's main short-term energy source, but also as the long-term fuel of diabetes complications, mainly in the form of oxidative, pro-inflammatory AGEs. Food commonly consumed after exposure to heat contains a significant amount of pre-formed AGEs, a fact that offers a new perspective on food as a major environmental risk factor. It may be necessary, for instance, to restructure our guidelines to include methods of food preparation along with or in addition to routine recommendations about food quantity and composition." [xxvi]

An illustrative study published in the Proceedings of the National Academy of Sciences found people with diabetes who consumed foods cooked at lower temperatures, which therefore had fewer AGEs, had lower AGE and inflammatory protein levels in their blood compared to those who ate the same amount of food cooked at higher temperatures.

In fact, among those who ate foods cooked at higher temperatures, blood levels of AGEs rose by almost 65 percent after two weeks while levels dropped by 30 percent in those who ate the low temperature foods.

Results were even more telling after six weeks. Those who ate the high temperature foods had increased levels of two inflammation messengers, TNF and CRPs. However, the levels of both these indicators decreased among those who ate the low temperature foods.[xxvii]

Indirectly, high sugar intake could be one of the most significant causes of aging, an interesting thought when one considers all the money, time, and anguish spent on trying to retain youthfulness!

Anyone can measure glycated red blood cell levels by taking an A1c test, also known as a Glycohemoglobin Assay. Diabetics usually have their AGEs measured at least twice a year to give a more accurate picture of blood sugar stability over time. Six percent or less is normal and levels below seven percent indicate good control. Only 36 percent of diabetics reach this goal. AGEs can perpetuate ill effects, especially oxidation, long after blood sugar levels are brought under control. Self-testing kits are readily available. See how easy it is @ http://www.a1cnow.com/Professionals/A1CNow-Overview/Procedure.

---

* The chronic inflammatory conditions to which AGEs contribute are: colitis, nephritis, asthma, and heart muscle inflammation (shortness of breath or fluid retention). Oxidative stresses to which AGEs contribute are: heart disease, high blood pressure, cancer, acute respiratory distress syndrome, asthma, inflammatory bowel disease, arthritis, diabetes, autism, stroke, Huntington's, Parkinson's, and Alzheimer's.

"AGE complexes are particularly troublesome for poorly controlled diabetics. Because they accelerate inflammation as well as cellular death, gum disease is almost a given. AGEs:

- Interfere with collagen, the body's critical structural protein in bone, joints, skin, ligaments, tendons, and fascia. AGEs disrupt collagen's formation and accelerate its breakdown. For instance, AGEs are responsible for the sagging and wrinkling of aging skin. In fact, this is how AGEs first came to my attention! AGEs also build up in the collagen of bone to impair its mechanical properties. It destabilizes the structure of bone collagen,[xxviii] which provides yet another blow to the oral pocket tissue's balance between health and destruction. They also interfere with bone remodeling during both during the destructive and rebuilding phases. Even though diabetics sometimes have higher bone densities than non-diabetics, they have an increased risk of fracture. As mentioned in the osteoporosis chapter, fracture risk is not solely dependent upon bone density.
- AGE accumulation in joints disrupts normal cell function that leads to stiff, painful, and brittle joints. AGEs here interfere with the normal degradation of aging cartilage. Sound like arthritis?
- AGEs damage DNA and RNA.
- AGEs promote inflammation throughout the body. They bind to the oral pocket tissue and smooth muscle cells, such as those of the heart. They eat away at nerve and sensory cells and they increase blood vessel leakage by binding to cells lining the blood vessels.[xxix] [xxx xxxi] (Again, picture a tennis court-sized area!)
- Increased blood vessel leakage can ultimately lead to clot formation.
- Besides the atherosclerosis to which diabetics are prone, AGEs also cause blood vessel walls to thicken, which further narrows the inside diameter. When clots do form, these blood vessels are more easily blocked.
- AGEs in tissues significantly increase the rate of free radical activity. Free radicals accelerate aging.

"Now you see why gum disease, heart disease, and diabetes are a trio. These disease states feed off each other and themselves in complex ways. There is much we don't yet know about the biochemical dance between these diseases. I know it is frustrating."

MARK: "Well, it is a lot of diseases to manage at once. And it is more complicated than I thought. I think I understand it better. No wonder it's going to take a while to see which medications work for me and to learn how to care for myself, find the right exercise routine, and learn to eat right. As difficult as it is, I guess I'm glad you sent me off in the right direction before too much destruction could occur.

"But can you clear up one thing? You once mentioned that controlling my gum disease could help control my blood sugar levels. Can you clarify?"

## Inflammation Increases Insulin Resistance

CAROL: "Again, I appreciate how seriously you're taking this. The emotional side of this disease is initially difficult to handle, which means some take longer to accomplish consistent good results. It requires a lot of personal courage and power to accept a chronic disease and make necessary changes. I admire you. And remember this great news. Each lifestyle change you make doesn't affect just one disease; it improves them all.

"But yes, I mentioned the oral link to blood sugar control only in passing, so I'm glad you asked. Many studies back these links. Once a diabetic has established gum disease, controlling blood sugar levels is more difficult because the reservoir of bad germs hiding in those hidden pockets cause constant low grade infections and inflammation. I won't elaborate, but one study is worth mentioning. In a two-year period, those with bad gums had *six times* the chance of worsening their glycemic control![xxxii]

"When we first talked, I mentioned how researchers believe circulating infection messengers encourage insulin resistance. This is because several studies showed increased insulin resistance and difficulty in controlling blood sugars in patients who had recently suffered severe bacterial or viral infections unrelated to gum disease.[xxxiii] [xxxiv] The insulin resistance remained for a long time after they recovered from the original infection. Since they subsequently improved, it is likely the infection was what caused the insulin resistance.

"Likewise, there have been several recent studies showing improved long term sugar control after gum disease therapy, both when antibiotics have been used[xxxv xxxvi] and when they haven't. [xxxvii]

"You know I can wrap this all up in an animal study, right?"

MARK: "Oh yeah, here we go. What have they done with the pigs this time?"

CAROL: "Well, actually this time they were rats. Gum disease can be induced in animals by putting a ligature like a rubber band around teeth at the gum line. Researchers did this to half of some lean rats and half of some rats on a high fat diet. How do you think that worked out, Mark?"

MARK: "Gee. Let me think. I'm guessing the rats with gum disease couldn't handle their sugars as well as those without gum disease, and the fat rats handled it worse than their lean counterparts with gum disease. Is that pretty much it?"

CAROL: "You have it! [12] [xxxviii] To sum it up in human terms: as an uncontrolled diabetic, you had about eleven times the risk of oral bone loss as someone without a blood sugar problem. As you gain control over blood sugar levels, your risks decrease from eleven to two times. That is a substantial benefit for your mouth alone.

"Your doctor and other sources may alert you to various strategies that reset how your body processes and stores energy so you can step up your metabolism, lose weight, gain energy, and reduce your vulnerability to degenerative diseases. These strategies may include:

- **Alpha Lipoic Acid (ALA).** ALA is an antioxidant known to lower blood sugar. It also recycles other antioxidants. Diabetics often use it to treat nerve damage. ALA increases the number of energy generators, called mitochondria, in each cell. Mitochondria are your body's furnaces and can make up about ten percent of your body weight. The more mitochondria your body has, the more it will burn sugar to create energy. ALA also reduces triglycerides and improves insulin sensitivity. To improve mitochondrial function and number, your health care provider may suggest timed-release doses of R-alpha lipoic acid in conjunction with methylated

---

12 In a 2007 study, periodontal disease was induced in half of all study rats. (Just as with the pig study of Chapter Four, half the littermates were lean and half had a high fat diet.; in half of each group, gum disease was induced.) Those with gum disease, in both the fatty and lean groups had increased glucose intolerance. Furthermore those in the group of lean rats with gum disease showed higher fasting glucose, insulin, and insulin resistance compared to those without gum disease. There was significantly more bone loss in the fatty rats with gum disease compared to lean rats without gum disease.

resveratrol[13] and quercetin,[14] which extends the life of resveratrol. **Note:** CoQ10 in the reduced form (ubiquinol) is also important to mitochondrial function. It recycles the critical antioxidants vitamin C and E. Oxidation rates increase as the mitochondria in each cell generate energy. Adequate CoQ10 minimizes oxidation. Together, these are a powerful combination for diabetics. Choose a high quality gel-cap CoQ10, oil-based and crystal-free.[15]

- **Acetyl-L-Carnitine (ALC).** ALC helps transport fatty acids into the mitochondria. These fatty acids also help maintain healthy mitochondrial membranes.

- **Chromium.** Found in whole grains, nuts, and particularly broccoli, chromium activates insulin and changes cell membranes to allow sugars to pass through cells for use or storage. Many adults are chromium-deficient. One reason is that chromium, essential for sugar metabolism, has been stripped from refined sugars and grains. Another is that diets rich in sugars accelerate chromium excretion.[xxxix] This means that every time you eat refined carbohydrates you deplete rather than build chromium stores. According to Oregon State University's Linus Pauling Institute Micronutrient Information Center, "Because chromium appears to enhance the action of insulin and chromium deficiency has resulted in impaired glucose tolerance, chromium insufficiency has been hypothesized to be a contributing factor to the development of type 2 diabetes." [xl] The center also states, "Individuals with pre-existing kidney or liver disease may be at increased risk of adverse effects and should limit supplemental chromium intake." [xli] (See glossary.)

- **Zinc.** Excessive sugar consumption also depletes zinc. Zinc is a component of the insulin molecule that moves sugar out of the blood stream. Zinc combats cold and flu viruses. It also aids wound healing and supports the immune and reproductive systems, especially the prostate. Zinc also supports healthy liver function. (See glossary.)

---

13 Resveratrol helps control obesity and improve insulin sensitivity in cells.

14 Quercetin is an antioxidant found in small amounts in onions, tea, broccoli, and apples.

15 Xymogen is an example of a reputable company that carries these products. Since ALA has a limited lifespan (about 30 minutes), they offer a timed release ALA supplement called ALAMax CR. Resveratin is their product that provides resveratrol and quercetin together.

- **Limiting caffeine and chocolate.** Both raise blood glucose, cholesterol, and uric acid. They decrease chromium, magnesium, and zinc levels.
- **Limiting alcohol consumption.** Alcohol also raises levels of blood glucose, cholesterol, and depletes magnesium, manganese, potassium, and folic acid Alcohol, caffeine, most meats, and many other foods need to be buffered with alkalizing foods, as discussed in, "Environmental, Non-Estrogen Related Risk Factors for Osteoporosis."
- **Enjoying egg yolks, milk, poultry broccoli, and fish** often. They are rich in biotin, an important B vitamin. Biotin contributes to many steps of energy metabolism.
- Your doctor may suggest a **vanadyl sulfate supplement**. Vanadyl sulfate and insulin each move glucose out of the bloodstream. Because they use different pathways, vanadyl supplements may help lower insulin levels. It may also help protect pancreatic beta cells that produce insulin. Research continues.

  **L-glutamine** (or glutamine peptides, which are more stable and better-absorbed and utilized) can reduce sugar, alcohol and other carbohydrate cravings. Improved insulin signaling in liver and muscle cells is one of its many benefits.[xlii] Glutamine is the most abundant amino acid, but is often depleted in those with constant high metabolic stress or the yeast overgrowth that often accompanies excessive sugar intake. Food hinders glutamine absorption; therefore take supplements on an empty stomach. Meat, eggs, and dairy are glutamine-rich foods. Vegetarians find it in legumes, raw cabbage, beets and some seeds like hemp and chia. [**Note:** Those with kidney disease or severe liver failure should not take glutamine. Many diabetics have kidney damage and should take it only under a doctor's supervision.] There are many other strategies for reducing sugar cravings. See "Sugar, An Unrecognized Addiction" in the "Food as Medicine" chapter.
- **Glutathione.** Alternatively, consider strategies that raise glutathione levels, explored in Chapter Fourteen and "Menu for Immune System Boosting" in Appendix X. Diabetics are almost always deficient in glutathione and benefit from boosting strategies.
- **Leptin.** Learn more about leptin resistance and leptin signaling. Just as you can restore the sensitivity of fat, muscle and liver cells

to insulin's signals, you can restore sensitivity to leptin sensitive neurons in the hypothalamus. There are several books available on the subject. Dr. Rosedale's books and web articles are good starting points. Dr. Rosedale is a leptin metabolism expert.

- **Nutrition.** Learn more about food, nutrition, and the essential fatty acid balance between omega-3 and omega-6 fatty acids. Consumed in the proper balance, these fatty acids lower triglyceride levels[xliii] and reduce overall inflammation. They are briefly introduced in Chapter Twelve. Avoid all trans fats, such as margarine.

- **Raw Apple Cider Vinegar.** To even out blood sugar spikes after a high-carbohydrate meal, take 1 to 2 tablespoons of raw apple cider vinegar, perhaps in a salad dressing before meals. Vinegar may even out blood sugar spikes and help insulin ferry sugar into cells. [xliv xlv xlvi xlvii] [In one study, pre-diabetic subjects who took apple cider vinegar prior to eating a meal, cut blood glucose concentrations by 34 percent. These levels were superior to those of the healthy controls who did not have pre-diabetes. Type 2 diabetics improved their glucose levels by 19 percent when they consumed apple cider vinegar.]

  Raw apple cider vinegar also provides gut colonizing probiotics and minerals that help buffer acidifying foods. Read more about this important principal in Chapter Seven, "Environmental Non-Estrogen Related Risk Factors for Osteoporosis." Many diabetics suffer osteoporosis and arthritis.

- **Herbs.** For those interested in Ayurvedic remedies, the National Institute of Health says, "There is evidence to suggest that the single herbs Coccinia indica, holy basil, fenugreek, and *Gymnema sylvestre* and the herbal formulas Ayush-82 and D-400 have a glucose-lowering effect and deserve further study. Evidence of effectiveness of several other herbs is less extensive (*C. tamala, Eugenia jambolana,* and *Momordica charantia*).[xlviii]

- **Vitamin C.** Vitamin C competes with sugar for absorption, so diabetics often have low levels of the antioxidant vitamin C. High blood sugar levels increase the oxidative stress that damages cells and creates disease, so diabetics often take mega doses of vitamin C. However, it is best to get this and other antioxidants as part of a well-balanced diet because high supplemental vitamin C intake by diabetics, as with smokers, paradoxically increases oxidation, rather than reducing it. Supplemental C may also create

AGEs.[xlix] [See Chapter Two: Immune System Sings the Sugar Blues.] Keeping sugar levels low prevents a lot of oxidative stress.

- **Mushrooms/Adiponectin.** Enjoy mushrooms regularly. It may be that button and portabella mushrooms increase adiponectin levels. Adiponectin is a protein-signaling molecule that regulates fat and sugar metabolism. Fat cells produce adiponectin, just as they produce leptin and the inflammatory messenger TNF. However adiponectin levels actually decrease as body fat accumulates. Like leptin, adiponectin signals your brain when you are full. It is known to suppress diabetes, atherosclerosis, and fatty liver disease through its anti-inflammatory effects on blood vessel walls. "Higher adiponectin levels are associated with a lower risk of type 2 diabetes across diverse populations, consistent with a dose-response relationship."

- **Exercise.** Exercise is probably the most effective strategy. Exercise increases insulin sensitivity because muscles must have sugar to burn for energy. Aerobic exercise also multiplies the number and function of mitochondrial furnaces in each cell, especially of muscle cells. When human cells are packed with mitochondria, oxidative stresses diminish and the body becomes highly energy efficient. [Interesting note: skeletal muscles produce nitric oxide (NO) as they contract. NO relaxes and opens blood vessels, encourages muscle cells to accept blood sugars, and fuels the mitochondria with oxygen. NO also activates mitochondria production.

"I know this kind of lifestyle adjustment can be overwhelming. Just remember, there is a lot of support out there for you, and I think the lift you get from feeling more energetic will help you continue to work on positive changes. Pretty soon, all the wonderful energy you create will far outweigh the difficulty of changing some of your favorite habits. People have expressed this over and over. To paraphrase Dr. Oz, we recalibrate our bodies and brains.

"I hope this knowledge empowers you. For now, let's be sure we meet every three months. This will keep your mouth's contribution to the biochemical dance positive. As you have probably already learned, if you are able to keep your blood sugar levels under tight control, damage to your tissues – including those anchoring your teeth – will likely be minimal. And keeping your gums healthy will help keep your blood sugar under control, thereby reducing your insulin needs."

Mark is still at the beginning of the journey to regain his health. His oral story is largely unwritten. I suppose his path will be similar to Jack's, with many great attempts, and not a few setbacks, including some periods where his health needs lose priority. He may experience times where his symptoms are so obvious they will scare him into redoubling his efforts at control. I hope he takes advantage of help from many of the available sources. I do know his positive attitude will take him farther and faster than most.

## HENRY
## Needed: Guidance, Attention to Detail and Consistent Professional Care

Henry's need was not uncommon. After he was diagnosed with diabetes years ago, he diligently worked to control it. He knew a little about how his oral health interacted with his condition, but this knowledge was incomplete. As a result, despite earnest efforts, much of his self-care was ineffective.

The first time I met Henry, his blood sugar had been kept fairly well controlled for many years. His most recent A1c reported was 6.6. Physicians prefer it be around 6 or less, but his control was better than most.

It took some time for him to trust me, but by the end of our first appointment I realized why. He is a man who keeps much to himself and was just "there to get his teeth cleaned" according to commonly understood health myths. (He "had them cleaned" every six months. For decades, this has been the mantra of preventive dental care in America, despite evidence showing that everyone should have intervals of care based on medical history risks and their personal response to professional and personal care. While many dental offices recommend care intervals that reflect individual client needs, this mantra is still firmly entrenched. It is also reflected in the insurance industry's lagging schedule of authorized reimbursement, )

Henry had scheduled preventive dental visits as often as was recommended to him. He frequently sought care through the Veterans Health Administration (VA), but sometimes he visited private offices. He flossed often and as well as he could, but I shared his disappointment at the condition of his mouth and by what he knew about the relationship between it and diabetes. He had heard of the oral connection to heart disease and knew gum disease was "the sixth complication of diabetes" because someone at the VA had mentioned it. He did his best to control his gum disease at home and with routine dental visits.

He was also pleased to be asked about his morning's glucometer (blood sugar) reading. He happily and proudly delivered it. Diabetics like to know all their health care professionals understand their disease and consider it in treatment. They immediately understand we are thinking in terms of their integrated health picture and not just an isolated element of their health.

He was surprised when I asked him about his last A1c. This test reflects general blood sugar control over several months. I could tell he did not expect me to know of it and, further, could not imagine what I would gain from it. Just as many clinicians do not go beyond their local focus in health care, Henry did not know the full bidirectional nature of his diabetes and oral care. I believe my query was what allowed Henry to open up to the mutual trust that would become a necessary part of his treatment and recovery.

## Lack of Basic Information

After a lively discussion about diabetes and oral health, I asked Henry if his physician had ever mentioned he could improve his blood sugar control with good oral care. He told me the subject had not surfaced. I told him A1c readings have been known to drop up to two points after gum disease therapy. I mentioned I was surprised at how obscure this information remains, and that sometimes a diabetic needs less insulin after gum disease clears. I shared with him that even after an extensive search of the American Diabetes Association (ADA) web site, I failed to come across the information links I expected. (This was in 2008. There are now extensive links on the ADA web site and many others, as information about systemic connections roll out. Nonetheless, we have a long way to go to raise public awareness about oral health and its impact on the rest of the body.)

More concerns arose during Henry's exam. His gums at first seemed healthy, but deep pockets measuring a depth of 6mm were found between the back molars. Whenever I see this pattern, I suspect flossing is a challenge. Clients can manage front teeth moderately well, but have difficulty tackling molars. Because teeth are widest between the molars, the potential "wound" area is largest here. Because of Henry's diabetes, it was particularly critical for him to be able to clean them well.

Henry needed individualized coaching to help him develop effective cleaning techniques, which we did. For future reference, I told him diabetics' fingertips often suffer nerve damage. I suggested if he ever found manual flossing too difficult, he could switch to floss holders or other ideas we would develop.

My last concern was that Henry did not believe he could improve his care by developing a relationship with a single professional care provider who could track progress and setbacks and share new information. I was afraid he did not see the value in finding a provider who understands his particular health issues, cares about him, and helps him manage his health. And somehow, in all that bouncing around from dentist to dentist, no one ever recommended a shorter professional care interval. The blanket recommendation of regular six-month checkups in no way fit his needs.

I enjoyed getting to know Henry and his background. We talked about his time in Vietnam and his exposure to Agent Orange, among other things. While his stories were colorful and helped me learn more about his personality and character, I was also scavenging for health-related clues. It is likely his chemical exposure had significantly challenged his immune system and likely ushered him into his diabetic condition sooner than would otherwise have happened.

**Note:** Three months later, a follow-up appointment showed excellent results from his improved flossing technique. All deep pockets resolved (from 6mm to 3mm) and his gums reflected complete health. Gum tenderness had disappeared.

## DIANA
## Needed: Early Preventive Intervention

Diana is another client whose daily mechanical oral care became optimal over the years. Because her gums always bled too freely despite her great home care, she scheduled quarterly wellness visits. Years ago, over the course of two successive appointments, I suggested she have her blood sugar levels checked as I suspected she might be diabetic. On a following visit, she informed me her blood sugar levels tested normal. I nodded, surprised, and then listened as she happily shared something exciting to her. She had lost 40 pounds since she last saw me! She enthusiastically discussed her diet plan, which basically excluded all white foods: all sugars, white refined flour, rice, potatoes, and similar starches that quickly convert to sugars. She was ecstatic about her new body and renewed energy from the weight loss and improved nutrition.

I added my assent as we talked. I have been a whole food enthusiast for many years and avoid refined and processed foods. This includes fruit juices, from which most essential nutrients and fiber have been removed. People often overlook the importance of enzymes and other micronutrients that allow for optimal nutrient absorption. They are also largely unaware that the fibrous complex carbohydrates of whole foods slow absorption of fruit sugars.[16]

## Glycemic Index

Sugars are just one kind of simple carbohydrate. Simple starches like white rice, white potatoes, white bread, and white noodles convert into sugars in the mouth as a result of enzymes in saliva. A food's glycemic index, or GI, is a measure of how fast starches raise blood sugar. Glucose is the fastest simple carbohydrate to enter the blood stream, so it sets the standard against which all other foods are measured. It has a value of 100. Foods with numbers less than 55 are considered low GI foods, while numbers above 55 are high GI foods. The more saturated a diet is with high glycemic foods, the more likely there will be blood fat abnormalities, high blood pressure, cardiovascular diseases and obesity from high blood sugar and insulin's harmful effects.

The index reflects not only simple carbohydrate content, but also texture and density. For instance, the finer a grain is ground, the more surface area is exposed to digestive enzymes. The glycemic index will be higher because sugars enter the blood stream faster. Overcooking

---

16 Yale University's Griffin Prevention Research Center developed a "Shopping by the Numbers" food evaluation sheet that ranks, by number, many supermarket products based on nutrients, vitamins, sugar, and salt as well as their general impact on health. On a scale of 1 to 100, oranges rate a 100, orange juice only a 39. Whole Foods has just adopted the ANDI system, rating aggregate scores of foods based on: Calcium, Carotenoids: Beta Carotene, Alpha Carotene, Lutein & Zeaxanthin, Lycopene, Fiber, Folate, Glucosinolates, Iron, Magnesium, Niacin, Selenium, Vitamin B1 (Thiamin) Vitamin B2 (Riboflavin), Vitamin B6, Vitamin B12, Vitamin C, Vitamin E, Zinc, plus the ORAC score.

also raises the glycemic index. In this case, food components break down faster, so their glycemic index is higher. GI values are meant only to give people an idea of how various foods compare to each other in their ability to raise blood sugars.

Listed in the following box are the average GIs of a few favorite foods. There are many databases and books available online where you can find the GI of most of the foods you enjoy.

| Carrots | 49 | Corn Chips | 72 |
|---------|----|-----------|----|
| Brown Rice | 55 | White Rice | 72 |
| Basmati Rice | 58 | Rye Bread | 76 |
| Colas | 65 | Pretzels | 83 |
| Beets | 69 | Gatorade® | 78 |
| Bagels | 72 | White Baked Potato | 93 |

While Diana and I were discussing how whole foods function as perfect packets of enzymes and nutrients, it struck me – her gums were neither bleeding, nor inflamed. Obviously, her healing processes were finally outweighing the destructive processes.

We were both elated. Ruling out other changes, I asked if she was doing anything new to support her immune system. We specifically discussed stress, exercise routines, sleep habits, new medications (many influence blood sugars), and other possible dietary changes. These factors had remained stable.

Although she had tested normal on the fasting blood sugar screening test, I knew her significantly improved oral tissue health was likely related to her abstention from simple carbohydrates. I realized then she was more likely pre-diabetic/insulin resistant (IR) and that asking her doctor for a fasting glucose tolerance test would have been more appropriate. Fasting blood sugar level and HbA1c tests can be wildly misleading. These screening tests fail to diagnose damaging post-meal blood sugars. The fasting plasma glucose test identifies only half as many people with abnormal blood sugars as the glucose tolerance test. Significant nerve damage and up to 70% loss of pancreatic beta cells occurs before a fasting blood sugar test begin to show impairment.

CAROL: "It is good you changed your diet now. You are likely in an early phase of metabolic difficulty called insulin resistance, which can persist for at least a decade before it tips into type 2 diabetes. During this time, there is no apparent sugar metabolism problem, but gum disease, erectile dysfunction, high cholesterol levels and high blood pressure begin to show. Insulin resistance also decreases nitric oxide levels. Nitric oxide keeps blood vessel walls healthy and able to dilate. Those with IR have less blood flow to the heart.

"Insulin resistance occurs when liver, fat, and muscle cells become insensitive to insulin. You can still move the sugar out of your blood into those cells, but your body has to pump out massive amounts of insulin to do it. In other words, your glucose screening was normal, but that only proved your pancreas is still healthy enough to make sufficient insulin for the job. It does not tell you how much insulin your pancreas had to secrete to move the sugar.

"Two hour glucose tolerance tests, not as popular as they should be, provide earlier information about energy metabolism, especially when combined with information that puts a person in the category of what we call "metabolic syndrome". We say someone has metabolic syndrome and likely IR when they have any three of the following conditions:

- A waist measurement of 40 inches or more for men; 35 inches or more for women
- Triglyceride levels of 150 milligrams per deciliter (mg/dL) or above, or taking medication for elevated triglyceride levels
- HDL, or "good," cholesterol level below 40 mg/dL for men; below 50 mg/dL for women, or taking medication for low HDL levels.
- Blood pressure levels of 130/85 or above, or taking medication for elevated blood pressure levels.
- Fasting blood glucose levels of 100 mg/dL or above, or taking medication for elevated blood glucose levels.

"It is good you are changing your diet now because high insulin levels bring other sets of problems. For instance, people who have metabolic syndrome or insulin resistance have three times the risk of a stroke. In fact, eighty percent of those with insulin resistance die from a heart attack or stroke. This is a great time to start building your future!"

This conversation about something Diana thought was unrelated has helped her understand more about her changing body and possible health risks. She is more motivated than ever to continue educating herself about nutrition and lifestyle.

Diana was concerned about stabilizing her weight and asked me if I had any ideas about a fast acting energy food that did not spike her blood insulin. I mentioned that surprisingly, coconut oil added to the diets of diabetics and pre-diabetics does seem to help stabilize weight thus improving one's chances of avoiding Type 2 diabetes.[xli xlii]

## Oxygen Radical Absorbance Capacity (ORAC)

Since oxidation is a major component of uncontrolled diabetes and other inflammatory diseases, knowing and consuming foods with high antioxidant value is a good strategy. The National Institute on Aging developed a unit of measurement to describe the antioxidant capacity of foods, called a food's oxygen radical absorbance capacity or ORAC. The higher the ORAC value of a food or herb, the greater the ability to neutralize free radicals.

The following list of selected ORAC values is derived from the 2007 Nutrient Data Laboratory, Agriculture Research Service, of the US Department of Agriculture.

| HIGH ANTIOXIDANT FOODS | | HIGH ANTIOXIDANT FOODS | |
|---|---|---|---|
| Item | ORAC Value | Item | ORAC Value |
| Spices, cloves, ground | 314,446 | Spices, paprika | 17,919 |
| Spices, cinnamon, ground | 267,536 | Chokeberry, raw | 16,062 |
| Spices, oregano, dried | 200,129 | Tarragon, fresh | 15,542 |
| Spices, turmeric, ground | 159,277 | Ginger root, raw | 14,840 |
| Unsweetened cocoa | | Elderberries, raw | 14,697 |
| powder | 80,933 | Peppermint, fresh | 13,978 |
| Spices, cumin seed | 76,800 | Oregano, fresh | 13,970 |
| Spices, parsley, dried | 74,349 | Nuts, walnuts, english | 13,541 |
| Spices, basil, dried | 67,553 | Nuts, hazelnuts or filberts | 9,645 |
| Unsweetened baking | | Savory, fresh | 9,465 |
| chocolate | 49,926 | Cranberries, raw | 9,584 |
| curry powder | 48,504 | Pistachio nuts, raw | 7,983 |
| Chocolate, dutched | | Currants, black raw | 7,960 |
| powder | 40,200 | Spices, garlic powder | 6,665 |
| Maqui berry, juice* | 40,000 | Blueberries, raw | 6,552 |
| Sage, fresh | 32,004 | Blackberries, raw | 5,347 |
| Yellow mustard seed | 29,257 | Garlic, raw | 5,346 |
| Spices, ginger, ground | 28,811 | Raspberries, raw | 4,882 |
| Spices, pepper, black | 27,618 | Basil, fresh | 4,805 |
| Thyme, fresh | 27,426 | Nuts, almonds | 4,454 |
| Marjoram, fresh | 27,297 | Strawberries, raw | 3,577 |
| Goji berries | 25,300 | Cherries, sweet, raw | 3,365 |
| Spices, chili powder | 23,636 | Broccoli raab, raw | 3,083 |
| Candies, chocolate, dark | 20,823 | Apples, raw, with skin | 3.082 |
| Flax hull lignans* | 19,600 | Broccoli, cooked | 2,386 |
| Semisweet chocolate | 18,053 | Juice, Pomegranite, 100% | 2,341 |
| Nuts, pecans | 17,940 | Tea, green, brewed | 1,253 |
| *values derived from Brunswick Labs | | Orange juice, raw | 726 |

## Common Symptoms of Insulin Resistance

- Fatigue
- Brain drain, i.e., impeded memory and lack of focus
- Agitation
- Weight gain
- Intestinal bloating from carbohydrate overabundance
- High triglycerides/cholesterol
- High blood pressure
- Depression
- Osteoporosis.
- A skin change called *acanthosis nigricans*. At the neck (often the back of the neck), the armpits, and underneath the breasts skin begins to darken and takes on a velvety, mossy, sometimes flat warty-like appearance. Almost 90% of women with these skin changes have insulin resistance.

At a minimum, suspect insulin resistance where there is a history of diabetes in first-degree relatives; those with a personal history of gestational diabetes, polycystic ovary syndrome, or impaired glucose tolerance; and those with abdominal obesity.

## Classic Symptoms of Type 1 Diabetes

Survival for type 1 diabetics depends on carefully controlled insulin intake. Without it there is an escalating risk of entering acidotic comas, which can lead to death. The most immediately recognizable symptoms are: excessive thirst, hunger, and urination.

Type 1 diabetics have little to no insulin available to process glucose. Instead, muscles burn glycerol derived from body fat. When glycerol is burned, the free fatty acids released into the bloodstream from fat breakdown convert into large molecules called ketones. To eliminate these ketones, the person must drink massive amounts of water. This is why a type I diabetic will experience excessive frequent thirst accompanying frequent urination. When ketones reach a critical level in the bloodstream, coma and death can result. Many receive no warning signs but others exhibit a mix of the following signs:

- Constant fatigue
- Blurred vision
- Unexplained weight loss
- Slow healing of cuts and bruises
- Burning or dry mouth
- Itchy, dry skin
- Numbness or tingling in the hands or feet
- Absence of menstruation
- Nausea and vomiting
- Abdominal pain
- Trembling and weakness
- Confusion
- Dizziness
- Lack of coordination
- Convulsions or unconsciousness

## Classic Symptoms of Type 2 Diabetes

- Inflamed gums
- Patchy skin on the elbows and back of the neck, also often seen in the earlier stages of insulin resistance. Some schools check the back of the neck of children interested in participating in sports, since diabetics are prone to complications including more broken bones.
- Slightly excessive thirst and need for urination
- Frequent hunger signals, even one to two hours after a large meal

Type 2 diabetics rarely produce ketones, since their metabolic difficulties are different from type 1 diabetics. For them, high blood sugar levels silently destroy organs and tissues years before diagnosis.

**Post-meal blood sugars of 140 mg/dl (7.8 mmol/L) and higher and fasting blood sugars over 100 mg/dl (5.6 mmol/L) cause permanent organ damage and cause diabetes to progress.**

All blood sugar levels discussed in this book refer to plasma calibrated meter readings used by all meters sold in the United States. In other parts of the world where blood calibrated meters are still in use, including the UK, users should divide the numbers given by 1.12 to get the blood calibrated equivalents.

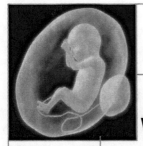

# 6

# WOMEN, SEX HORMONES, AND GUM DISEASE

**Explore:**
1. How do sex hormones affect women's mouths?
2. Do fertility drugs contribute to inflamed gums?
3. Can gum disease affect a woman's ability to become pregnant?
4. What are the connections between gum disease and the risk of having a pre-term low birth weight baby, gestational diabetes, preeclampsia, and other pregnancy complications?
5. What health risks might a pre-term baby face?

Can hormones influence our healthy smiles? Most women intuit the answer to this question. They know their sometimes surging, sometimes ebbing hormones demand attention. There are hundreds of estrogen receptor sites all over a woman's body. Estrogen, the female hormone, activates these sites as a woman journeys through puberty, monthly cycles, pregnancy, and menopause.

Women's mouths are loaded with estrogen receptors, so female gums reflect estrogen's influences. Often the balance of power between healing and destruction shifts. When it does, it triggers a series of far-ranging responses.

## Some Known Oral Effects of Female Hormones

- When estrogen levels peak just before ovulation – in the middle of a cycle – and again, just before a cycle, women often note mild burning sensations in their gums, easy gum bleeding, and associated gum tenderness. These symptoms reflect an exaggerated inflammatory response to plaque, which causes the gums around the teeth to become red and puffy with gingivitis.[i] As estrogen levels ebb during a period, these symptoms subside.

- Pregnancy amplifies monthly female responses. Due to elevated levels of progesterone, pregnancy gingivitis occurs in 60 to 75 percent of women during the second to eighth month of pregnancy. Occasionally, pregnant women experience "pregnancy tumors" or "pyogenic granulomas." The gums between the teeth swell substantially and bleed easily. These symptoms are benign and resolve after delivery and breast-feeding.

- Bacteria that destroy tissue, particularly *Prevotella* and *Bacteroides,* use estrogen and progesterone as food and growth factors.[ii]

- High estrogen levels cause blood vessel walls to become leaky.[iii] Fluids seep out into gum tissue and cause swelling.

- Just prior to ovulation, another hormone surge[1] adds to blood vessel dilation and leakiness. Swelling and congestion increase as fluids seep into surrounding tissues.[iv] This fluid is rich in inflammatory molecules like neutrophils, which is why many researchers call ovulation an inflammatory-like process. During ovulation, the ovaries also make VEGF (vascular endothelial growth factor). This glycoprotein (remember diabetes?[v]) is identified as a factor causing blood vessel leakiness even as it makes vessel walls thicker. VEGF assists new blood vessel formation in the failing diabetic retina described in the diabetes chapter. It also binds to receptors on the lining of blood vessel walls of gum tissues.[vi]

- While high estrogen levels contribute to tissue destruction, "normal" estrogen levels (typical of premenopausal, non-pregnant women, and postmenopausal women on hormone replacement therapy) generally protect tissues. At normal levels, estrogen helps wounds heal. Women with normal levels have significantly more collagen (a structural protein) and growth factors at wound sites compared to women with low estrogen levels.[vii] Growth factors aid cellular growth and wound repair. In this way, estrogen helps the body maintain fibrous collagen protein in its connective tissue. Healthy tissue with strong structure is less likely to break down under biological stress.

---

1 Luteinizing hormone

In gum disease management, those with normal estrogen levels have better Velcro-like tissue attachment to the tooth via fibroblasts.

- There is an optimal range for estrogen in this protective healing mode. Unfortunately, the chain reaction of inflammatory mediators surges as estrogen levels drop in postmenopausal women.[viii]
- The female hormones in oral contraceptives often result in folate (vitamin $B_9$) deficiency. Low folate levels delay healing after inflammation.[vii][2]
- As estrogen drops in menopause, osteoporosis causes loss of bone mass, including that of the jawbone that anchors teeth. An offshoot study from The Women's Health Initiative found three times the bone loss around teeth in women with osteoporosis, regardless of whether they had gum disease or not.[ix]
- Bisphosphonates, which include Actonel, Boniva, Didronel, Fosamax, Skelid, Aredia, Bonefos, and Zometa, are used to treat osteoporosis and bone cancers. Oral osteonecrosis, a serious, but uncommon oral side effect of these medications deserves increasing awareness.[x] Chapter Seven reviews osteonecrosis in more detail.

## ANALENA
## Hormone Surges

Analena is a strong, energetic, and intelligent woman. Born and educated in Cuba, she has lived in America for ten years. She came from a privileged family, which allowed her to receive a spectacular education. Judging from the stories of her arrival in this country, Analena has used her talent and audacity to forge an amazing career.

But her adventurous life exerted a price. She married late and waited several years before she considered having children. And so, at forty-one, her desire for a child collided with infertility. Her obstetrician wisely suggested a dental visit before he prescribed fertility drugs. He was familiar with research literature showing how periodontal disease may increase the risk of pre-term low birth weight (PT/LBW) delivery. The same research showed that gum disease may double the

---

2 Also, up to 72% of all spina bifida cases can be prevented with adequate doses of $B_9$.

risk for a life threatening condition called preeclampsia. In fact, gum disease probably accounts for more preeclampsia than any other cause. Analena's obstetrician noticed she had not had a dental check-up in years. If she had gum disease, he wanted to intervene early. Like most obstetricians these days, he encouraged his expectant mothers to have thorough dental check-ups.

Most women who are either trying to conceive or are already pregnant share an amazing attribute; they have a voracious appetite for learning about pregnancy and motherhood. I hoped Analena was one of these women. She chose our office because her husband is a client. From him, I learned most Cubans are unfamiliar with floss. (He once quipped this was the only good thing he could think of about Cuba!)

Now it was Analena's turn. She had been taking ovulation-stimulating hormones for about three months before she scheduled her first dental visit. Her exam showed her gums required immediate care. She was able to see on the camera monitor how puffy, red, and fragile they were. The pockets between her back teeth registered 5mm to 6mm of tissue destruction. There were few visible deposits because she was an attentive brusher, but there were heavy deposits under her gums, especially between her teeth. She had not noticed any symptoms.

CAROL: "Analena, looking forward to having a baby is so exciting. The crazy tricks female hormones play only add to the excitement. The rapid body changes and mood swings you will likely experience signal extraordinary surprises ahead. Your doctor has you on some powerful ovulation-stimulating hormones, which is like being on a period with steroids. *Everything* is exaggerated, including a heightened sensitivity to infections.

"I assume you usually notice fragility – bleeding and tenderness – in your gums during your monthly cycles. It shouldn't surprise you, but your gums are rife with estrogen receptors, which boost estrogen's influence on your gums.

"First, estrogen makes blood vessels leaky. Rather than fine filters, they become porous, which allows protein-rich fluids from the bloodstream to flood nearby tissue. I wish estrogen were the only hormone that causes the swelling and congestion we see in your gum tissues. Unfortunately, two more hormones prompt researchers to call ovulation an inflammatory-like process. They are luteinizing hormone (the hormone that prepares you to ovulate), and vascular endothelial growth factor, VEGF, a chemical signal produced in your ovaries.

## Ovulation Processes Exacerbate Gum Response

"In fact, VEGF can make blood vessels so profoundly leaky that occasionally, some women taking the same ovulation-stimulating infertility drugs you take, actually lose enough circulating blood volume to have problems with low blood pressure.[xi]

"We must also consider the other source of the swelling we see here." I showed her some of the hidden deposits under her swollen gums and repeated the principles of inflammation I presented to Claire, but tailored them for Analena. "When estrogen and progesterone levels are high, several destructive bacteria thrive. Right now, you have four factors likely causing elevated levels of inflammation messengers in your blood:

- The degree of gum disease you have creates a heavy load of inflammatory messengers all by itself.
- You have elevated estrogen levels, which encourage proliferation of destructive bacteria. Right now your body strongly responds to estrogen.
- Permeable blood vessels leak out more inflammatory messenger-rich fluid than usual.
- Fertility drugs that stimulate ovulation also exacerbate gum inflammation and bleeding. The longer you take these drugs, the more inflamed your gums will likely become." [xii]

ANALENA: "Wow! I suppose I should not be too surprised to hear any of this, but the information is still disturbing. Of course I want to regain my oral health. Still, I don't understand how inflammation could affect the outcome of a pregnancy. How could inflammation influence my delivery date to produce an underdeveloped baby?"

CAROL: "It sounds implausible, doesn't it? I'll explain in a minute. Your first concern is becoming pregnant. Several studies relate in vitro fertilization implant failure and unsuccessful embryo development to the presence of infection in the body, so we can presume periodontal disease affects the success of infertility treatment. Since this reflects recent research, it's hard to estimate an individual's risk."

## Pre-term/Low Birth Weight Babies and Gum Disease

"Researchers continue to investigate the links between inflammation and pre-term/low birth weight (PT/LBW) babies.

"One reason obstetricians repeatedly check pregnant woman for gastrointestinal tract and vaginal infections is because they know infections cause inflammatory messengers (the cytokines: IL-1, IL-6, and TNF-alpha) to circulate and enter the amniotic fluid. In turn, those messengers trigger prostaglandin release, another step in the inflammatory pathway. Prostaglandins stimulate labor. In fact, obstetricians and other caregivers often use it for that purpose. In its presence, the cervix softens, the fetal membrane ruptures, and labor contractions begin.

### Oral Infection and PT/LBW babies

Elevated hormones in pregnancy tip the scales of gum disease towards destruction.

Gum disease, with its heavy biofilm loaded with bacteria and virulent endotoxins, is no different from any other infection pathway.[xiii][xiv][xv][xvi]

- Simple gingivitis (gum inflammation without accompanying bone loss) can triple PT/LBW risks.[xvii] Researchers hypothesize that perhaps 40 percent of all pregnant women have some degree of oral infection; it may be the most common source of all infections in pregnant women.
- Studies show a three to eight times greater risk of PT/LBW delivery in mothers with moderate periodontal disease compared to women with healthy mouths. Researchers continue to look for additional explanations. For instance, it is possible some mothers have a suppressed immune response.[xviii]
- Researchers estimate that half of all neural defects in babies are due to PT/LBW.
- Asthma, poor vision, cerebral palsy, low IQ, poor motor skills, and hearing and neuro-developmental disabilities are linked to those born with extremely low birth weight, or less than 1,000 grams or about 2.25 pounds.[xix]

"Many wonder if successful gum disease therapy *after* becoming pregnant lowers risk. It appears possible,[xx][xxi] but right now we have an incomplete picture. Researchers think it is important to achieve gum health before pregnancy because once the inflammatory cascade has started, it may be too late to alter negative outcomes.

"Although you probably do not need any more motivation for controlling your oral infection while you are pregnant, you'll want to be aware of three further associations:

- Some studies suggest when a mother hosts an infection, it alters fetal brain structure.[xxii]
- Six of the destructive anaerobic bacteria known to contribute to gum disease are found at least half the time in placentas of mothers with preeclampsia, the most dangerous pregnancy complication.[xxiii] Preeclampsia affects both mother and fetus. While damage can occur to blood vessel walls, kidneys, and the liver, high blood pressure is the most visible sign.
- Recently, Dr. Han at Case Western Reserve showed a direct causal relationship between *F. nucleatum* and pre-term birth. This organism was chosen as an example of correlations between oral health and pre-term birth. This particular bacteria, found in simple gingivitis and advanced gum disease, targets the placenta and amniotic fluid in the sac. There is a significant association between *F. nucleatum* and complications in previous pregnancies including miscarriage, intrauterine death, neonatal death, pre-term delivery and premature membrane rupture. [3][xxiv]

"I don't say these things to worry you at this most exciting time of your life. I just want you to know the timing of your visit here is

3 From a recent report: "A case of stillbirth caused by *Fusobacterium nucleatum* originating in the mother's mouth." (Han Y, Fardini Y, Chen C, et al. *Obstet Gynecol.* 2010 February; 115(2 Pt 2): 442–445.)
Case — A woman with pregnancy-associated gingivitis experienced an upper respiratory tract infection at term, followed by stillbirth a few days later. *Fusobacterium nucleatum* was isolated from the placenta and the infant. Examination of different microbial flora from the mother identified the same clone in her subgingival plaque, but not in the supra gingival plaque, vagina, or rectum.
Conclusion — F. nucleatum may have translocated from the mother's mouth to the uterus when the immune system was weakened during the respiratory infection.

excellent. Perhaps therapy will slightly improve the odds of becoming pregnant and delivering a healthy, full-term baby. The best outcomes happen when therapy precedes pregnancy."

Analena actively participated in her care. After therapy, the markers for disease subsided substantially. Within two months she was pregnant with twins!  We worked closely together to find techniques she could use at home to keep her mouth healthy. She scheduled dental wellness appointments every three months. During these visits, she showed no signs of bleeding or swelling. Her gums were never tender again.

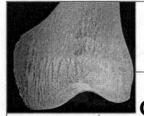

# OSTEOPOROSIS: WOMEN – AND OLDER MEN – AT RISK

**Explore:**

1. Osteoporosis is about bone density, right? ... *Right?*
2. Is it reasonable to think osteoporosis spares the jawbone that anchors teeth?
3. Does gum disease speed skeletal osteoporosis?
4. How does normal bone maintenance keep your skeleton strong?
5. When should men be concerned?
6. How does lifestyle reduce fracture risks?
7. What are the risks of taking bisphosphonates (Examples: Boniva, Actonel, and Fosamax)?
8. Are there alternative treatments to bisphosphonates?
9. How can you and your medical team work to assure a positive outcome?
10. Other than lifestyle changes, are there alternative strategies to minimize osteoporosis risks?

## Our Amazing Bones

Architects learn early what shapes make strong structures. They test how compression and tension forces distribute themselves throughout triangles, arches, and domes. Triangles impart strength. Arches use compression to provide strength. Arches and domes bear weight. Consider light yet strong corrugated cardboard shipping boxes. The key to their strength lies not in their flat exterior layers, but the consistent bends of the middle layer. These create architecturally strong alternating triangles.

So it is with our bones. They need to be light and strong, able to bear weight and handle the forces of compression (running and jumping) and tension (flexing). Our bones have strong exteriors, but their interiors – the bone matrices – are as light and airy as foam. The ability to withstand fracture is as much about architecture and what makes up the matrix as it is about mineral mass/density. Glass is denser than plastic but far more brittle and likely to shatter. Collagen is the glue that makes bones strong. Nutrients and minerals comprising the collagen matrix allow it to expand and contract without breaking.

Our bones are dynamic and always changing. Healthy people regenerate bone throughout life in a process called remodeling. New bone cells constantly replace worn cells. This cellular turnover allows our bodies to repair the micro-fractures that occur from daily living. It also allows the body to increase bone mass in response to increased mechanical loads such as those created during exercise. Complete turnover of bone in a healthy person takes from seven to ten years.

## Osteoporosis

### Osteoporosis Statistics

- Nineteen percent of women 65 to 72 years old have osteoporosis.
- By the time they are 85 years old, more than half of all women are diagnosed with osteoporosis.[i]
- At least a third of all women over 50 will fracture a bone due to osteoporosis, as will about 20 percent of men over 50.[ii]
- Every year, more than 300,000 Americans fracture a hip. Twenty percent die within three months.[iii] One in four die of complications within a year. Roughly half will never walk again. Those that do usually require long-term care.
- One third of all people who sustain a fracture are hospitalized.
- Over eight percent of those fracture victims are relegated to nursing homes[iv] due to serious and permanent mobility impairment.

These numbers will increase significantly as the U.S. population ages. The health costs of osteoporosis are staggering. The personal costs, tragic.

Osteoporosis leaves its victims' bones with low mineral density and flexibility, which makes the bones incapable of handling compressive and tensile pressures. They become fragile and riddled with micro-fractures, which change its architecture. Bone architecture matters orally because the quality of the bone anchoring the teeth affects whether they are retained or not. As we have seen, oral bone loss is related to inflammation and the formation of a large oral wound. Osteoporosis causes decreased bone density and decreased flexibility, which speeds bone loss around teeth.

Eighty percent of those diagnosed with osteoporosis are women. Before menopause, most women enjoy the protection estrogen provides bones:

- Estrogen bars an enzyme, caspase-3, from killing off bone-building cells called osteoblasts.
- Estrogen reduces levels of TNF, an infamous inflammatory mediator molecule. TNF increases the formation rate of bone-destroying cells called osteoclasts.
- Estrogen reduces blood levels of other inflammatory mediators, such as IL-1 and IL-6, which also increase osteoclast formation.

Subsiding estrogen comes with menopause, complete hysterectomies, suppressed menses in top-level athletes, stressed people with adrenal fatigue, and medications called gonadotropin-releasing hormone agonists, or GnRH agonist drugs, prescribed specifically to suppress estrogen. Endometriosis, ovulation suppression, and hormone sensitive cancer tumors, including some breast cancers, respond well to decreased estrogen levels. Aromatase inhibitors that reduce estrogen levels also induce osteoporosis.[1] With subsiding estrogen levels comes the threat of osteoporosis.

As a woman ages, one of the biggest health decisions she must make concerns whether or not she should supplement her subsiding hormone levels during and after menopause. Estrogen's role in promoting bone strength – among other benefits – must be carefully weighed against serious risks associated with hormone replacement therapy. Equivocal studies in recent years complicate the decision. A definitive study released in 2007 suggests hormone replacement therapy is a more attractive choice for women just entering menopause because

---

1 Aromatase is the principal way postmenopausal women maintain estrogen. It converts androgen, produced by exercise, into estrogen.

therapy affects their blood vessels differently than women long past menopause.[v]

Two potent osteoporosis prevention tactics are related to estrogen. The first – retain some body fat after menopause because fat stores estrogen. The second is exercise. Exercise releases testosterone, which converts to estrogen. Weight-bearing exercise activates bone-building processes.

When people think of osteoporosis and the threat of fractures, they think only of bone density and calcium. Flexibility is just as important. Collagen provides the structural framework, the matrix, for the mineral crystals that give bone density. Bone contains protein "glue" molecules with sacrificial bonds and hidden, coiled length that dissipate energy when pulled or stressed. These bonds rupture, but subsequently reform when bone is healthy. To keep bone healthy, the immune system, nutrition, and hormones work together.

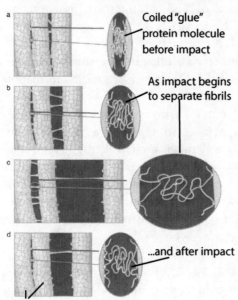

Coiled "glue" protein molecule before impact

As impact begins to separate fibrils

...and after impact

Mineralized collagen fibrils

Micro-structure of bone: Tiny mineral crystals only a few atoms thick coat bone collagen fibrils. A self-healing protein "glue" holds these mineralized collagen fibrils together. Think of the glue as being like coiled springs that uncoil when bone is stressed. This helps bone absorb shock. It takes more energy to stretch hidden length than it does to break a bond. When the stress is relaxed, the protein returns to its coiled state. (Based on the work of Paul Hansma and his research group/Department of Physics/ Santa Barbara, California.

Osteoporosis from low hormones also threatens men. Lupron and other GnRH drugs are prescribed for men with prostate cancer. The intended therapeutic effect is to keep sex glands from producing the sex hormone, testosterone. Less well-known – this is a leading cause of osteoporosis in men. These drugs decrease bone mineral density and increase fracture risk in men with prostate cancer.[vi]

## Environmental, Non-Estrogen Related Risk Factors for Osteoporosis

- **Heavy smoking.** Estrogen protects bone because it reduces powerful inflammatory mediators. Smoking counteracts estrogen because it increases inflammatory mediators. How long and how much a person smokes is an excellent predictor of inflammatory mediator levels.
- **Sedentary Lifestyle.** Exercise exerts a load on bones. Skeletal bones respond to loads by remodeling themselves. Only through remodeling does the human body make new, stronger, and more flexible bone. Sedentary lifestyles allow little opportunity for bone repair and remodeling.
- **Low dietary intake of calcium, magnesium, and vitamin $K_2$.** Inadequate sun exposure or supplementation leads to low **vitamin D** levels. Despite calcium's role in the spotlight for osteoporosis prevention, calcium is useless without these nutrients. Boron consumption also increases bone strength at levels substantially below those reported to be reproductively toxic.[vii]
- **Impaired thyroid function.** The thyroid gland makes calcitonin. Calcitonin aids calcium and magnesium deposition into bones.
- **Lack of adequate nutrition due to absorption problems.** Celiac disease, Crohn's disease, and gastrectomy (partial or total removal of the stomach) are a few digestive problems that elevate risk. Anorexia nervosa excludes dietary essentials, so also elevates risks.
- **High sugar intake/acidity.** Blood serum must be kept between pH 7.35 and pH 7.45. Diets high in refined carbohydrates like sugar, cereal grains, white rice, and white flour, are mineral poor and result in a need to buffer blood acidity. Skeletal bones release the necessary minerals, including calcium, to do this. These liberated minerals are then available to stiffen arteries as they calcify blood vessel plaques. Free calcium also calcifies oral plaques, produces kidney stones, and readily enters tumors. High calcium mobility is why many cancers show up in x-rays. Excessive sugar intake also reduces magnesium, so necessary for calcium absorption and utilization. Finally, the accumulation of AGEs in the collagen matrix of bone destabilizes its structure[viii] and interferes with bone cell regeneration and development. AGEs also accumulate in other areas of slow turn over, such as cartilage and tendons. In this way

unchecked AGEs lead to stiff, uncomfortable joints with impaired function. Arthritis anyone?

- **Acid-producing foods.** Meats (excessive phosphorus), some melons, soy beans and other legumes, salty processed foods, and hard cheeses create a need to buffer the acid load. Alkalizing minerals, pulled from bone is one way we buffer our systems. An abundance of fruits and especially dark green leafy vegetables help create a mineral balance. Raw apple cider vinegar, rich in minerals and probiotics, is well-known for being alkaline-forming. Potassium and sodium hydroxide change the acid of lemons and vinegar to a base, so they are fine. While working to understand the principals that can correct your diet, consider supplementing with a base that counteracts acid-promoting foods, such as potassium citrate. A 2006 study suggests that taking a potassium citrate supplement can help counteract the high acidity of modern diets. Subjects who supplemented their diets with potassium citrate, rapidly increased bone mass.[ix]

  I check my clients' acidity with pH testing strips, though saliva is only somewhat indicative of a body's buffering capacity. If too acid, I encourage them to monitor their own pH with pHion Diagnostic Test Strips (http://www.phionbalance.com). I counsel them on subjects covered in Chapter Twelve and Fourteen.

- **High intake of caffeine or alcohol**, defined as two or more drinks per day, create a need for bone to donate buffering minerals.
- **Most medicinal and mind altering drugs** as well as chemicals, pesticides and herbicides require mineral buffering.
- **Frequent soda consumption.** Ingesting 500 mg of phosphorus – the amount present in most sodas – adversely affects the important calcium/phosphorus blood serum ratio, which also creates acidity. Again, to balance the acidity caused by increased phosphorus blood levels, bones must release calcium. High phosphorus levels also drain magnesium from skeletal bones. Phosphoric acid found in diet and regular sodas erodes tooth enamel, even with minimal exposure. Soft drinks often replace calcium-rich milk, though modern dairy products have their own set of issues.
- **Elevated blood levels of the amino acid homocysteine** can double the risk of osteoporosis-related fractures. This might be because high homocysteine levels (again, derived from meat) interrupt the interlacing of bone's structural collagen fibers. These fibers

are key to bone flexibility.[x][xi] A diet rich in B-complex vitamins [folic acid ($B_9$), $B_{12}$, and $B_6$] is critical to homocysteine breakdown in the bloodstream.[xii]  Take B-complex vitamins separately from other vitamins. (See the discussion on $B_{12}$ under Celiac disease in Chapter Fourteen.) If you take birth control pills, please be aware they deplete folic acid and $B_6$.

- **Adrenal fatigue.** Women who chronically diet have inadequate nutrition, poor digestive function, and a low metabolic rate. Adrenal fatigue is the end result. This mimics the condition noted next regarding glucocorticoids (also called corticosteroids). For them, osteoporosis is the result – not the underlying cause – of other health conditions.

- **Long-term use of drugs like anticonvulsants, lithium, anticoagulants, and glucocorticoids.** Prednisone and Prednisolone are two glucocorticoids prescribed for anti-inflammatory and immuno-suppressive properties in autoimmune diseases like systemic lupus and rheumatoid arthritis. Again, they do cause osteoporosis.

- **Taking medications that treat stomach acidity for at least a year** may increase hip fracture risk by 44 percent. These drugs are classified as proton pump inhibitors. Some of them are Nexium, Prilosec, Prevacid, Zoton, and Inhibitol.

## Some Common Non-Environmental Risk Factors for Osteoporosis

- Female
- Lean body
- Caucasian or Asian ethnicity
- Systemic diseases such as rheumatoid arthritis, leukemia, and chronic obstructive pulmonary disease (COPD)
- Positive family history
- Premature menopause
- **Age.** As one ages, cells that break down bone are more active than cells that rebuild bone.
- **Hyperparathyroidism (secondary).** The parathyroid glands produce a hormone (PTH) that controls calcium levels in blood and bone, and helps intestines absorb dietary calcium. Low blood calcium levels trigger excessive release of this hormone. A vitamin D deficiency, absorption problem, or drug-induced metabolic

problem often exists.[xiii] In these cases, messages are sent to liberate calcium from the skeleton, possibly resulting in osteoporosis.

- **Serotonin use.** The neurotransmitter serotonin is known for its influence on brain activity. Prozac and other popular SSRI drugs boost serotonin and its mood-elevating effects. Most bone cells contain it and it seems to decrease bone-building activity. Eight percent of American adults take SSRIs for depression. Several studies found that postmenopausal women who take these drugs lose bone faster than those who do not, though there may be other common causes.[xiv xv] Men taking SSRIs also lose bone faster than those who do not.[xvi] Interestingly, 95 percent of serotonin is actually produced in the gut as enzymes create it from tryptophan. A protein called Lrp5 blocks this conversion. If you have plenty of Lrp5, your bones remain strong.[xvii] Stay tuned to see if this leads to future bone-sparing therapies!

### Bone Maintenance

Our skeletons face many challenges. Human bones suffer constant micro-damage and rely on their capacity to repair themselves. Also, as muscular activity (think exercise or active lifestyles) elevates, it heightens mechanical stresses on skeletal bones. To keep up with these stresses, bones undergo constant remodeling. Two processes are involved. Bone-gobbling osteoclasts remove aged, deteriorating bone. Bone building cells called osteoblasts replace the bad bone with new, good bone. Complete skeletal turnover takes between seven to ten years. Stated another way, ten percent of our skeleton turns over every year. To keep bones strong, it is important that bone breakdown and bone formation stay balanced. Estrogen helps promote this balance.

Decreasing estrogen levels trigger a cascade of events. First, special immune system cells, called T cells, proliferate. They activate infection messengers that stimulate destructive osteoclasts. Osteoblasts and subsequent re-mineralization cannot keep pace with the abundance of destructive osteoclasts. To further outstrip osteoblasts, osteoclasts stay in play longer. Their preprogrammed death occurs much later without estrogen's influences.

As estrogen levels decrease, so do bone growth factors. Osteoblasts become less sensitive to mechanical stimuli and micro-damage detection is impaired.[xix]

Is there an association between osteoporosis and oral health? This systemic disease does not spare jawbone. Both diseases are chronic degenerative diseases. Both involve bone density loss through inflammation and other imbalances wherein bone destruction overrides formation. Inflammatory mediators released in gum disease amplify oral and skeletal degenerative bone loss.[2] A sub-study of the Woman's Health Initiative showed tripled bone height loss around teeth in women diagnosed with osteoporosis, regardless of their gum disease status. A more recent study drew the same conclusion.[xviii]

## MOLLY

This petite, 97-pound woman in her late 60s vibrates with energy and determination. Molly routinely made the 450-mile drive into Austin for preventive dental care every three months. She was only delayed once, when she hit a deer while flying down the deserted roads of West Texas. Being the spirited woman she is, she took a deep breath, and picked up her cell phone to advise us she would be a few minutes late.

Her spunk that day exemplified a life fully lived. Molly is always busy and stressed from working long hours at the computer, usually with a cigarette dangling from her lips. That is until a few years ago, when health complications caused her to adjust her lifestyle. She gave up her cigarettes and evening scotches. She shifted her diet to include more organic, nutrient-dense foods and took up jogging. However recent pain from rheumatoid arthritis forced her to scale back her vigorous exercise routine. To help control the arthritis, her doctor prescribed Prednisone to suppress her immune system. She declined hormone replacement therapy (HRT) because of reported side effects.

Years of relationship-building finally erased Molly's fears of dental office visits, although she routinely dismissed my attempts to involve her in her own oral health. A joke led her to commit to meticulous self-care. Her story has inspired and encouraged more than a few other clients.

One day I teased, "Molly, I love you, but soon I'm going to quit pestering you. We've progressed beyond the days when you trembled your way through every visit. I know you enjoy your appointments now. I do, too. But I encourage daily care between teeth for about six years before I give up and move on." She laughed with me as I checked

---

2 Once again, inflammatory mediators IL-1, Il-6, Il-8, TNF-alpha, prostaglandins, and enzymes such as collagenase are implicated.

her chart to see how long I had been caring for her. A moment later I exclaimed, "Oh! Would you look at that! Molly, I completely made that up. But guess what! This particular visit actually completes six years of our association. I guess I'm done!"

She smiled and our conversation moved on to other things. But at the end of her visit, she returned to the subject of flossing. She peered into the mirror, smiled, and said, "I'm too much of a politician to promise I'll floss every day, but I'm going to give it a shot." I was mildly surprised, but did not give her comment another thought.

Three months later, Molly sank into my chair trembling again. I was perplexed until she exuberantly said, "Man! I *like* this flossing stuff! I don't care if you can tell whether it's doing me any good or not. I'm going to keep doing it! Is twice a day too much?"

I broke my initial stunned silence with a giggle. I lifted my forearm to my forehead in mock despair and said, "Jeez Molly, if I had known you were obsessive compulsive I would have used it against you years ago! You are the first person to ask if flossing twice a day is too much." [3]

How surprising to realize she was trembling with excitement. She could not wait to tell me about her success and to find out if her mouth was healthier. Ten years prior to that visit, Molly had generalized moderate gum disease. Easy bleeding and swollen tissues accompanied generalized 5mm to 6mm pockets between her back teeth. This meant she had lost about 2mm to 3mm of supportive jawbone, but thorough scalings and a three-month care schedule had allowed her gums to reattach to her teeth, which reduced her pockets to the 3mm to 4mm range. Her gums were still puffy because she lacked the self-care component, but she maintained moderate health and was happily avoiding surgery.

That day we raced through her wellness appointment. Afterward, she seemed startled as she sat up. "Are we done? It was so easy!"

CAROL: "Well, Molly. You didn't leave much for me to do. The swelling and bleeding are gone. And there were few deposits. This is actually the official definition of a "cleaning" – a simple procedure accomplished on an already healthy person that helps maintain that health." She was delighted and has never looked back or slipped in her care.

---

3 My daughter did several years later, while in braces! Much to my surprise, she waxed on about the glories of flossing. I took this as proof that kids can be brainwashed! Flossing twice a day while wearing braces is a significant commitment.

Several years ago, while reviewing Molly's health history, she casually mentioned her bone mass had decreased so much her doctor suggested she start taking Boniva. I frowned as I considered her health information and slight build.

I began slowly, "You know, I wish I knew then what I know now. All those years ago, I should have had the foresight to discuss with you your risks for developing osteoporosis. You have so many of them. I'm sure you know some of them. You are Caucasian. You have the petite frame everyone covets. But I don't know if you are aware that some of your past lifestyle choices also contributed to your risk. Your history of heavy smoking definitely comes to mind. I am thrilled you quit, but all those years of smoking kept your body's inflammatory response active. It negated the bone protection estrogen would have otherwise provided during that time. Your daily drinking also contributed to your risk picture. Now your body has stopped producing estrogen and, to compound its lack, you just started taking Prednisone. I notice you are not yet suffering any of the puffiness and weight gain normally associated with glucocorticoids, but I'm sure your doctor knows Prednisone adds a potent risk factor for bone density loss[4] as does the arthritis it's designed to treat.[xx] Last, you are now sedentary because of joint pain. You are not getting the exercise that brings the mechanical load your bones need to stay strong and flexible.

"I want to congratulate you again on controlling your gum disease. Many women don't realize they have it, or that the inflammatory cycle it creates contributes to local and systemic bone loss. I could compare it to your rheumatoid arthritis. You might have active arthritis in a particular joint, but joints distant from that joint can also erode. It's a difficult concept, but at least not one you have to worry about. I am so proud of how healthy you keep your mouth now, and that you quit smoking and most simple carbohydrates like sugars, alcohol, and grains.

---

4 After initiating corticosteroid therapy, bone loss occurs quickly during the first three months. It is thought these steroids reduce the rate of bone formation, interfere with calcium balance, and interfere with protective sex hormones. Risks increase with dosage. There is significant bone loss with doses above 7.5 mg/day of prednisone or its equivalent. Significant bone loss is also reported after prolonged steroidal inhalation therapy and prolonged potent topical steroid therapy. Further, all steroids depress immune function in a multitude of ways and exacerbate diseases such as diabetes, high blood pressure, GI ulcers, TB, etc.

## Bisphosphonates: Boniva, Actonel, and Fosamax

"I worry about you because I know half of all women in the U.S. eventually break a crucial bone due to osteoporosis.[xxi] Boniva has helped a lot of people. It belongs to a class of drugs you will likely hear a lot about. Has your doctor described how it works?"

MOLLY: "No, but I remember reading a newspaper article some time ago about possible side effects. It scared me, but I can't quite remember how it goes. What do you know?"

CAROL: "You may be recalling an article in *The Wall Street Journal*. [xxii] When it was published, Boniva's association with jaw osteonecrosis was still unclear. There are still many uncertainties, but I'll tell you some of what we know to date.

## Osteonecrosis of the Jaw

"First, you should know what osteonecrosis is. Bone is a living tissue with its own blood supply. If normal blood supply is lost, the tissue easily becomes infected and dies, which causes the bone to collapse. Orally, this situation usually occurs after an invasive procedure. In this case, symptoms would include a non-healing extraction site or exposed jawbone. Oral osteonecrosis is often painful, so you would likely call us. In its early phases, osteonecrosis can mimic the symptoms of gum disease or a tooth abscess. We'd see tissue swelling and redness that normally indicates infection, but the area may or may not be infected and probably would not respond to normal dental therapies. Over time, some teeth may become loose, or we would notice drainage from infection. Eventually, you would be left with exposed bone that does not heal, thus we call it "osteo" (bone) "necrosis" (death).

"Bisphosphonates suppress blood supply to bone. Having a good blood supply helps retain bone vitality. This is because blood carries important nutrients and infection-fighting immune system molecules to all parts of the body, including the bones.[xxiii] It could be said bisphosphonates kill bone to "save" it. They are also a quick fix for what is essentially a nutritional issue.

"This is a good time to mention you do have two known indicated risks for developing jaw osteonecrosis. One is your age. "Bone death" seems to happen most often after age 65. Unfortunately, the Prednisone – or any corticosteroid – that contributes to your osteoporosis risk also adds to your risk picture for taking Boniva. In fact, the complication of rheumatoid arthritis coupled with your need to take Prednisone might be the biggest consideration in your decision of how to treat your osteoporosis. In a recent study, one in twelve people who took corticosteroids followed by Boniva-like drugs experienced osteonecronosis in their jaws. Another study showed 11.4 percent of patients who were prescribed oral corticosteroids developed osteonecrosis.[xxiv]

"Right now, we should be happy you eliminated a strong risk indicator years ago, which was your level of gum disease. You are so healthy now!

"When considering any drug, you have to decide whether the benefits outweigh the risks. As the saying goes, 'You can't get something for nothing.' Patients and lawyers often think in black and white terms, but all health therapies carry some risk for some people. I'm pleased you came to see us before you started bisphosphonate therapy because there are a few dental needs we haven't yet addressed. If you choose to take one of these drugs, you will have to take care of them first. Do you know what dental needs I'm referring to?"

MOLLY: "Oh, no. Don't tell me I have to confront my darned wisdom tooth!"

CAROL: "Molly, it's half submerged! You *know* it's an impossible-to-clean bacterial sink, which is only half the reason you need to take care of it. Hang on for this one and you'll see what I mean.

## Alternatives to Bisphosphonates

"Beyond balancing your diet by reducing grains and grain-fed meats, there are several choices you could discuss with your doctor to help your body regulate bone remodeling and increase bone mass. Boniva is one of them.

"Do you remember when I talked about collagenase, the enzyme released by inflammatory messengers? You may remember my saying it irreversibly destroys bone and tissue structure. Well, it is just one of several kinds of tissue destroyers whose presence was partly to blame for causing the breakdown of the gums and bone around your teeth years ago. These tissue destroyers, called MMPs, also destroy skeletal bones.

"Several prescription drugs slow bone destruction by reducing MMP levels. Low-dose doxycycline hyclate, or LDD, also known as

Periostat, is one.[5] At sub-microbial doses – doses less than what is required for use as an antibiotic, i.e., 20 mg of doxycycline twice a day – these LDDs can favorably tip the balance toward bone building without many of the side effects present with higher antimicrobial doses. The LDDs inactivate tissue-destroying MMPs and slow down the destructive behaviors of osteoclasts and neutrophils. This therapy improves the outcome of patients with periodontal disease and osteoporosis. (See next section: Vitamin D/Marshall Protocol.)

"Some doctors prescribe a calcitonin nasal spray. (Calcitonin is also produced in the thyroid). It is most effective for women who suffer osteoporosis as a result of glucocorticoid use. It stabilizes high calcium levels by inhibiting bone destroying osteoclast cells. An osteoclast's job is to destroy old bone so new bone can be laid down. Unfortunately, side effects of calcitonin can be nasal irritation, headaches, depression, joint pain, and heart attack. This is obviously not ideal for you.

"SERMS, or selective estrogen receptor modulators, are a class of drugs shown to help some women. SERMS activate estrogen receptors in some kinds of tissue and block estrogen receptors in others. Familiar examples of SERMS are Femarelle and Evista. SERMS block inflammatory messengers before they can activate MMPs or bone-destroying osteoclasts. Bone mass increases because osteoclasts remain dormant. Side effects can be: stroke, blood clots, and hot flashes.

"Gene therapy to increase OPGs, or osteoprotegerins, might soon be available. It would provide a double benefit for you. OPG is a cool little cell that helps keep bone building and destruction in balance. As with all body tissues, your skeleton renews itself constantly. It takes seven to ten years to completely rebuild a new skeleton. It is how your body repairs the accumulated micro-fractures caused by daily living and the way it responds to the demands of an active lifestyle.

"Normally, bone-making osteoblasts release a cell called RANK-L, that docks onto its receptor, or RANK, which is found on destructive osteoclasts. It signals the osteoclasts to produce the acid that removes old bone so osteoblasts can begin to lay down fresh bone. Removal of old bone by the acids osteoclasts produce is called resorption. It's a great recycling process! But OPGs are also involved in the process.

---

5 Periostat is now available generically, though to protect its market position, it is reformulated as Periostat MR, a once-daily tablet. Oracea is a newcomer to the market, with benefits substantially similar to Periostat. Its marketing efforts have shifted towards dermatology – specifically as a treatment for acne and rosacea. Nonetheless, it is important to note that Periostat lowers hs-CRPs and A1C levels also.

They act as a decoy receptor. In other words, they can snatch the RANK-L before it docks onto the osteoclast, so the osteoclast never gets the signal to start destroying.

"If one increases OPG levels, usually by injection, bone formation overrides bone resorption. Gene therapy to increase OPGs is still in clinical trials, but researchers hope it will be successful.[xxv] This option might be a great choice for you because informed conjecture suggests it will help reduce bone degeneration from both rheumatoid arthritis and osteoporosis!

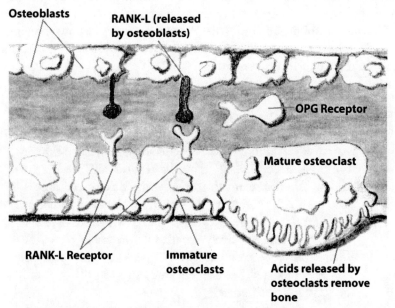

**Osteoblasts**

**RANK-L (released by osteoblasts)**

**OPG Receptor**

**Mature osteoclast**

**RANK-L Receptor**

**Immature osteoclasts**

**Acids released by osteoclasts remove bone**

"Finally, doctors in the United Kingdom use strontium as an alternative to bisphosphonates. This mineral gives a two-for-one punch. It increases bone formation and slows bone resorption. Bisphosphonates, SERMS, and hormone replacement therapy are only anti-resorptive. Studies show those taking strontium ranelate, a synthetic, therefore patentable, form of strontium, have significantly less fractures and better bone density.[xxvi xxvii xxviii] Other forms of strontium are likely as effective, though they may create more digestive problems like irritation or diarrhea. Of the non-patentable forms, strontium citrate is well absorbed, well tolerated, and available as a supplement in the U.S. Strontium accumulates especially in actively remodeling bone. Strontium ranelate can cause nausea and diarrhea, blood clots, fainting, seizures, and memory deficiencies.

"Strontium taken with calcium or other foods may impair strontium absorption. For this reason, take it on an empty stomach. Note that strontium is much denser than calcium, so bone mineral tests may give artificially high results.

## Boniva

"Now let's discuss Boniva, a bisphosphonate. Your concerns involve osteonecrosis of the jaw reported with bisphosphonate use. An anti-resorptive unit, or AR, is a unit devised to describe the potency of various bisphosphonates. The IV-administered bisphosphonates, which include Aredia, Bonefos and Zometa, used to treat bone cancers are rated at 80 to 100 AR/month.

### Risks for Jaw Osteonecrosis with Bisphosphonate Use

The first association between bisphosphonates and jaw osteonecrosis occurred only recently, around 2003, so much is still unknown. Risk seems to correlate with dosage and time.

- The high AR potency ratings of intravenous-administered bisphosphonates are most associated with risk. Even so, those risks are relatively small. Of the orally prescribed forms, only one case per 100,000 person-years' exposure* has been reported, but a recent study suggests the rate could be substantially higher.[xxxi]
- Consider the fact that over 22 million prescriptions were written for Fosamax in the U.S. in a recent year.[xxxii]
- Consider, too, that osteonecrosis cases are probably underreported. It is uncertain how many doctors realize they should report known cases to MedWatch.** (Call 1-800-FDA-1088.)

* The number of people taking a drug multiplied by the number of years each person has taken that drug equals the total person-years' exposure.

** FDA Safety Information and Adverse Event Reporting Program. Available at: http://www.fda.gov/medwatch/.

"Boniva is also in the bisphosphonate group, as are Actonel and Fosamax. These three are oral forms, usually prescribed for osteoporosis. Their potency is more like two to six AR/month, so they're considered much safer. Still, they bind directly to bone and so, because of bone's ten year turnover cycle, the decision to take this drug remains with a person for a long time. One must carefully weigh the benefits and risks. The National Osteoporosis Foundation says, "Based on current information, the benefits of oral bisphosphonate medications outweigh the risk of necrosis in most patients." Bisphosphonates do target many bone-wasting processes. In the first place, they reduce the release of many inflammatory messengers. They also reduce osteoclast formation, function, and cell life[xxix] as well as MMP levels.[xxx] That can be an effective combination.

"Bisphosphonates bind rapidly to bone, especially in areas of high bone turnover. The jawbone qualifies as an area with one of the fastest rates of bone turnover. This explains why osteonecrosis has only been noted in the jaw and why more bisphosphonate-bound bone is found there.

"An American Dental Association, or ADA, position paper suggests another reason the jaw is singled out for osteonecrosis. Do you remember past visits when I encouraged you to let us fabricate a splint for you to wear at night? I mentioned the surprising pressures chewing and clenching put on your teeth and supporting structures. Chewing can exert at least 68 pounds per square inch. Your teeth might withstand between 134 to 202 pounds per square inch of pressure while clenching, particularly at night. Bisphosphonates significantly repress bone remodeling. Can you imagine clenching your teeth for hours at a time with that kind of force? Do you think any micro-damage or micro-fractures might occur in your already osteoporotic jawbone? The American Dental Association suggests that bisphosphonate-bound bone is brittle and under supplied by blood vessels that keep normal bone alive and well nourished. Since this bone does not undergo normal robust remodeling, this micro-damage is left unrepaired and damage becomes cumulative. It could possibly set the stage for osteonecrosis.[xxxiii]

"If you consider trauma more serious than clenching forces, chances for complications expand. You already know the mouth can be one of the most infected places in the human body. What if you add further issues, such as a failed root canal, or a broken, infected, or submerged tooth sitting in a pool of anaerobic germs?

"Unfortunately, most osteonecrosis cases occur at tooth extraction sites.[6] Currently, there are no recommendations for special dental treatment of those who have taken oral bisphosphonates for less than three years or those about to begin oral drug forms. However, the FDA suggests appropriate preventive dentistry for those with other risk factors such as cancer, chemotherapy, corticosteroid use, or poor oral hygiene. A thorough oral consultation, a completed dental treatment plan, and release from a dentist are important steps to take prior to taking prescribed bisphosphonates with high ARs.

"I know you are health-conscious, so you may want to consider addressing some of these concerns before bisphosphonate therapy.

"I don't believe you need a clearer picture for why you should extract your wisdom teeth.

### General dental considerations prior to bisphosphonate use:

- Remove all questionable teeth after implementing good immune system support principals. Perhaps choose a biological dentist who will be certain all surrounding diseased soft tissue and bone is removed and who may choose to apply ozone gas to the socket to kill germs and stimulate healing.
- If you contemplate dental implants, results are better prior to bisphosphonate therapy, though bisphosphonate therapy does not preclude implants. A promising study unrelated to bisphosphonates shows treating an implant fixture with bone marrow-derived stem cells prior to implantation may lead to improved retention and function.[xxiv]
- Be certain partials fit well and do not pinch your gums.
- Complete all necessary gum surgery and other necessary therapies. Keep gums healthy!
- If you clench day or night, consider having your dentist fabricate a splint – and wear it as prescribed.

---

6 According to the National Osteonecrosis Foundation, "… the many risk factors for osteonecrosis can be divided into two categories: definite and probable. Definite risk factors include major trauma, fractures, dislocations, Caisson Disease, Sickle Cell Disease, post-irradiation, chemotherapy, Arterial Disease and Gaucher's Disease. Probable risk factors include corticosteroids, blood clotting, alcohol, lipid disturbances, connective tissue disease, pancreatitis, kidney disease, liver disease,

"It is also time to decide if or how you want to replace your missing tooth. A small partial is always an option, but mechanical trauma could be a problem if the fit isn't perfect or a clasp bends. We could always fabricate a bridge, but I know a bridge isn't your first preference.

"We've discussed implants, and osteoporosis doesn't make implants as impossible as you might think. Several studies show no increase in implant failure rates for people with osteoporosis compared to the general population. This is true even though implant fixtures don't integrate with bone as completely for those on bisphosphonates. The bone to implant contact is less, but it doesn't seem to affect longevity. Incidentally, a study showed decreased contact of implant to bone far more often when osteoporosis began after implant placement, rather than before.[xxxv] You may also want to consider that glucocorticoids are used to induce osteoporosis in study rats.

"We'll have to consult with your periodontist after he evaluates your jawbone. Long-term implant success is better judged by the bone density in your jaw as opposed to density measured far from your jawbone. It is possible he will also suggest removing those bony growths you have on the tongue side of your lower arch, your tori. These are frequent osteonecrosis sites.

"Regardless of whether you choose to have an implant, there is one more thing you should revisit. Any idea as to what I am referring?"

MOLLY: "As you talked about bone remodeling, I realized how important it is for my jaw to repair accumulating micro-fractures from clenching. I never thought of it that way before. I didn't want to "own" my nighttime clenching before, but I'm going to have to jump on this. I know what you are referring to and, yes, I'm ready. I want to make a splint now, whether I decide to take Boniva or not – whether I get the implant or not. When can we start?" (Caveat: Read Chapters 12-13)

CAROL: "Molly, that's you all over again. As with most of us, sometimes you're not ready to act on new research. But when you are, you're on it! Let us put together our team, formulate an optimal plan, and start moving."

---

lupus, and smoking. The FDA recognizes additional risk factors associated with the development of osteonecrosis (not limited to the jaw): cancer patients, female gender, advanced age, edentulous regions, combination cancer therapy, blood dyscrasias/ metastatic disease, anemia coagulopathy, surgical dental procedures, and prior infection." http://www.fda.gov/ohrms/dockets/ac/05/briefing/2005-4095B2_02_12-Novartis-Zometa-App-11.pdf

This information was the catalyst Molly needed to take care of her outstanding dental needs. An oral surgeon removed her half-buried wisdom tooth and a periodontist completed Molly's implant. Molly finally received her splint, which she wears nightly.

She wanted sufficient healing time between dental treatments and bisphosphonate therapy in case she chose that option. In the meantime, she started taking pharmaceutical-grade mineral and vitamin supplements[6] to build strong skeletal bone.

The supplements included calcium citrate, strontium citrate, essential fatty acids including omega-3 fatty acids, vitamins A, $B_6$, $B_{12}$ sublingual drops, $B_9$ (folic acid), and magnesium.[7] She also added vitamin $K_2$, which anchors calcium to bone's framework. It also directs calcium away from blood vessel walls where it contributes to atherosclerosis, and into skeletal bone. It is a fat soluble vitamin, so if you are on a low fat diet, you may not absorb it. Natto, a fermented soy product, is a superior choice for obtaining this vitamin. It is also an excellent source of gut probiotics. Choose a non-GMO, organic source.[8] Curd cheeses from pasture-raised animals are another good source.

---

6 Pharmaceutical grade supplements lab-certify that labels reflect listed ingredients, they are pure, and in a form easily absorbed by the human body.

7 Under appreciated and often processed right out of foods, magnesium is critical to bone maintenance. Magnesium depletion decreases bone-forming osteoblasts, increases bone-resorbing osteoclasts, and stimulates inflammatory activity in bone with loss of trabecular interior bone – that part that looks like foam. In pre-agrarian days when humans evolved, calcium to magnesium intake was about 1:1. Diets today usually reflect a skewed ratio. In dairy products it's about 12:1. As magnesium and calcium compete for absorption in the gut, modern diets are often deficient in magnesium. High sugar intake depletes magnesium for instance. With inadequate magnesium, absorption of vitamin D, calcium, and phosphorus is impaired. If you supplement with these vitamins, be sure you also supplement with magnesium.

8 Soy is a "scrubber" crop. When farmland has become saturated with pesticides and herbicides, farmers know that planting soy or rapeseed (aka canola oil) will clean the soil. These crops pull the toxins out. They sell the crop and voila! You acidify your body with toxins. Additionally, Round-up Ready GMO crops are sprayed with Round-up. The active ingredient, glyphosate, binds to minerals making them unavailable to the plants or the humans eating them. Do you see any in this list of minerals glyphosates chelate that would be good for bone strength? They are: iron, chromium, manganese, calcium, magnesium, zinc, copper, sulfur, and boron. It also looks as though glyphosates drive estrogen receptor mediated breast cancer cell proliferation within the infinitesimal parts per trillion concentration range. Combined with the naturally occurring phytoestrogens found in soy beans, it could contribute to breast cancers in postmenopausal women.

## Vitamin D as a Paradox

Current thought is that vitamin D is as critical to bone health as vitamin $K_2$ is. Vitamin D is actually not a vitamin at all, but a steroid hormone, influencing more than two thousand genes in the human body. Biologically active vitamin D is produced in the skin as a result of exposure to UV radiation, usually from daily sun exposure. Some people produce enough vitamin D because they spend adequate time outdoors. But roughly 85 percent of Americans may be vitamin D deficient, which means they absorb calcium poorly. Testing vitamin D levels may be important for everyone. Because it is stored in fat tissues, toxic doses can accumulate. Some dentists offer in-office or in-home vitamin D testing.[9] If you choose to supplement, the best-absorbed form of the vitamin is vitamin $D_3$. If sprayed or dropped under the tongue, it bypasses the digestive system and enters the bloodstream directly.

**The paradox:** It may be "optimal" vitamin D levels are really optimal only for healthy people. For those with autoimmune diseases, surfacing research muddies the conversation. Once again we see that very little in medicine leads to clear choices.

We have discussed how the human body hosts multiple microbe ecosystems – in the mouth, stomach, intestines, joints, blood vessel walls, amniotic fluid and brain (both thought once to be sterile), and many other locations. In fact, microbial cells outnumber human cells by a factor of ten. Taken together, they contain millions of genes compared to the 23,000 genes in the human genome. Microbial profiles in healthy people significantly differ from the microbial profiles of those with health issues. Obese people have germ populations that tend to create methane.[xxxvi] Diabetics have significantly different bacterial profiles than non-diabetics. One difference is they have far less of the class of microbes called Firmicutes and Clostridia than healthy people. [xxxvii] Not surprisingly, the same is proving true for those with irritable bowel syndrome, Crohn's disease, autism, rheumatoid arthritis, and many other autoimmune diseases.

As you know, bacteria are survivors. One of their survival tactics is to subvert vitamin D receptors. If vitamin D does influence two

---

9 One source for kits that independently monitor both Vitamin $D_2$ and $D_3$ is: Healthy Life Labs at: www.healthylifelabs.com. Currently there is no test for adequate $K_2$ levels.

thousand genes, yet can't because these bacteria have downregulated its receptor, it may prove to be one of the most clever evasion maneuvers yet discovered. Dr. Trevor Marshall's work with bacterial biofilms, and that of others, has shown just such vitamin D receptor (VDR) dysregulation. This also plays into cancer origination.

Vitamin D receptors themselves are important to health. They help make important antimicrobials and as Dr. Marshall interprets it, successive infections have the ability to continuously diminish the immune system. The process snowballs, shifting bacterial populations more and more to disease-causing species. In this way, inflammation continues uninterrupted as the immune system struggles to control them.

## Herkzheimer's Crisis

Those trying to regain health need to understand a very important idea. Once referred to as the "crisis" of an illness, after which people either get better or die, it occurs when the immune system is operating at peak efficiency. Disease-causing microbes die off in high numbers, but as they do they release massive amounts of bacterial toxins and other debris into the bloodstream. This is called the Herkzheimer response. The toxic load usually makes the host feel the sickest, even while it indicates their immune system is working its best. This is why many people don't take aspirin or other fever-reducers during an illness. They understand the immune system is using heat to kill off microbes. Our culture has a difficult time with the idea that periods of remission, when a person feels best, may equal times when the immune system is exhausted. Paradoxically, when the immune system gets a boost may be when these people feel worst. Any of us would surely die if their body's entire bacterial load along with their toxic end products were to die off and be released into the bloodstream at once.

Dr. Marshall's successes in treating victims of Lyme disease, sarcoidosis, rheumatoid arthritis, Hashimoto's Thyroiditis, IBS, and osteoarthritis, has piqued the interest of forward-thinking dental practitioners. These practitioners understand his protocol could be valuable in treating patients whose bodies may be riddled with any of the fifty-three known spirochetes that originate in the mouth.

Spirochetes have a large number of plasmids. Maybe half of a spirochetes' genes reside on these plasmids. These plasmids do not share genes sexually. They self-replicate and can share these genes between species. Since antibiotics do not target plasmids, it is important to activate the immune system, rather than dampen it. All too often, traditional modalities aim to suppress the immune system.

In brief, the Marshall Protocol involves:

1. *Removing* all supplemental sources of Vitamin D.
2. Activating the VDR with Olmesartan (licensed for sale as angiotensin receptor blocker, also VDR activation off label).
3. Administering specified types and subclinical doses of pulsed antibiotics for months or years. Subclinical doses are doses too small to function at the levels of an antibiotic. They function by inhibiting bacterial ribosomes and do not cause common side effects or antibiotic resistance.

## More Strategies for Combating Osteoporosis

Molly also alkalized her diet by adding foods rich in minerals known to alkalize the body. She takes a tablespoon of raw apple cider vinegar before or with meals and eats far more vegetables – especially leafy green vegetables – and fruits. She uses what she learned about how certain antioxidants trigger osteoblast bone-building activity and that the polyphenols found in foods like olives and citrus fruits supercharge bone building. She also substituted water for sodas and coffee.

She stopped jogging and started rebounding on a trampoline and now lifts weights four times a week to relieve stress and give her bones and muscles the mechanical work they require to retain strength and flexibility. She is still considering her options for pharmaceutical intervention to control her osteoporosis.

She recently asked if osteoporosis was likely to weaken the bone around her teeth. She wanted to know if her gum disease would advance if she didn't treat her osteoporosis.

## The Association Between Osteoporosis and Periodontal Disease

CAROL: "As with so many other diseases, bone loss is a two-way street. Osteoporosis definitely does not spare oral bone. The Woman's Health

Initiative showed tripled bone height loss around teeth in women diagnosed with osteoporosis, regardless of gum disease status.

"And yes, the converse is true. Remember when I told you the encouraging news about OPG trials?  All those inflammatory messengers[10] released in gum disease also increase RANK-L production, so as gum disease recruits more and more osteoclasts throughout the body, bone destruction outweighs rebuilding. Good gum health definitely correlates with increased bone mass."

I reminded her to be hyper aware of her oral conditions if she ever decided to choose bisphosphonate intervention and to notify us of any oral changes. I emphasize a three-month wellness schedule for all clients taking bisphosphonates. This allows for close monitoring and infection control. If problems do develop, we can implement an early intervention strategy and ozone therapy.

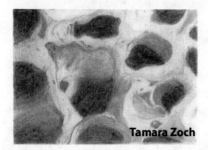 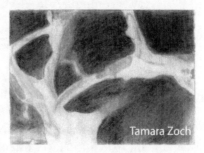

**Healthy bone**          versus          **Osteoporosis**

---

10 Prostaglandins, cytokines, TNF-alpha

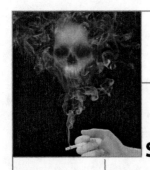

# 8

## SMOKING INFLUENCES

*"I kissed my first girl and smoked my first cigarette on the same day.
I haven't had time for tobacco since."*

~ **Arturo Toscanini** ~

**Explore:**
1. Background for the under-thirty crowd.
2. How does smoking change oral pocket tissue to create specific risks for gum disease?
3. How do these changes obstruct healing?
4. How does smoking mask clues to gum disease?
5. How much healing can smokers and non-smokers expect? Do expectations differ?

Three decades ago, the scientific literature barely recognized tobacco's strong negative influence on gum disease. However, in my first fledgling specialty practice geared to treat gum disease, it was clear heavy smoking prevented healing after surgery. Our most important goal – making the oral pocket shallow enough to be cleaned at home – often failed. Smokers' positive results were usually short-lived. We conjectured smoking contributed to the disease, since the percentage of smokers in our practice was far higher than numbers in general dental practices.

We puzzled over our smoking clients' poor healing responses. The most notable differences we found between smokers and non-smokers were the scar-like fibrousness of smokers' gums and lack of typical disease symptoms despite their advanced bone loss. Smokers rarely exhibited swelling, redness, or easy bleeding.

How far we've come! In 1988, I attended a ground breaking seminar whose goal was to teach dental professionals improved gum disease diagnosis and treatment. Equally important, we learned new insurance codes for "innovative" gum disease treatments. But these non-surgical, first-line procedures were not new. What was new was that insurance companies finally recognized treating gum disease required more time and advanced skills than those required for brief, healthy mouth preventive appointments. They knew it was time to compensate for the additional expertise and time required to treat gum disease.

Financial realities prompt most of us to allow insurance companies to dictate which health needs we treat, and how. Before the mid-1980s, insurance benefits covered either healthy mouth preventive "cleanings" or surgery for advanced disease. Obviously most clients' conditions lie somewhere between these two extremes. Many people initially need multiple non-surgical visits and more intense management than those with no disease.

I was dismayed the lecturer did not address the subject of smoking and its relation to gum disease, so I quizzed him before a break. Uncomfortably, he suggested there were no clear scientific links between smoking and gum disease. Surprised, I watched him dash off – and light up. Ah denial, easy for all of us.

### Research clarifies smoking's influence on gum disease

- More than half of all gum disease is directly attributed to smoking.[i]
- Smokers are three times more likely to develop gum disease than nonsmokers.[ii]
- The odds of developing gum disease increase with the number of cigarettes smoked per day.[iii]
- Even with regular professional dental care and good daily oral home care, smokers have comparatively more frequent and severe periodontal destruction than non-smokers.[iv]
- Gum surgery patients who smoke are twice as likely to lose teeth in the first five years after surgery as non-smokers.[v]

These risks are reversible if a person quits smoking. There is a direct correlation between risk and number of years since quitting. Oral health differences between former smokers and non-smokers seem to disappear at around eleven years.[vi]

## JACK

Jack and I traveled a long and difficult road together. An attractive and gregarious man, he first sought treatment in our office about seven years ago. I could never remember what he did for a day job because his sideline as a popular musician was more memorable. As is often the case with musicians, alcohol and smoking accompanied Jack's lifestyle. Did health care concerns cross his mind? Not so much. In fact, personal and professional dental care was not on his radar for many years. I presumed he knew he had a winning smile – and no clue about the complicated road ahead of us.

## Major Complaint: Aesthetics

Jack scheduled a dental appointment because he was concerned about a drifting front tooth. He wondered if he should consider braces to improve his smile.

According to his health history, Jack started smoking two packs of cigarettes a day when he was 18 – 23 years prior to our first visit. He had not seen a dentist in about eight years. During the oral cancer exam, I noticed Jack's gums had receded and exposed tooth roots in many areas. When I picked up my measuring probe to evaluate gum disease, I crossed my fingers and hoped I would not find the degree of destruction typical for a smoker.

Unfortunately, Jack was typical. Many areas showed he had lost from half to nearly three-fourths of the bone and soft gum tissue that supported his teeth. After learning the implications of his gum disease, Jack was aghast. He knew he had smoke stains on his teeth but really had not noticed other visible deposits. He experienced no pain, no bleeding, and no loose teeth. How could this be? Why had he not noticed?

## Smoking Masks Clues

CAROL: "Jack, it's sad, but your heavy, long-term smoking is largely to blame for both your disease and your lack of symptoms. Smoking is the single most important risk factor for developing gum disease. I'm sorry no one knew that back when you started.

"I realize this diagnosis is a shock. Your tissues dramatically changed because they were exposed for years to the heat and chemicals of the cigarettes you smoke. For most people, bleeding is typically the first worrisome symptom of gum disease. It encourages them to seek professional help. But there is a strong dose-dependent relationship between smoking and its suppressive effect on bleeding.[vii] Smoking cuts the blood supply to your gums by about a third. Therefore, the effects of smoking masked your disease.

"The same is true about why your gums didn't swell. Your gums mimic a scar's fibrousness. Once you know the middle of a lit cigarette tip burns at almost 1300° Fahrenheit (700° C), it suddenly makes sense hot smoke would cause thermal damage to oral tissue. The same tissue is also negatively affected by the chemical additives and nicotine in cigarettes.

"It is tragic the signs and symptoms of gum disease are painless and unremarkable until the disease reaches its end stages. This holds especially true for smokers. Jack, even experts often guess smokers have excellent gum health at first glance. While evaluating tissue health, I also catalogue color, tissue tone, and swelling. I've learned appearances can be deceptive, especially in smokers, so I withhold comment until I've gathered all the data.

"Occasionally, a smoker who has developed the characteristic thick, fibrous tissue that looks pink and doesn't bleed has not yet experienced jawbone degradation. In these cases, I still find dense, crusty deposits under the gums. Only upon removing these deposits does the tissue slightly ooze. This reminds me of how little blood actually nurtures that tissue – how stagnant the wound area must be. It reminds me humans respond differently to similar circumstances. Host response, lifestyle, genetics, and immune system strength all play variable roles.

"You are apparently susceptible to gum disease. Given your particular set of genes, you have all the wrong risk factors.[viii] It's not fair, but it's what we have to work with."

Jack was visibly shaken, but exceptionally curious. Most smokers are defensive and, understandably, do not want to be told any more about the negative impacts of smoking. They already face incredible social pressure and most have tried to quit. At least 70 percent of people who smoke wish they didn't. But it is such a strong addiction that quitting is a high hurdle.

JACK: "How, other than heat, has smoking changed my mouth?"

CAROL: "I'll share what I know. Some of it is technical, but I will do my best to relate current information in understandable terms." I began by reviewing the fundamentals of wound management and inflammation theory before specifying risks particular to smokers.

## Fibroblasts: A Velcro Zipper

CAROL: "First of all, Jack, let's explore our treatment goals. Initial therapy cannot restore the lost bone around your roots, but together we can explore non-surgical ways to achieve a certain level of health. The British imaginatively call the first stage of therapy a 'detox.' Your detox will consist of several treatment sessions devoted to removing the mineralized deposits cemented to your roots. This will disrupt the biofilm. Under the right circumstances, the gums will shrink and the tissue lining will reattach to the teeth. Because it will not be supported by new bone, this attachment will be fragile. Depending on nutrition, stress, and self-care, among other things, the tissue lining could possibly detach from the teeth. If we make the pocket shallow enough to permit careful daily cleansing, though, we can possibly control the disease.

"The best way I can describe this reattachment is to have you think of the pocket lining as Velcro. This lining actually has countless little fibroblast cells that can decrease the depth of the crevice by zipping themselves onto the tooth like Velcro. This kind of reattachment is not perfect because it relies on many things.

- First, it takes at least three to six months for gums to hook onto teeth. Home care must be meticulous during the attachment phase. Then it has to be meticulous to stay attached.
- Second, it relies on a strong immune system. When we are young, we think we are bulletproof. We generally do not think about behaviors that weaken our immune system and contribute to disease. You should evaluate life stressors and your style of stress management, reevaluate your nutrition philosophy, and make sure you are getting adequate sleep and exercise.

- Third, we are talking about a fragile attachment. Gums easily detach when the immune system is challenged, general health slides, or bacteria are allowed to re-colonize the pocket. To be realistic, Jack, detachment is bound to happen occasionally while you try to redefine your lifestyle. It takes time for healthy practices to become habits. Don't be overwhelmed by your need for immediate perfection. Approach it in steps and remember: every detox presents you with a new opportunity to heal.

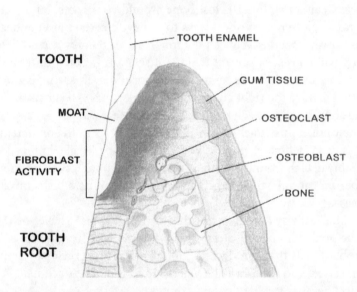

**Fibroblasts from infected tissue next to the root need to attach to the root. If wound depth can be reduced to 3mm or less, and the client keeps it properly cleaned, anaerobic germ populations may not repopulate the area.**

## Smokers Face Extraordinary Healing Challenges

"I realize this is a formidable list. Regretfully, I must add a further challenge smokers face during the healing process. The real deal killer for smokers is that nicotine is actually stored in and released from fibroblasts.[ix] Further, nicotine inhibits production of several substances (fibronectin and collagen) that are critical to the zipping that takes place during reattachment. Smoking also increases collagenase production.[x] You may remember collagenase is the enzyme that helps destroy the gums and bone around your teeth in the first place. Last, smoking challenges your immune system with an incredible load of free radicals. Regardless of the mechanism, nicotine significantly and irrefutably inhibits the attachment and growth of the fibers you need.[xi]

"I suppose you know where this is headed. If you want to keep your teeth, smoking is your biggest obstacle. At this point, you want to do everything you can to support your immune system, and smoking is a major challenge to it. I'm sure this is discouraging. It is a steep path. No one reinvents himself overnight. We are here to coach and to help you. Every time you have a preventive dental visit, the balance of bacteria shifts in your mouth. Every detox provides a new chance to take another healing step.

"You asked if smoking did anything besides mask the symptoms of gum disease. It does. In fact, smokers suffer more gum disease than non-smokers and tend to not heal as well after treatment as non-smokers. Extensive data explains why both cases are true.

## Heat and Chemical Reactions and the Immune System

"Because you smoke, blood flow to your gums is sluggish. This means your gums receive less oxygen and other nutrients necessary to maintain good health. Because they aren't carried away from the wound, powerful endotoxins from bacteria build up. This and a dry mouth is why a smoker's bacterial load is heavier than a nonsmoker's bacterial load. Because you smoke, your immune system is already depressed by the free radicals you generate. All these factors produce high levels of inflammatory messengers in your body, which further increase destruction. Cadmium in tobacco may also contribute.[xii] To make matters worse, your pocket tissue has difficulty healing because your tissues don't reattach. Finally, you are less able to rebuild a healthy blood supply to the area after treatment because you smoke. That's the quick version. Does all this make more sense now?"

JACK: "I never knew smoking had so many far-reaching effects. The connection between smoking and heart health is also much clearer now. I knew how smoking related to cancer and lung health, but this is unbelievable! I never would have thought I could lose my teeth over this. I just wanted them straight, like they used to be. I guess we'll have to see how things settle out later, huh?"

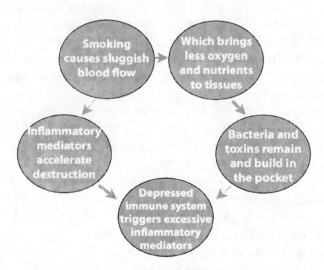

### Smokers face almost inevitable destruction

- Constant heat diminishes oral blood supply. Without adequate blood supply, the tissue is robbed of proper nutrients and oxygen.
- Chemicals in tobacco smoke slow healing. They depress many of the body's defense mechanisms that fight bacterial infections.[xiii]
- Because their immune systems are less efficient, smokers have double or triple the odds of hosting three of the anaerobic germs commonly found in deep pockets compared to former smokers or non-smokers.
- The circulation of inflammation messengers increases because extra germs near the wound area cause inflammation.[xiv xv xvi xvii xviii xix] The increased prevalence of inflammatory messengers in the body is mirrored in the oral pocket tissue site. How long and how much a person smokes is an excellent predictor of inflammatory mediator levels.
- The infection rate is related to heat and chemical dose. More cigarettes correlate to increased disease.[xx]
- Smoking releases enormous numbers of free radicals into the bloodstream. This puts an additional burden on the immune system.

CAROL: "Yes. It will be a journey and we will be partners in your health. Most people cannot remake their lifestyles overnight. Take it in steps. As your health improves, each step encourages the next one. We are your coaches and will provide therapy, guidance, and support. Remember, every appointment offers you a new opportunity to change some habit and make a difference."

It is common for clients to want to avoid surgery. They often opt to try to control disease without it. Still, they are advised at the outset that specialists might need to be called in to assist.

In an attempt to improve healing, some dental offices prescribe adjunctive therapies designed to boost the immune system prior to non-surgical therapy. Scaling imposes a heavy bacterial load on the circulatory system; boosting the immune system helps the body handle that load.

Taking pharmaceutical-grade supplements is another helpful therapy. Many product lines provide immune system support. One company that markets products specifically for gum disease care is Pharmaden Nutraceuticals. To view a bibliography of studies and a nutritional summary go to: http://www.pharmaden.net/research-resources/periodontal-nutritional-summary-and-bibliography.html. Also visit Appendices IX and X in this book.

Another proven adjunctive therapy involves taking subclinical doses of doxycyclines as mentioned in the last chapter (LDD therapy/Periostat). Taken in doses too small to function as antibiotics, the doxycyclines inhibit important mediators from creating destruction in gum pockets. They also tip the balance of bone remodeling towards building rather than destruction, important throughout the body. At these subclinical doses, doxycycline has not been found to interfere with the effectiveness of birth control pills and does not cause the common doxycycline side effect of photosensitivity.

Some doctors prescribe non-steroidal anti-inflammatories (NSAIDs). Because a number of negative side effects have been linked to NSAID therapy, other doctors use a more targeted approach to dampen inflammation: synthetic lipoxins, protectins, or resolvins. These omega-3 fat-based mediators strongly modulate the duration and magnitude of inflammation. In fact, one of the negative side effects of some NSAIDs (like COX-2 inhibitors) is that, though they curtail the mediators that accelerate inflammation, they also curtail the production of lipoxin, protectin, and resolvin compounds that turn off the response. Thus, paradoxically, they prolong the inflammation they are prescribed to inhibit. Aspirin seems to be the one NSAID that both curtails inflammation and stimulates inflammation-resolving lipoxins. Long-term use has disadvantages such as stomach bleeding, ulcers in the digestive tract, and ear ringing.

The natural building blocks for resolvins and protectins are the omega-3 essential fatty acids called EPA and DHA, so eating foods high in omega-3 fatty acids or supplementation is best.

## MPO Marker

Some doctors measure myeloperoxidase (MPO) levels. Myeloperoxidases (MPOs) are released during inflammation and may irreversibly modify proteins and fats. MPOs promote high levels of oxidized LDLs, thus atherosclerosis. Smokers with gum disease have significantly elevated MPO markers – in other words, smoking shifts their immune response. Recent studies suggest MPOs may both help develop atherosclerotic lesions and keep them unstable. [xxi xxii]

## It is Always a Journey

Jack began his journey to better health. We detoxed his teeth and referred him to a gum surgeon. As with most journeys, it has taken years to work through various steps. These steps usually mirror the maturation of the person who commits to taking them. Although Jack knew smoking was the most detrimental factor to his healing response, it was the last factor he addressed. Change requires self-respect, courage, and power.

At first, Jack was happy to "let the professionals do it." He opted for surgery after initial therapy and scheduled maintenance visits with me at three-month intervals. At each visit, we measured his progress and offered him a renewed chance to improve. He made huge progress in caring for his mouth at home. He began to realize if he did not take better care of himself, he could not take care of those he loved.

While Jack still enjoys music, he no longer plays professionally. This has positively affected his sleep schedule and stress levels. He prepares most meals at home and focuses on healthy nutrition. He understands "food is medicine" and rarely eats processed foods. He is comfortable and secure at his job. Several years ago, he and his wife started running three miles a day. The running helped him finally eliminate cigarettes.

In the beginning, his endurance suffered. He made a pact with himself to run one mile for every cigarette smoked. Between the pact and his feelings of responsibility for his newly adopted child, he was sufficiently motivated to change.

After seeing his mouth via the intraoral camera, Jack made serious adjustments to his daily oral care routine. He now has a sparkling smile. While his smile is flashy, he knows its foundation is weak. He realizes braces are not the answer to his oral health issues. The front tooth that motivated him to come see us in the first place is still splayed. Jack thinks he would eventually like an implant, but he is not ready. He has become comfortable enough with himself to realize he is loved for who he is.

## RONNIE

I want to share part of Ronnie's story since I appreciated how he responded to his periodontal condition and its ties to his smoking habit. It shows one never knows what the motivation to quit will be.

When I broke the news about his condition, he said, "I always knew lung cancer was a risk and I really never cared. I've always been comfortable with the risk. But this! That I might lose my teeth surprises me. This might just be the straw that breaks the camel's back. I had no idea I could lose my teeth because I smoke. I've been thinking about quitting anyway. You see, I have two sweet Weimaraner dogs and they're very susceptible to asthma. I was holding one of my "little girls" on my chest the other day and heard and felt her wheezing against me. I just can't rationalize smoking around her anymore. I guess I need to figure out how to quit."[1]

Note: News from MSNBC February 24, 2011: "The U.S. Justice Department wants big cigarette manufacturers to admit they lied about the dangers of smoking. This would force the industry to set up and pay for an advertising campaign apologizing for their past behavior, or face charges for contempt of court.

The move comes as part of a 12-year-old lawsuit against the tobacco industry. The government released 14 "corrective statements." At the time of the printing of this second edition, it appears we will be seeing

---

1 See appendix I for Quitline support information.

stark images on cigarette packages and maybe other places, along with statements such as:

- "A federal court is requiring tobacco companies to tell the truth about cigarette smoking. Here's the truth: Smoking kills 1,200 Americans. Every day."
- "We falsely marketed low tar and light cigarettes as less harmful than regular cigarettes to keep people smoking and sustain our profits. Here's the truth: We control nicotine delivery to create and sustain smokers' addiction, because that's how we keep customers coming back."
- "We told Congress under oath we believed nicotine is not addictive. We told you smoking is not an addiction and all it takes to quit is willpower. Here's the truth: Smoking is very addictive. And it's not easy to quit."
- "Just because lights and low tar cigarettes feel smoother, that doesn't mean they are any better for you. Light cigarettes can deliver the same amounts of tar and nicotine as regular cigarettes."
- "The surgeon general has concluded" that "children exposed to secondhand smoke are at an increased risk for sudden infant death syndrome, acute respiratory infections, ear problems and more severe asthma."

The FDA won the authority to regulate tobacco in June 2009. The law does not let the FDA ban nicotine or tobacco, just regulate what goes into tobacco products, require the ingredients be publicized, and limit how tobacco is marketed, especially to young people.

**Smokers are the ultimate mouth-breathers.**
**See Chapter Twelve!**

# ORAL CANCER

*"Growth for the sake of growth is the ideology of the cancer cell."*

~ Edward Abbey ~

**Explore:**
1. How common is oral cancer?
2. Why is early oral cancer diagnosis critical?
3. Smoking, alcohol, and... What's sex got to do with it?
4. Does smokeless tobacco really contain a radioactive ingredient?
5. What other factors increase oral cancer susceptibility?
6. Nutrition allies.
7. New diagnostic tests.
8. Signs and symptoms to watch for.

## Oral Cancer? Who, Me?

Oral cancer has the highest fatality rate of all cancers among Americans. Yet despite its frequency, it never occurs to most people that oral cancers *exist*. According to a 2007 article by Donna Mager, Robert Haddad, Lori Wirth, and Anne Haffajee, "Each year, nearly 30,000 Americans are diagnosed with oral cancer, and 90 percent of these lesions are oral squamous cell carcinoma (OSCC). Despite advances in surgery, radiation and chemotherapy, the five-year survival rate is 54 percent, one of the lowest of the major cancer sites, and this rate has not improved significantly in recent decades."[i] There are two major reasons for the low survival rate:

- Oral cancer is routinely discovered late in its development. At best, treatment outcomes are terribly disfiguring. At worst, treatment is unsuccessful.
- Those oral cancer patients who do survive have 20 times the risk of developing a second cancer five to ten years after their first diagnosis. The same factors causing the first cancer have usually caused considerable harm to oral tissues in general, so they are more susceptible to cancers. Often, contributory habits have not been modified.

As cells copy themselves, mistakes, called mutations, often occur. Cellular mutations are common in everyone, but many biological mechanisms cope with these mistakes. Malignancies arise when roughly six to ten genetic mutations have occurred and cellular death has not ended their mutations. The faster cells regenerate, the higher their chances for "copy" errors. This is why cancers appear more readily in tissues with rapid cell turnover. Oral cells turnover rapidly.

As malignant tumors form, faulty cells multiply out of control. They use available nutrients, especially blood sugars, to feed the tumor to the exclusion of healthy cells. These tumors can invade and damage nearby tissues and organs. Cancer cells can also break away from the original mass and enter the bloodstream or lymph system to begin a secondary tumor elsewhere in the body.

## Origins of Cellular Mutation

Epigenetics is the study of how the environment shapes specific gene expression. The epigenetics of oral cancer is fascinating. Nutrition profoundly influences gene expression and these traits are passed on to subsequent cell generations. When these changes affect cell growth or differentiation, cancer can result. Repetitive chemical exposure, oxidation from smoking, exposure to frequent high heat or UV sources, and copy errors due to rapid multiplication are other environmental factors that impact cellular mutation.

Adult stem cells are present in many tissues, including blood, bone marrow, tooth pulps, muscles, retinas, and brain tissue. These tissue-specific immature cells can differentiate into many kinds of cells. Stem cells gather and multiply at damaged sites in order to repair them. As an example, scientists hope that eventually, the extremely plastic stem cells – those cells easily manipulated to grow into different cell types

– saved from pulps of "baby" teeth will be able to regenerate motor nerves lost due to stroke, injury,[ii] or Parkinson's disease. Dental stem cells also hold promise for damaged blood vessel regeneration,[iii] giving those with heart disease another chance to modify their lifestyles. Recovering and banking stem cells from baby and extracted teeth, especially those of young adults (most commonly the "wisdom teeth"), may be an excellent strategy for protecting the future needs of an individual as they age or as health fails and science advances. (See: www.ndpl.net/)

Chronic irritation requires constant stem cell-driven repair. The resulting rapid reproduction of stem cells increases chances of stem cell mutations. Many researchers suggest this can translate into cancerous tumors. Could chronic inflammation be another driver? Dr. F. Marinacola, Chief Infectious Disease and Immunogenetics Section at the Clinical Center, of the National Institute of Health, has said, "Everybody knows inflammation induces cancer." This startling statement refers to the fact that microorganisms have evolved to persist inside cells by knocking out a particular receptor, the VDR nuclear receptor. This is the Vitamin D receptor introduced in Chapter Seven. In this way, microorganisms interfere with how genes are copied as new cells are made, again, leading to copy errors.

**Oral cancer statistics:**

In the U.S., 34,360 new oral/pharyngeal cancers are diagnosed and 7,500 deaths occur annually. That is almost 24 deaths every 24 hours.

- Ninety percent of those diagnosed with oral cancer are tobacco users.
- Ninety percent of oral cancers are squamous cell carcinomas.
- Most people are diagnosed over the age of 45. The exceptions are smokeless tobacco users and those with the human papilloma virus in the oropharynx. These patients are considerably younger.
- In 1950 the male/female risk ratio was six to one. Women have almost caught up. In 2002 the ratio was two to one.[v] Other than that there has been little change in early detection of oral cancer or in 5-year survival rates.
- Survival rates among races are unequal. The five-year survival rate for whites is 56 percent, while the five-year survival rate is 34 percent for African-Americans.

Dentists have long recited the follow oral cancer mantra: If it is detected early (Stage I), there is a 77 percent survival rate. If it is detected late (Stage IV) – as most are – survival chances flip; there is a 20 percent survival rate.[1] This is often due to metastasis into the lymph nodes of the neck or invasion of deeper tissue structures.[iv] Survivors suffer dreadful impairment. Worse yet, roughly 30 percent of those who do survive will develop a new primary tumor within ten years.

## Primary Cause: Tobacco

Oral cells exposed to the heat caused by smoking and the chemicals in both tobacco products and alcohol have a high chance of replication errors. Combined use causes about eighty percent of oral cancer in the United States. Together, both habits exponentially increase individual risks. A 35-fold increase was found among those who smoked two or more packs of cigarettes daily and consumed more than four alcoholic drinks/day.[vi] Milder habits divide that risk in half. These numbers reflect the dose dependence consistently noted between the two habits and cancer. Poor nutrition adds further synergy.[vii] Since alcohol and smoking risks are dose dependent, risks reduce as dose reduces.[viii ix]

Alcohol per se is not the culprit for higher oral cancer risks, but acetaldehyde is. Acetaldehyde is alcohol's first breakdown product and the toxic and carcinogenic chemical responsible for hangovers. Numerous and varied additives added to alcoholic beverages by manufacturers are also implicated. These additives are absent from most labels.[2]

Those who drink six or more whiskey equivalents a day are at greater risk for cancer than two-pack-a-day smokers. This is due to systemic and local effects of alcoholic beverages. Systemically, drinking alcohol causes nutritional deficiencies and decreases the liver's ability to detoxify cancer-causing agents. Alcoholic beverages are known to

---

1 Oral cancer stages are classified I-IV. The 20 percent survival rate reflects a Class III oral cancer. The average five-year survival rate for all four classes is 59 percent.
2 Many also point to the mycotoxins molds and fungi use to inhibit or prevent the growth of other organisms. Mycotoxin exposures in small amounts over long periods of time are implicated in health problems across the spectrum and include cancer, heart disease, asthma, multiple sclerosis and diabetes. Alcohol is the mycotoxin of brewer's yeast. Other mycotoxins are introduced into these beverages through the use of mold-contaminated grains and fruits. Some suggest producers often use grains too contaminated with mycotoxins and fungi to be used for table foods.

have many contaminants. Locally ethanol has a solvent action on the gums: it alters the metabolism of the protective shield.

**Relative smoking and drinking risks:**

Minimum smoking and minimum drinking = risk factor of 1
Heavy smoking and minimum drinking = risk factor of 8
Minimum smoking and heavy drinking = risk factor of 23
Heavy drinking and heavy smoking = risk factor of 100

Smokeless tobacco, used regularly by six percent of all U.S. adult males and some females, is not as risk-free as the industry would have young people believe. There are at least 28 known carcinogens in smokeless tobacco, including nitrosamines. Nitrosamine levels are regulated in bacon and other processed meats because of their carcinogenic potential. In smokeless tobacco, they are present at many times the levels allowed in meat and beer. Nitrosamines are formed in the growing, curing, fermenting, and aging of tobacco. A few other carcinogens present in the leaves and absorbed by humans are formaldehyde, arsenic, nickel, cadmium, benzopyrene, acetaldehyde, and polonium-210.

This is a largely self-explanatory list of toxins, but many people are particularly curious about polonium 210. This carcinogen is the highly volatile, radioactive, uranium-derived metal responsible for killing Russian ex-spy, Alexander Litvinenko, in 2006. For the high-energy alpha particles to cause damage, polonium has to be ingested or inhaled. Could this be problematic for smokeless tobacco users? Because the penetrating particles are of such short range, only nearby tissues are harmed by polonium 210. This would mean only the oral tissues and cells in contact with saliva as it is swallowed are at risk for mutation. How, you might ask, do these products remain legal?

Smokeless tobacco users absorb three to four times the amount of nicotine as cigarette smokers. The chemical also stays in the bloodstream longer.[x]

That smokeless tobacco users are hit with cancer at younger ages than cigarette smokers is hardly a surprise. Although associated lung cancer rates do not equal smoker's risks, oral and pancreatic cancer rates are higher, as are gum disease rates for those who use smokeless tobacco. Further, gum recession around teeth is likely. Scientists continue to study smokeless tobacco use and its association with health problems like diabetes, heart disease, and reproductive problems.

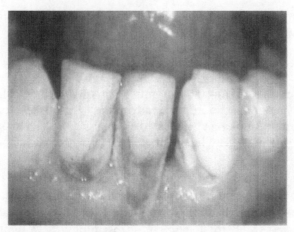

**This person has long since given up smokeless tobacco but still lives with the root exposure (gum recession) it caused.**

## Other Oral Cancer Risks:

- **Viruses**. For years, many have thought viruses played a role in oral cancers. In 2007, a new report implicated the Human Papilloma Virus (HPV). HPV 16 and 18 are sexually transmitted viruses and represent two of the four viruses of their kind against which the controversial vaccine Gardasil is said to protect.[3] HPV 16 and 18 cause about 70 percent of cervical cancers. HPV viruses may now account for about half of all oral cancers.

    One percent of the 40 million Americans who have HPV are infected with the HPV-16 strain implicated in cervical, vulval, vaginal, anal, penile and oral cancers. The rates of oral cancer from HPV-16 increase in a line consistent with numbers of lifetime vaginal sex partners and oral sex partners. An 8.6 times risk was associated with a lifetime history of more than 26 vaginal sex partners or more than six lifetime oral sex partners.[xi] Some suggest other viruses such as Epstein-Barr and the Herpes Simplex viruses may also play a role in oral cancers.

---

3 *The New England Journal of Medicine* (Human Papillomavirus Vaccination – "Reasons for Caution." 2008; Aug 21;359(8):861-862.http://content.nejm.org/cgi/content/full/359/8/861) points out we are far from knowing what real impact this vaccine may have on cancers, how long protection lasts, and how it will affect natural HPV immunity since most cases of HPV are cleared by the immune system anyway. It is far from being the "safe sex" vaccination many young girls commonly refer to it as, and is not without serious side effects.

- **Obesity.** Obesity increases the risk for many kinds of cancers, such as those of the colon and rectum, breast, uterine lining (endometrium), and kidneys. Obesity also raises rates of esophageal cancer. There is an increased opportunity for DNA replication errors because an overweight person's cells metabolically divide faster.
- **UV Exposure.** Lip cancer is considered an oral cancer and one most people do not consider. Those most at risk are, of course, alcohol and tobacco users; those accustomed to leaving a lit cigar or cigarette on the lip have the highest risk. But early and cumulative sun exposures have additive effects. Those with light-colored eyes seem to have skin more susceptible to damage. It is equally important to shade our lips, eyes, and the rest of our skin from sun damage.[xii] The incidence of lip cancer increases by a factor of ten for every ten degrees closer to the equator a person lives.
- **Heat.** Frequently consuming very hot drinks and foods probably increases the risk for cancers of the oral cavity, pharynx, and esophagus.[xiii xiv] Recently, the inhabitants of Iran's Golestan province were studied because confounding risk factors for esophageal cancer such as smoking tobacco and drinking alcohol, are uncommon habits here, yet this population suffers an unusually high occurrence of esophageal cancer. In Iran, the drink of choice is tea served at a temperature of 140° F or higher. In this study, esophageal cancer was eight times as common among people who drank tea hotter than 149° F, compared to those who drank tea between 140-147° F. Those that drank tea at between 140-147° F had two times the chance of esophageal cancer as those who drank it at 140° F or less. The researchers believe the high esophageal cancer rates could be related to chronic inflammation from constant esophageal burning.[xv]
- **High alcohol mouthwashes.** Some implicate high alcohol mouth rinses as carcinogens. Many scientists no longer think alcohol is the agent. Studies are equivocal. Product additives may well be the culprits. Most commercial mouthwashes and toothpastes are acidic, a negative.

Note: Particularly people with tooth-colored resin fillings,[4] dry mouths induced by pharmaceutical or other drugs, inadequate water intake, or those with oral cancer should abstain from alcohol mouthwashes. Tissues of those with oral cancer are extremely fragile; alcohol's drying effects exacerbate their vulnerability.

---

4 Alcohol etches these resin "aesthetic" white filling materials.

Some doctors prescribe a chlorhexidine rinse for temporary oral bacterial control. They contain less alcohol, but people find the taste alteration and staining they cause unacceptable. Worse, chlorhexidine rinses and Listerine interfere with fibrobasts, the mechanism by which the gums reattach to tooth roots.[xvi xvii xviii] Also, Peridex and Colgate's Periogard both have 11.6 percent alcohol. Closys® may be a better choice. It is alcohol free, has about the same bacterial "kill rate", and does not interfere with the fibroblasts that heal. It is also over-the-counter instead of a prescription.

**Note:** Those undergoing cancer treatments often suffer candida yeast overgrowth in their mouths and intestines. Most mouthwashes on the market remove natural bacterial competitors of candida yeasts, so this fungus can thrive. Worse, mercury vapors from silver-colored fillings naturally migrate to yeast cell walls. Yeasts bind roughly their own weight in mercury.[xix] Biological dentists often suggest careful filling replacement, followed by heavy metal chelation, then anti-fungal and immune system support therapies with continued chelation as dying yeasts give up bound mercury. Many people substitute essential oil mixtures such as Thieves, containing clove and cinnamon oil to freshen breath, rebalance germ populations, and create an unfriendly environment for others by changing pH balance. Some essential oils also build collagen.

- **Periodontal disease.** As with infection links in other cancers,[5] people with serious gum disease have double the risk of a pre-cancerous lesion and four times the risk of an oral tumor of any kind compared to those without serious gum disease. There is a 5.23-fold increase in the risk of tongue cancer with each millimeter of bone loss. Periodontal viruses and bacteria are toxic to surrounding cells and produce changes that lead directly to oral cancer or could indirectly contribute to cancer via inflammation.[xx] Oral bacteria normally produce the carcinogen acetaldehyde, but the bacteria of heavy smokers and drinkers produce far more of it.

  Another study found that men who had gum disease had 14 percent higher cancer risk overall compared to those who did not. Risks varied, depending on types of cancer. Dr. Dominique Michaud of the Imperial College of London and colleagues wrote in the journal Lancet Oncology, "After controlling for smoking and

---

5 Examples of cancer associations with specific bacteria: H. pylori and stomach cancers, human papillomavirus and cervical and oral cancer, cytomegalovirus and Kaposi's sarcoma.

other risk factors, periodontal disease was significantly associated with an increased risk of lung, kidney, pancreatic and hematological (blood) cancers." [xxi]

Currently there is an association between the two diseases. Cause and effect is not firmly established. Extracting teeth with a poor prognosis, treating gum disease, and subsequently maintaining healthy gums, helps support the immune system and likely helps avoid several kinds of cancer.

- **Electrogalvanism.** Defined as the flow of electric currents between two different metals in an electrolyte solution, electrogalvanism occurs in the mouth because the mouth is a perfect battery. Two different metals – a mercury filling and a metal crown, for instance – provide the current. Saliva, with all its minerals, is the electrolyte. The current runs to the path of least resistance, or into oral tissues. A repetitive current could initiate mutations.
- **Age.** A lifetime exposure to all the above increases a cell's risk of developing cellular mutations. The previously mentioned phrase, "People visit dentists when they are well and doctors when they are sick" usually means the dental community sees the general population more often than physicians. This gives them the opportunity to offer many kinds of screenings and preventive care. However more than half of those over age 65 have not seen a dentist within the past five years. They are generally the ones in the "ill" category, busy visiting physicians an average of six times more often than the under-65 population. It is imperative they receive routine oral examinations that include an oral cancer screening.
- **Lack of protection afforded by dietary fruits and vegetables.** Fruits and vegetables contain antioxidants that neutralize harmful molecules and decrease the risk for oral and other cancers.
- **Chronic iron deficiency.** An association between squamous cell carcinoma and iron deficiency exists, perhaps because the enzymes necessary for differentiation of shield cells (epithelium) require iron.

## It Always Comes Back to the Immune System

Our immune systems can be a powerful ally. Though we continually unveil secrets of the origins and individual expressions of cancer, one thing is certain: if we care for ourselves and maintain a strong immune system, we increase our cancer-fighting abilities.

Excellent nutrition probably reduces risk for all cancers. A diet rich in fruits and vegetables certainly helps prevent cancers of the digestive tract, including oral, esophageal, stomach, and colorectal cancers. Diets high in carotenoids, bioflavenoids, vitamins C and E, iron, selenium, folate, ubiquinone, and other trace elements are particularly cited. If you supplement, be sure to use a reliable source. Many insist on pharmaceutical-grade vitamins to ensure accurate labeling, purity, and an easily assimilated form.

- **Carotenoids** (Vitamin A and its relatives are contained in highly pigmented red, yellow, orange, and dark green plant foods.): Plant pigments protect plants from the oxidation that would otherwise occur when they are exposed to UV light. Carotenoid anti-oxidants protect you when taken in the balance in which they occur naturally. **Note:** In particular, just as with vitamin C, smokers and ex-smokers who take carotenoids out of their naturally occurring context – real food – experience higher rates of lung and colorectal cancers. As with vitamin C, these carotenoids presumably act as pro-oxidants rather than antioxidants for this group.
- **Bioflavonoids** (apples, onions, oranges – especially the white part of the skin – tea and red wine): Bioflavonoids are powerful antioxidants. They protect vitamin C, help prevent mutations, slow aging, and improve connective tissue structure among other things.
- **Ubiquinol** (the reduced form of Coenzyme Q10): Our bodies produce CoQ10 to help transport oxygen and help cells use oxygen to produce energy. The more cellular energy you generate, the more calories you burn, and the more you need CoQ10. CoQ10 also increases the competence of your immune cells and recycles antioxidants like vitamins C and E. The antioxidant function reduces DNA damage, especially to the body's energy furnaces, the mitochondria. It helps maintain an efficient heart, normalizes blood pressure, and lowers blood sugar levels and cholesterol. Dietary sources of CoQ10 are limited and poorly absorbed by the body, but you can augment your stores of this fat soluble compound by eating beef, herring, pork, salmon, sardines, anchovies, nuts, and red palm oil.

  If you choose to supplement, you may want to invest in the reduced form (ubiquinol). Ubiquinone is the already oxidized form. Once oxidized, it does not have the free electrons available to quench oxygen-free radicals. It is primarily the young who can return oxidized CoQ10 to the reduced state. We begin to lose that ability by our late 20s.

Note: If you are uncertain about which form of CoQ10 you have, break open a capsule. If orange, it is already oxidized. Otherwise, the powder will be white. Companies making high-grade products are oil-based, crystal-free, enclosed in gel-caps, and incorporate ingredients to protect the ubiquinol from oxidizing. Most of the damage produced by the heavy metals mercury, plutonium, and lead stems from proliferation of free radicals they cause and the resultant decrease in cellular energy production in the form of ATP. If you suspect you have heavy metal toxicity, if you have mercury-laden filings, strongly consider supplementing with CoQ10.

We produce less CoQ10 as we age or suffer diseases like heart conditions, cancer, diabetes, HIV/AIDS, Parkinson's, or muscular dystrophies. CoQ10, cholesterol, and dilochol are all end-products of a particular synthesis reaction in the body, so if you decrease cholesterol via statin drugs like Lipitor, Levacor, Zocor, Pravachol, or Crestor, or even the "natural" substitute, red rice yeast, which is essentially the same thing, you reduce CoQ10. You also reduce squalene – a potent antioxidant, precursor to cholesterol, and possible anti-cancer compound – and dolichol. Dolichols are intracellular messengers that direct newly synthesized proteins to their appropriate destinations. They also help make the neurotransmitters called beta-endorphins that regulate cellular activity and feelings of wellbeing.

- **Vitamins C and E** (Rich vitamin C food sources are: broccoli, parsley, bell peppers, strawberries, cauliflower, citrus fruits, and dark green leafy vegetables. Food sources abundant in vitamin E are: avocados, fresh sunflower seeds, nuts – especially raw almonds, unrefined oils like palm and coconut oils, and turnip greens): These antioxidants prevent and possibly repair damage at the DNA level. Foods are the best source of vitamin E because they provide the full spectrum of vitamin E, unlike most supplements. As with many nutrients, vitamin E must be taken with fats to be absorbed. Vitamin C is water soluble. In general, 0.5 g of vitamin C saturates the body. Mega doses may only be partly absorbed, quench ozone activity, act as an oxidant and, most likely be rapidly eliminated with highly acidified urine. If in poor health, your doctor might suggest this dosage can be doubled.

- **Selenium**: Toxic in high doses, selenium can prevent some cancers. In animal studies, dietary supplements of selenium were shown to prevent viral and chemically induced cancers. Selenium seems to reduce the toxicity of chemotherapy drugs and increase their efficiency. It may fortify DNA against aging and environmental factors. Finally, selenium assists the body to make glutathione peroxidase, an important antioxidant enzyme.

  Glutathione peroxidase reduces inflammatory mediators. Glutathione also binds directly to toxins like organic and inorganic cancer-causing agents, mold toxins, and heavy metals. It prepares them for elimination. For example, two glutathione molecules remove one atom of mercury. If you suspect mercury toxicity, selenium becomes more important, if only to protect the energy furnaces (mitochondria) of each cell in your body. Deficiencies are seen in conditions of high oxidative stress such as some cancers, cataracts, asthma, Parkinson's, and Alzheimer's disease.

  The inorganic form of selenium, selenite, is often offered in supplements because it is cheap. This form is more toxic, however, and it reacts with vitamin C to form elemental selenium that humans cannot absorb. Scientists use L-selenomethionine, the organic, bioavailable form, in studies. Plants that provide us with cereal grains and nuts convert inorganic selenite to L-selenomethionine. Two Brazil nuts equal 100 micrograms of L-selenomethionine supplementation.[xvii]

  Mushrooms and sunflower seeds are also excellent sources if grown in non-depleted soils. Animal proteins and eggs also provide this source. Plants in the onion and broccoli families might provide the most important cancer-protective and bioavailable form of selenium, L-Se-methylselenocysteine.

  As always, the dose makes the poison. High levels of plasma selenomethionine may be linked to diabetes. Further studies need to clarify selenium's role.

- **Folate** ($B_9$ – found in spinach, asparagus, legumes, beef liver): $B_9$ helps produce and maintain new cells. The mouth and other areas of rapid cell division have a high $B_9$ requirement because it is used in DNA replication. Folates also help prevent DNA changes that can lead to cancer and are involved in the breakdown, use, and creation of new proteins. Heat from cooking easily destroys $B_9$, so eat some foods raw.

- **Vitamin D** (called the "sunshine vitamin", but actually a steroid hormone with far-ranging influences on health through its interactions with thousands of genes): Vitamin D can reduce cellular proliferation, a key problem with cancers because the more cells reproduce, the higher the chance for copy errors or mutations. When researchers from the European Institute of Oncology in Milan, Italy and the International Agency for Research on Cancer in Lyon, France reviewed 18 trials of more than 57,000 people, they concluded people who took vitamin D supplements had a seven percent lower risk of death from life threatening conditions (including cancer, cardiovascular disease, and diabetes) compared to those who did not take vitamin D supplements. The average dose was 528 IUs.[xxiii] A wide variety of cells have vitamin D receptors. Scientists are assessing whether vitamin D supplementation protects against many kinds of cancer, including esophageal cancer. If you do supplement with vitamin D, use the form $D_3$ (cholcalciferol). $D_2$ is less expensive but poorly absorbed.

  Beyond cancer protection, vitamin D is the body's main calcium regulator. It maximizes calcium absorption, which encourages strong bones. Just as importantly, if blood does not maintain proper calcium levels, the parathyroid hormone signals bones to release calcium, which exacerbates osteoporosis. Anything that causes bone loss is generalized to the jawbone, causing gum disease to accelerate. Vitamin D may also help prevent falls by making muscles stronger and improving coordination. Preliminary evidence suggests vitamin D may also fight inflammation, which in turn helps control gum disease.

  In fact, vitamin D's role in reducing many health conditions may be crucial. The Public Health Agency of Canada is investigating whether optimal vitamin D levels diminish flu severity.[6] Vitamin D can also protect against respiratory infections and stroke.

  Again, the dose makes the poison. Vitamin D is fat soluble, therefore it is stored in fat tissues. Toxic doses can accumulate, so check blood levels before you supplement. DiaSorin, Inc. recently developed an automated immunoassay called Liaison, which provides clinically accurate results.

---

6 Note the U.S. FDA has decided to threaten reputable doctors like Andrew Weil with jail time if they suggest the use of herbs or supplements to boost the immune system will ward off or improve symptoms of influenza viruses and other ailments.

**Note:** Particularly if you have autoimmune problems, please review Chapter Seven about possible negative consequences of vitamin D supplementation.

- **Iron**: (Iron from animal sources is more available for absorption than from other sources. Clams, mussels, beef, shrimp, sardines and turkey are good sources.) People with Plummer-Vinson syndrome have iron deficiency anemia. This syndrome is associated with an increased risk of oral and esophageal cancer. Symptoms can include a smooth, shiny red tongue that has a burning sensation. The corners of the mouth can also be cracked and dry. It may be difficult to swallow. Treatment is correction of the iron deficiency.
- **Curcumin** (found in the spice, turmeric): Inhibits the transformation of cells into tumor cells and inhibits tumor cell proliferation. It helps the body destroy cancer cells so they can't metastasize and helps blunt blood supply formation in tumors so they can't grow. Turmeric decreases inflammation and may help reduce beta-amyloid plaques in the brain, but it is poorly absorbed from foods, though heat helps to release its benefits. Researchers at UCLA developed Longvida® capsules to provide significant amounts of bioavailable turmeric.

## Diagnosis

Dentists and hygienists should provide an oral cancer exam at least annually. However, if you notice any of the following symptoms, it is urgent you seek a professional exam:

- A sore or lesion in the mouth that does not heal within two weeks
- A lump or thickening in the cheek
- A white or red patch on the gums, tongue, tonsil, or lining of the mouth
- A sore throat or feeling like something is caught in the throat
- Difficulty speaking, chewing or swallowing
- Difficulty moving the jaw or tongue
- Pain, paresthesia, or numbness of the tongue or other areas of the mouth
- Swelling of the jaw that causes dentures to fit poorly or become uncomfortable

An oral cancer exam includes a visual and tactile exam of all oral tissues including the tongue. The throat neck, and lips are also examined. If anything abnormal is discovered, the clinician will refer you to a specialist or may perform an Oral CDx preliminary test.

**Oral CDx** is a cytology test similar to a Pap smear. A tiny brush twirled gently in a suspicious lesion gathers a sample of questionable cells. The cells are slipped into a liquid preservative and then sent to an oral pathologist for computer lab analysis. This simple and painless test has been used successfully since the late 1990s.

## Diagnostic Screening Tools

Not all lesions are visibly evident. Since early diagnosis is the key to successful treatment, the following screening tools are sometimes used:

- **ViziLite Plus[7] with Tblue**. Squamous cell carcinomas make up 90 percent of all head and neck cancers. This screening technology is based on the principal that increased nuclear content of malignant cells reflects light in a specific spectrum.[8] The client rinses with a mild one percent solution of acetic acid. This makes squamous cells look white under a blue luminescing "wand." If a suspicious lesion is noted, the area is swabbed with acetic acid and marked with a blue dye. Lesions are then documented for a two-week follow-up or a referral is made. **This technique does not illuminate red abnormalities, and, though rare, they are far more frequently malignant than white lesions.**

- **VELscope (Visually Enhanced Lesion Scope)** is a luminescing device. Normal oral tissues fluoresce green as the light of VELscope's wand reaches them. Suspicious lesions do not fluoresce and appear dark. The VELscope, identifies both white and red lesions early, an advantage over the ViziLite Plus.

---

7 This is a Chemiluminescent Light.
8 In the 430, 540, and 580nm range.

- **MicroluxDL** is a screening device that uses LEDs to illuminate the oral cavity. It is used after a one percent acetic acid rinse, similar to the ViziLite but without the dyes.

## Saliva As a Promising Tool

Saliva has been used successfully for pathology and drug testing for many years. Although testing for oral cancers is still in the discovery phase, some trials are promising. Medport World Wide News reported in May 2007, "The University of Florida is among those searching for cancer tags in saliva. A protein called CD44 is involved in normal body cell function. In cancer however, it mutates slightly and is found in elevated numbers. When the mouth is rinsed with salt water, these cells are flushed out with it and can be detected. Their findings showed CD44 was significantly higher in 170 patients known to have oral cancer." [xiv]

In 2005, Dr. David Wong, director of Dental Research at the University of California, Los Angeles looked at identifying four particular messenger DNA molecules in a combination associated with malignancy. Preliminary tests show it could prove extremely accurate. Saliva tests of 300 oral cancer patients showed better than 90 percent sensitivity and specificity for oral cancer.[xxv] Clinical trials in tandem with the US National Cancer Institute should show results by 2011. A similar molecular signature in saliva has been discovered for some breast cancers. Oral DNA Labs now has a test to check for HPV viruses, called the "OraRisk HPV Salivary Diagnostic Test."

Oral cancer exams are an important component of routine dental visits. If lesions are found and treated, the dental team maintains its vital place in the medical team. We are often the first part of triage. From what you've learned in previous chapters, you should recognize excellent gum health and extraction of teeth with a poor prognosis is a critical first step in localized immune system support.

## Managing Post-Treatment Complications

Head and neck radiation therapy slows or stops saliva flow. Since saliva helps maintain tissue integrity, cancer patients often say saliva loss is the worst side effect of therapy. Since tissues become sticky, rough, and may even tear and become infected, these people often become depressed and have trouble sleeping. Low saliva flow increases the risk of severe tooth decay and chances of bone death at extraction sites. It is imperative cancer patients work closely with an informed dental professional.

Before initiating chemotherapy or radiation therapy, begin a regimen of the artificial saliva Caphosol.[9] This prescription is a supersaturated calcium phosphate rinse. It helps alkalize and lubricate the mouth and avoid sores by maintaining tissue and tooth integrity. The minerals mobilize into tooth structure, at risk for serious decay because oral dryness leads to an inability to buffer acids. (See also Appendix V-D.) Both minerals also help maintain and repair tissue. Calcium may also help with blood clotting.

The last chapter, "Solutions," has many suggestions for coping with a dry mouth. Over-the counter remineralizing toothpastes like CariFree CTx3 Gel with nano particles of hydroxyapatite or Dr. Collins Restore toothpaste containing NovaMin® (see Chapter 16, Shifting the Balance From Destruction to Reconstruction) are wonderful for helping with tooth sensitivity and decay induced by a dry mouth. NoveMin® is available in other pastes sold around the world. Check online for shifting availability. Prescription toothpastes like MI paste are helpful. Additionally brushing with baking soda in the evenings to alkalize your mouth helps.

Oral yeast infections are common in those with dry mouth. Systemic yeast infections are tenacious and sometimes need a three-pronged attack: antifungal agents, enzymes, and probiotics. Oral infections should probably be treated as aggressively as systemic infections.

Almost all pharmaceutical anti-fungals have a down side and one has to weigh these with the benefits. Nystatin rinse contains up to 50% sugar (sucrose), not the best choice in a medicine developed to fight yeast infections, especially for those with cancer, dry mouth, and the resulting tendency towards cavities. Diflucan, a systemic tablet, has a fluoride-based component (quinoline) that has come under question lately, plus many strains have developed a resistance to it. Clotrimazole contains the sugar dextrose and also magnesium stearate, but may be superior to the others mentioned. (Refer to Appendix V-D.)

---

9 Compounding pharmacies can also prepare this for you. I use Annie's Apothecary. They send it to my clients at about a tenth the cost of the brand name. (lagrasso@ anniesrx.com. PHONE: 830-4774/FAX: 830-981-4775.)

A functional medicine approach may include rinsing often with a few drops of essential oils mixed into yogurt or kefir. Anti-fungal oils include tea tree, chamomile, oregano, lavender, geranium, and/ or patchouli. Rotate the oil type every 4-7 days, since fungi quickly adapt to all anti-fungals. Another choice is to rinse with regular Lugol's solution: 10% total iodine (from 10% potassium iodide and 5% iodine in water). This strength is hard to obtain these days due to regulatory efforts, but it is still available.

A biologically compatible approach would also include a diet high in omega-3 fatty acids and saturated oils like virgin coconut oil. Orally and systemically, the medium chain fatty acid called lauric acid is anti-fungal. It also kills fat (lipid)-coated bacteria, while leaving good intestinal bacterial intact. Rinse a small amount for as long as possible, several times a day. A derivative of lauric acid, caprylic acid, is available in tablets, though without saliva, they are difficult to swallow. Grapefruit seed extract, natto, and garlic are also systemic anti-fungals.

Ozone is strongly anti-fungal and so fast-acting, fungi cannot develop a resistance to it. Swabbing the oral cavity with ozone-saturated oil several times a day would alone likely resolve a fungal infection. (Ozone Gel/Ozene by Premier Research Labs is one option. Available online, they use pure medical grade oxygen and organic olive oil to make their highly saturated gel. O3 Skincare is my preferred brand because they use organic jojoba oil. Clients seem to prefer the taste.) Swab partials or dentures or have your dentist bag and gas them. Follow an hour or so later with an oral probiotic like Evora. Fungal infections invade tissues, so continue to apply for several days after the infection seems to be resolved.

Routinely passing ozone gas over the teeth by means of a specially fabricated ozone tray helps prevent cavities resulting from a dry mouth.

There is an old saying, "Sugars feed cancers." Likewise, sugars also feed yeast infections. Neither thrive when people alkalize their bodies systemically. Refer to chapters seven, twelve and thirteen to learn more about alkalizing your body through diet, breathing, and other means.

## BARBARA

At this point I would like to relate an aspect of one client's care before she succumbed to cancer.

Barbara was another feisty woman. I did not realize this at first, because for years her dental phobias obscured her personality. It took a long time to establish a trusting rapport with her. Her oral health issues included gum recession, chronic inflammation, and extensive exposed and sensitive root surfaces covered with heavy deposits.

As the years passed, Barbara began to understand why and how I wanted her to care for herself at home. I was so pleased when she began to floss daily and courageously decided to commit time and money to quarterly wellness visits. She constantly worked at conquering many psychological and oral challenges and was satisfied when she slowly began to regain her oral health.

When breast cancer struck, her visits became highly irregular. Eventually, the cancer metastasized to her tongue and she had to visit us again. Although her body was bombarded with difficult treatments that left her frail and exhausted, she never gave up on the thorough home care routine we had established together. Her oncologist – like many others at the time – believed her oral tissues had became too delicate to floss and asked her to refrain from the practice. Barbara was dismayed by the advice and considered the doctor so uninformed she did not even consider adhering to his advice.

I clearly remember her first visit after her oral cancer diagnosis. She was outraged. "Can you believe I was asked not to floss any more? I had just gotten my mouth healthy! No way was I going to take a step backwards!" As I said, she was a courageous, smart woman.

I was pleased she had taken our discussions to heart and understood the importance of cleanliness and a strong immune system. She knew many of her chemotherapy drugs seriously reduced her white blood cell count, which negatively affected her immune system. She knew ignoring her oral health would only hinder the healing process and further stress her immune system.

Barbara's cancer treatments kept her from visiting our office for more than a year, but when she returned her teeth were nearly spotless and her gums, though fragile and dehydrated, reflected health as nearly as they could under the circumstances. She knew she had to be extremely gentle and slow in her meticulous efforts.

Oncologists have reversed their position on flossing in most cases. Cancer patients are now asked to follow this general guideline: Brushing and flossing are allowed when platelet counts are above $50,000/mm^3$. Flossing should be curtailed when the count falls below $50,000/mm^3$. Brushing should stop if platelet count falls below $20,000/mm^3$.

The Oral Cancer Foundation web site is a useful resource.

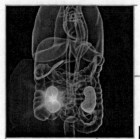

# 10

## KIDNEY TRANSPLANTS

## Why Should You Care?

Roughly 101,000 people waited for a donor organ in the U.S. in 2009. More than three quarters of them waited for a kidney.

According to the National Kidney Foundation, twenty-six million Americans, or one in nine adults, live with chronic kidney disease. An additional 26 million Americans are at increased risk – largely because of high blood pressure, diabetes and obesity.[1] The Centers for Disease Control suggests the numbers are far greater. That organization suggests that Chronic Kidney Disease (CKD) affects nearly 17 percent of adults over the age of 20. As with so many silent diseases, an estimated 75 percent[i] of those afflicted are unaware they have it, so don't seek treatment during early stages when medication and lifestyle changes could alter the disease's course. And not surprisingly, studies indicate gum disease influences kidney disease.[ii] [iii] Gum disease is

---

1 The estimated probability of chronic kidney disease was 98 percent for an older, non-Hispanic white toothless former smoker, who has had diabetes for more than ten years, has high blood pressure, high cholesterol with low HDLs, high CRPs, albumin spillover into the urine, with a lower income, who was hospitalized in the past year. (Fisher MA, Taylor GW. "A Prediction Model for Chronic Kidney Disease Includes Periodontal Disease." *J of Perio.*2009:80(1): 16-23. http://www.joponline.org/doi/pdf/10.1902/jop.2009.080226 (Accessed September 26, 2009.)

"prevalent, severe, and under recognized in chronic kidney disease patients," [iv] yet it decreases the survival of those with end stage kidney disease on dialysis.[v]

About half a million Americans have suffered complete kidney failure requiring an organ transplant or dialysis – triple 1983 statistics. This number is expected to quadruple within the next 25 years.[vi] They cannot build dialysis clinics fast enough. As with most chronic degenerative diseases, irreversible degradation quietly steals health during most of the disease's course. Only as systems fail and symptoms demand attention do people seek treatment. Refer to the appendices for a list of common symptoms of chronic kidney disease.

## Kidney Transplantation

Nearly half of all kidney failures, are due to diabetes. One third of diabetics will eventually develop chronic kidney disease. Blood sugar levels consistently out of the range of 70-150 can damage kidneys. Gum disease is a predictor of end-stage kidney disease for those with Type 2 diabetes.[vii]

High blood pressure accounts for another 23 percent of kidney failures. Any blood pressure reading higher than 130/80 can cause kidney damage. Less frequent causes include: autoimmune diseases, systemic infections, frequent urinary tract infections, urinary stones, lower urinary tract obstruction, cancers, certain drug exposures and low birth weight.

Clearly many of these conditions converge with gum disease and the integrative health model. For that reason I will spotlight this particular organ transplant and the complicated two-way path between oral conditions and kidney failure. Much of the information generalizes to all organ transplants.

## What Do Kidneys Do?

Healthy kidneys clean blood by removing wastes and excess minerals and fluids. In this way, they regulate fluid volume and the body's acid-base balance. This controls blood pressure and blood's mineral content, especially the minerals sodium, potassium, phosphorus, and calcium. Kidneys make hormones that keep blood healthy and bones strong. Malfunction can result in a low red blood cell count, which in turn leads to anemia and accompanying exhaustion. Other conditions that surface affect bones, nerves, and skin.

Doctors routinely use three blood measures to screen for kidney function: The Creatinine Serum test, the GFR, and the BUN. Refer to the appendices for details.

## DIALYSIS

Waiting for an organ transplant after kidney failure can be difficult. No one in this position has any doubt as to his compromised health status. Some of these patients choose to undergo a process called hemodialysis, which involves going into a hospital setting every two days for blood cleansing by machine with a special filter. This option causes wide swings in day-to-day body fluid levels. These fluctuations stress the circulatory system. It is said the heart of a 20-year-old on dialysis is as aged as that of an 80-year-old.

To even out swings in fluid retention and for added schedule flexibility, many choose to clean their blood at home – often several times daily – with peritoneal dialysis. Using an abdominal catheter, the patient injects a special solution into the abdominal cavity and allows it to "dwell" there while it pulls wastes and excess fluids from the blood. The solution is drained four to six hours later. Oral complications can arise from an inflammation of the peritoneum, the membrane that lines the abdominal cavity. This inflammation is called peritonitis.[2] A close relationship with one's dentist will help manage these possible oral complications.

### Dentistry and Kidney Failure

The rest of this chapter is not for everyone. It introduces details many people with end-stage kidney disease, now called Stage 5 chronic kidney disease (CKD), may not know.

---

2 Anemia and peritonitis are closely associated; both often cause a pallor of the oral tissues. Saliva flow can diminish – a dry mouth and parotid salivary gland infections can happen. The parotid duct secretes saliva near the upper molars. Loss of the thin bony plate that lines the tooth socket (lamina dura) and demineralized bone may occur as well as localized radiolucent jaw lesions, where bone density is equal to that of air or near air. Because urea levels may be high in the blood, saliva may smell like ammonia. If taking the anticoagulant heparin, as most dialysis patients do, blood clots abnormally. Be aware heparin is usually prescribed to thin blood, so it compromises blood clotting.

Prospective organ transplant recipients on dialysis should work toward a dental clearance as part of a pre-transplant work-up for the same reasons addressed in the chapter about "bacterial showers," though there is an additional complication. External infection sources are a major consideration. Dental office aerosols add a burden. Untreated dental problems can prevent or delay a kidney transplant.

### Treatment the dental team should address:

- Extract all hopeless teeth whether due to gum disease or decay.
- Repair teeth that can be restored.
- Aggressively treat gum disease.
- Excellent home and professional care are not an option. They are mandatory.
- Sometimes other dental complications should be addressed. As a result of dialysis, those with end stage kidney disease have an impaired ability to excrete phosphorus. These people can develop the mineral imbalance of secondary hyperparathyroidism referred to in the osteoporosis section. To maintain the phosphorus to calcium blood ratio balance, calcium is readily extracted from skeletal bones. Not only does this osteoporosis generalize to bone loss around teeth, often the free calcium is re-deposited into the tooth pulps. This chokes the blood supply that keeps teeth vital. Teeth become brittle and can spontaneously fracture. People who put continuous excessive forces on their teeth by clenching or grinding should seriously consider dental splints.

This mineral imbalance can cause other dental complications, such as an enlarged tongue or as benign tumors, called Brown tumors. These can be seen anywhere in the body, including the bone and tissues of the mouth.

In fact, end stage kidney failure with its increase in blood phosphorus levels, high calcium mobilization from skeletal bones, and decrease in vitamin D levels, can lead to spontaneous fractures, jaw osteonecrosis, and tooth loss due to gum disease. Implants are not a consideration. These are matters of no small concern to the dental team.*

* Modest improvement in blood phosphorus levels can be achieved by decreasing foods high in phosphorus. Those with kidney disease should be aware that phosphorus-containing food additives are on the rise in processed and restaurant foods.

Considerations For the Dental Team and CKD client:

- The dental team must consult with the patient's kidney specialist before all treatment.
- Pre-medicate all dialysis patients before dental treatment. Schedule appointments on the day their bodies retain excessive fluids. This is not on the day of their dialysis session unless patient has an afternoon dialysis session. In that case, they can schedule a morning dental appointment.
- Treat dental infections aggressively. Watch for fungal infections.
- Check salivary glands thoroughly.
- Take blood pressure on the arm opposite of that prepared for the cannula, to avoid cellulitis,
- Reduce oral bacterial loads prior to dental treatments with an antibacterial mouthwash, such as CloSYS, ozonated water, etc.
- Keep dental appointments brief and stress-free.
- If required by the nephrologist, check creatinine levels after dental surgery.
- Remember, drugs that compromise circulation or blood cleansing will not work as efficiently as they would in other patients.[3]
- Be aware heparin is usually prescribed to thin blood, so blood clotting is compromised. Additionally, Stage 5 CKD causes red blood cells to be more fragile than those found in healthy people.
- Emphasize gum health.
- Be aware that kidney disease increases one's susceptibility to fluoride toxicity. Healthy adults are able to excrete about 50 to 70 percent of ingested fluoride. Kidney disease reduces that to about 10 to 20 percent excretion rates, thus toxic doses of fluoride bioaccumulate.[viii] Even at the "idealized" 1ppm fluoride content in fluoridated drinking water, a quadruple increase in skeletal fluoride content is common in those with ESRD [End Stage Renal Disease].[4] This increases risk of spontaneous bone fracture and seems akin to skeletal fluorosis.[ix x] Since the kidney accumulates more fluoride than all other soft tissues except the pineal gland, and fluoride is

---

3 Those within the dental domain are the vasoconstrictors in some anesthetics.
Nephrologists usually do not allow vasoconstrictive anesthetic use and allow a maximum of 5-6 anesthetic carpules. NSAIDS like ibuprofen are completely off limits.
4 As discussed later in the book, fluoride is bone seeking, therefore it increases bone density. Nonetheless, skeletal bone undergoes degenerative changes including increased brittleness. Fluoride also increases the skeletal requirement for calcium, resulting in a general state of calcium deficiency and secondary hyperparathyroidism.

thought to cause kidney damage, there is concern this creates a vicious cycle.

**Rules for a clean toothbrush:**

Though everyone should follow these guidelines, dialysis and transplant patients must follow them scrupulously. A wet toothbrush provides a bacterial breeding ground. Do not cover your toothbrush head. Isolate toothbrushes from each other. Do not store them within six feet of a toilet. Close the lid when flushing to prevent aerosols from settling. Replace brushes at least monthly. A new toothbrush is essential after a fungal, viral, or bacterial oral infection. UV sanitizing toothbrushes, like the Sonicare version, are an excellent idea. Mouth Watchers makes inexpensive manual and spin brushes that are gentle on gums and have nano-silver impregnated bristles to give you extra protection against germ growth on bristles.

## RECEIVING AN ORGAN TRANSPLANT

Organ transplant patients cannot follow the redundant references about boosting the immune system presented in this book because transplant patients cannot take anything to boost their immune system. Doing so can lead to organ rejection. It is the immune system that recognizes a transplant as being foreign to the body and therefore something to be attacked and rejected. This mimics the body's natural response to parasites, fungi, bacteria, and viruses, so low resistance to infection is a common side effect of all of the following listed drugs typically prescribed to suppress the immune system. However, when taken in the combination and manner prescribed, outcomes for most organ recipients are almost always positive. The side effects arise when patients do not follow the treatment plan.

### Critical Immune System Depressants: Cyclosporine A

Cyclosporine's advent in 1971 opened the doors to organ transplantation. The difficulty until then was organ rejection by the immune system despite careful matching. Interestingly, cyclosporine works partially by reducing the production of interleukins, one of the inflammatory messengers often alluded to in this book. *Everything must be done to keep the immune system suppressed to prevent organ rejection.*

- Vitamin C is off limits. Grapefruits are particularly harmful as they erratically boost cyclosporine blood levels and contain chemicals that interfere with the breakdown of certain drugs in the digestive tract. High levels are maintained in the blood.
- Erythromycin class and sulfa class antibiotics increase cyclosporine levels, so must be avoided. Some anti-fungal medicines must also be avoided.
- Ibuprofen is not only toxic to kidneys; it decreases blood flow to the graft.
- Herbs are not recommended. For instance, St. John's Wort reduces cyclosporine levels.
- Ironically, the drug that makes transplants possible also leads to kidney dysfunction. That is, cyclosporines are toxic to the kidney transplant.
- Vomiting: Repetition of acids in the mouth can dissolve teeth and are of dental concern.
- The gums often enlarge as oral cells proliferate, just as with some anti-seizure and blood pressure drugs.
- Elevated potassium blood levels (hyperkalemia) – This serious potential side effect is not surprising, since part of the kidney's job is to maintain the balance of potassium and other electrolytes. When cyclosporines cause excess potassium retention, it shifts the delicate balance of this electrolyte that is the base of most body functions. For this reason acute hyperkalemia can lead to cardiac failure.[xi]
- Diarrhea: Avoid laxatives.
- Cholesterol and triglyceride levels increase.
- Pregnant and nursing mothers should avoid cyclosporine.

Other occasional side effects are: convulsions, peptic ulcers, an inflamed pancreas, fever, confusion, breathing difficulties, hair growing in unwanted places (hirsutism), numbness and tingling, and high blood pressure. Careful monitoring and dose adjustment usually control side effects.

## Prograf:

Prograf is sometimes used in place of Cyclosporine. Possible side effects: high blood pressure, tremors, nausea, and kidney toxicity. Instead of excessive hair growth, hair may fall out. Gum overgrowth is not a side effect of Prograf as it is with Cyclosporine. Again, careful monitoring and dose adjustment help mitigate side effects.

## Prednisone:

Most organ transplant recipients also take the steroid Prednisone to reduce inflammation, though many kidney centers attempt to minimize doses because of its serious side effects:

- It compromises the critical endocrine glands, the adrenals. These glands produce the stress hormone adrenaline, androgens like testosterone, glucocorticoids, and dopamine. Dopamine is important to nerve transmission. For instance, those with Parkinson's disease need to boost dopamine levels.
- Further, the adrenal gland regulates electrolyte concentration. Prednisone often causes sodium retention. Sodium and potassium are the two main electrolytes that regulate our body's water metabolism. Since prednisone interferes with sodium regulation and Cyclosporine interferes with potassium regulation, one can see the potential for difficulties in keeping water metabolism balanced, especially since the kidney is the challenged transplanted organ.
- The fungus Candida (yeast) can become deeply embedded in various organs while taking this drug. Deep-seated candida oral infections are often present. Sleeping with a humidifier helps, as does keeping the tongue scrupulously clean. Avoid simple carbohydrates such as sugars and breads since they promote candida infections. Candida infections are addressed elsewhere in this book.
- Prednisone masks infections.
- As discussed in Chapter Eight, corticosteroids like Prednisone contribute to osteoporosis.

## Cellcept:

Cellcept is generally well tolerated, but can have a few side effects such as:

- Diarrhea: Probably a sign of an out-of-whack sodium/potassium electrolyte balance.
- Vomiting: Again, tooth erosion from acids is a dental concern.
- Leucopenia: A decrease in the number of white blood cells such as phagocytes increases infection rates.
- Sepsis: A condition associated with a bacterial infection of the blood.
- Lymphoma: A tumor of the lymph nodes.
- An increased susceptibility to certain types of infections.

## Rapamune

Rapamune is sometimes taken in combination with other immune system suppressing drugs. Side effects are:

- High blood pressure
- Swelling of the extremities
- Depression of blood platelet counts
- Urinary tract infections
- Joint pain
- Increased susceptibility to lymphoma
- Elevated cholesterol levels
- Elevated creatinine levels
- Diarrhea
- Acne
- Interaction with other drugs and grapefruit juice, similar to Cyclosporine A.

Minimizing doses moderates side effects of all the drugs mentioned above.

## Gum Disease and a Suppressed Immune System

One can see how gum disease would complicate an already delicate balance: the immune system must be depressed to prevent organ rejection, but the drug regimen allows all kinds of undetected and therefore unresolved infections to persist. Yet if diabetes, autoimmune diseases, or circulatory system failures were the precipitating causes for kidney failure, these chronic inflammatory diseases combined with gum disease can make all kinds of metabolic mischief.

Organ transplant recipients should schedule quarterly dental wellness visits, primarily to minimize oral infections and to keep them from becoming systemic. If an infection becomes deeply seated, the organ runs the risk of being rejected. Transplant patients with gum disease have elevated levels of the infection mediator IL-6; loss of gum and bone tissues around teeth are predictors of IL-6 levels.[xii]

Once again, gum disease and CKD influence one another. When researchers from Case Western Reserve studied 12,947 adults from the Third National Health and Nutrition Examination Survey (NHANES), they discovered that subjects with gum disease were twice as likely to have CKD as subjects with healthy gums. They also noted that the risks for chronic kidney failure were greater as the severity of gum disease increased, independent of overall health.[xiii] Conversely, CKD patients are at increased risk for gum disease because they have weakened immune systems and are more prone to infections.

Further, calcium imbalances and poor vitamin D levels[5] result in osteoporosis. Osteoporosis does not spare the bones securing teeth. Remember, immunosuppressive drugs mask infections, so oral tissues may not appear as inflamed as they are. The mouth needs rigorous, yet gentle care.

A transplant patient's oral bacteria balance usually shifts. The first year usually brings a reduction in cavity rates; subsequent years usually see increased decay rates and more biofilm, stain, and hard deposits.

Transplant recipients need dental teams to carefully monitor them for cavities, schedule comprehensive, frequent wellness visits,

---

5 Vitamin D deficiencies develop as early as Stage 3 of CKD, when the body loses its ability to effectively produce it. To compound the lack, CKD causes there to be fewer vitamin D receptors in the body. Those that remain are more resistant to the vitamin's actions. Several studies show an association between vitamin D administration and improved survival rates for those with CKD.

and provide personalized self-care coaching. Because dry mouth conditions and frequent vomiting strongly influence cavity formation, cavity prevention strategies are crucial. Prescription lubricants like Gelclair help. Rinsing with coconut oil may lubricate as well as help unseat fungal candidiasis infections. Many recipients keep ice chips available for hydration and tissue soothing. Dentiva or Salese[6] lozenges help with hydration and cavity protection. Other xylitol products would also help. Xylimelts are now available on Amazon and elsewhere. Since they do not contain Sucralose, I now recommend them instead.

The brittle fragility of oral tissues combined with stressed immune systems causes transplant clients to be prone to oral infections that never previously affected them. The most threatening viral infection for these patients comes from the herpes simplex group (V). This family of cytomegaloviruses specializes in attacking salivary glands. Though all dental infections are serious, immediately refer an infection with a cytomegalovirus because it is a major cause of organ rejection and is therefore life threatening.

Dialysis and transplants, though challenging to manage, prolong lives. Careful teamwork between patients and their doctors is critical. Dental professionals are an important part of that team.

---

6 Addressed in Chapter Fourteen: Solutions. Order at 877-530-9811 or www.nuvo-rainc.com

# 11

# THE NIGHTLY GRIND

*"Keep your jaw relaxed and the rest of your body will follow."*
**~ André Previn, pianist and conductor ~**

**Explore:**
1. What *is* the temporomandibular joint (TMJ)?
2. What is bruxing?
3. How might a dysfunctional TMJ affect me?
4. How might the dysfunctional TMJ of a loved one affect me?

Temporomandibular joint (TMJ) problems limit how comfortably and well the mouth works. Many people are familiar with the frustrating symptoms associated with jaw joint derangements but do not know the cause of their suffering. These symptoms include:

- Stiffness in the muscles that control the jaw "hinge," including neck and upper shoulder muscles
- Chronic headaches and pain in the neck and upper shoulders
- Tense muscles that limit the mouth's ability to open during activities such as eating, yawning, dental exams, and sexual intimacy
- Cracked or worn teeth
- Jaw joint popping or clicking when the mouth opens and closes
- A jaw joint that sometimes locks
- Hearing difficulties or ringing in the ears
- Muscular fatigue while chewing, especially firm foods
- Changes in how the teeth fit together
- Sleep apnea

Upper and lower teeth are only supposed to touch each other for the few minutes a day spent chewing food. However many people tightly clench or grind their teeth together for much longer periods of time. This is called bruxing. Some people do it during periods of high stress or anger. Others spend excessive time on computer keyboards that are positioned too high. This creates tension in the shoulder and neck muscles that transmits to the jaw joint. As a result, clenching teeth while working on the computer is common. Still others take in too much caffeine or too little vitamin B complex. However most people that tap, clench, or grind their teeth do it while they sleep. In this common instance, it is classified as a sleep disorder. Almost all people who brux are unaware of their habit unless a dental professional or sleeping partner points it out.

Analyze your mouth. Are the biting edges of your lower front teeth flat across the top? Can you see the soft, yellow body of the tooth inside a ring of hard white enamel? Are your back teeth flat? Do you or your doctor see wear facets? Do you see small v-shaped grooves (abfractions) on teeth at the gum line? Are these exposed roots sometimes cold sensitive? These are signs you clench or grind your teeth. They may or may not lead to some of the listed symptoms. If you notice any of these signs, seek knowledgeable professional help to relieve symptoms, tension, and future complications. Treatment will not only relieve symptoms, appropriate treatment just might save your life.

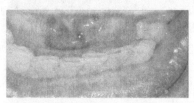

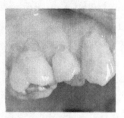

**Far from benign, clenching can destroy both teeth and their support structure.**
**Top left:** A ring of hard enamel surrounds the softer understructure of tooth, the dentin. A common sign one clenches, the person is often unaware.
**Top Right:** Gum recession and v-shaped grooves are not from brushing incorrectly as once thought, but from clenching or grinding. Brushing hard horizontally can aggravate it, but it is not the main driver.
**Right:** Severe abfraction led to extraction. Note the horizontal fracture beginning just under the notch. This is clearly no brushing injury! (Right image: Dr. Brian Palmer)

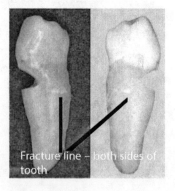

Fracture line – both sides of tooth

Jaw joint disorders favor females and are linked with other disorders like chronic fatigue syndrome, sleep disorders, irritable bowel syndrome, chronic rhinitis, and fibromyalgia. These diseases share an increased sensitivity to pain. There is still much we do not know about TMJ disorders, but there seem to be many influences – gender, genetics, estrogen, parasites, anti-depressant usage, and nervous system function to name a few.

Increasingly, TM disorders are equated with improper jaw development from mouth breathing, a lower tongue resting position, and other incorrect oral postures. The ramifications of partial airway obstruction and acidity that often result are so central to whole body health that the subject deserves its own chapter, following.

## Damage from Clenching or Grinding

Human teeth must bear hundreds of pounds per square inch while clenching – the small cusp tips withstand enormous pressures. People who fail to address clenching problems early in life often seek help from dental professionals when their teeth have flattened, fractured, or otherwise changed their relationship to each other. In these cases, the relationship of their lower jaw to their upper jaw have changed. Since teeth flex when pressure-loaded, supporting gums and bone tend to recede and V-shaped chips appear at the gum line. These areas are sometimes acutely sensitive to cold.

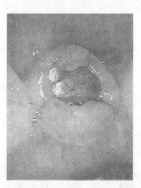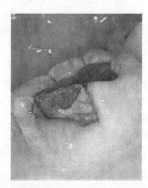

**Flattened teeth pre-weakened by old fashioned fillings. The tooth in the left image will likely break soon and needs treatment. (See "Death Spiral" Chapter.) The tooth in the second picture definitely needs repair. Note corrosion deep into the mercury amalgam filling material. The surface mercury and much of the deeper mercury has migrated out of the filling.**

Compare your jaw hinge and teeth to a three-legged chair. Imagine one leg of stability represents the way your teeth fit together while closed. The other two legs represent each jaw joint. People often clench or grind their teeth when the jaw is malpositioned or because their teeth are misaligned; the top teeth do not interlock well with the lower teeth. It seems these people try to force their teeth to fit by grinding them as they sleep. Other people have right and left jawbones of slightly different lengths. In this case, one leg of the stool is shorter.

When teeth significantly wear, the lower jaw over-closes and two legs of the stool have changed. These changes stress the other leg(s). A clenching habit often begins with an imperfect relationship between the three legs. Those with a dysfunctional bite or whose jaw relationships have changed or were never right to begin with (often due to poor oral posture, discussed in the following chapter), can suffer pain where this particular joint lies, just in front of the ears. They notice pain when the jaw ligaments loosen and distort, which causes the protective disc between the two bones to pop out of the joint.

It is not unusual for other damage to occur, particularly if teeth have been restored. Through the 1990s, mercury fillings were not bonded into teeth. In order to retain these fillings, the bulk of the center part of the tooth was drilled away – the walls flared at the base. Far more tooth structure was removed than was decayed.

Construction workers know not to cut into the middle third of a load-bearing board because it weakens its structural strength. It is the same with teeth. These old-style molar filling preparations remove the middle third of a tooth from five directions! This poor engineering design compromises a tooth's ability to withstand biting forces and has been unnecessary since the advent of Minimally Invasive Dentistry (see Chapter Thirteen, "Death Spiral").

Despite technique changes some dentists have adopted, many people still operate with vastly reduced tooth strength from older fillings. Years of high-stress active service crack teeth compromised by large fillings. Sometimes these teeth break in an unfortunate direction and require either extraction or root canals, an option that may endanger health. (Minimally, only consider having a root canal if it can be in conjunction with ozone therapy.) Something else you may not have considered about root canals: once a tooth has undergone a root canal, it lacks the hydrated organic material that helps it stay flexible. Cracks form with just one-third the force of that required to fracture a hydrated tooth.

Clients who clench and take bisphosphonates – including Fosamax, Boniva, Actonel, and other drugs of that class outlined in Chapter

Seven – should be concerned about how these drugs affect bone health. Clenching causes jawbone micro-fractures and bisphosphonates slow bone remodeling and repair. They also make bones brittle. At the very least, one should consider a protective splint for nighttime wear.

## Therapy Considerations

Symptoms associated with TMJ-related problems are temporary when conditions that cause clenching ebb and flow throughout a lifetime. If this is you, try conservative therapy – apply ice packs, eat soft foods, stretch and exercise gently, seek proper postural and breath training, and meditate. Obtain a correct diagnosis and carefully evaluate root causes since causes and treatments vary widely. Diagnosis and treatment of this jaw joint syndrome is no longer strictly relegated to one's dentist. Many people seeking relief also consult with physical therapists, neurologists, acupuncturists, rheumatologists, allergists, cranial/sacral therapists, osteopaths, or orofacial myofunctional therapists (OMTs). OMTs, by behaviorally and functionally changing oral posture, can vastly help those with TMJ problems stabilize their jaws and become comfortable.

Dental solutions that treat symptoms include wearing a splint or "guard." Some dentists recommend a relaxation deprogramming splint followed by an equilibration.[1] The point of single splints is to break the clenching habit and relax jaw muscles. Splints also provide a larger surface area over which to spread clenching forces. These can provide both protection and relief to the teeth and jaw. Often however, the cause is related to undiagnosed airway obstructions that can be life threatening. A typical splint usually makes these obstructions worse. Read the following chapter before you choose a therapy.

The main jaw muscle is called the masseter. Its upper attachment occurs across a few inches of cheekbone and continues down across the cheek to wrap around the lower jawbone. This roughly rectangular muscle provides cheek structure. Knotted jaw muscles are obvious in people under stress. When Clint Eastwood played detective Callahan in the 1983 film, *Sudden Impact,* he delivered the famous line, "Go ahead. Make my day," with strongly clenched jaws. You would not want to cross this man. Directors and actors know how to heighten drama this way. Viewers are edgy about how and when that tension will release.

1 An equilibration is the process of selectively correcting the bite through minute adjustments in tooth shape. Be aware muscles constantly change these relationships.

Everyone who clenches should consider an inexpensive home sleep-study that correlates well with those performed in sleep study labs. My favorite is the Watermark Ares. For many people, sleep lab studies for initial diagnosis are too uncomfortable to be accurate and too expensive.

Often, bruxing occurs at the end of a sleep apnea episode. The small home recording devices described in the next chapter often show people clench their teeth to bring their jaw, thus their tongues, forward and off their epiglottis. Tightened muscles also help open and stiffen the airway. They clench or grind their teeth, and then they start to breathe. Put another way, people sometimes clench to stay alive. This may not describe you, but wouldn't you want to know? Please read the next chapter to assure good health and longevity!

This may not describe everyone. People whose bites are not fully functional sometimes internalize stress by clenching. Their cheek muscles become so overbuilt they thicken noticeably. Beyond the obvious thickening, clenching causes these muscles to shorten, suffer tiny tears, and fatigue easily. The fatigue leads to limited oral opening, pain, and tension.

Limited opening ability and muscles so tense they feel like a spring-loaded trap are a troublesome combination. Intimacy is a particular minefield because it requires relaxed orofacial muscles. TMJ-related issues can frustrate both partners. Many doctors hesitate to address this facet of jaw-joint dysfunction. Decades of practice have led me to understand what a deep-seated concern this is for couples seeking solutions.

Anyone with TMJ-related symptoms should seek a well-trained dentist and myofunctional therapist,[2] perhaps also a physical therapist, cranio-sacral massage therapist, or other specialist with training in myofascial therapy.[3] Everyone has a stake in the management and treatment of jaw-joint dysfunction.

---

2 To access a database of orofacial myofunctional therapists, go to: http://www.myo-academy.net/myofunctional-therapist

3 To learn more about muscular therapy and trigger point therapy, read *Myofascial Pain and Dysfunction: The Trigger Point Manual* by David Simons, MS, PT. Physical therapists, massage therapists, and dental personnel with specialized training in myofascial training can be identified at: www.myofascialtherapy.org. Programs are accredited through the National Association of Myofascial Trigger Point Therapists.

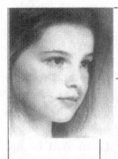

# THE SECRET: BEAUTY, BRAINS, AND BODY BALANCE

*"The Divine Proportion is an indicator of good health."*

**~ Chris Norton, D.D.S., orthodontist ~**

**Explore:**
1. How does oral fitness help a child grow his most attractive face?
2. How can we influence our body's acid-base balance?
3. What is the connection between sleep disturbances, mouth breathing, and a host of diseases and problems including high blood pressure, acne, poor blood sugar control, memory loss, reflux, and erectile dysfunction?
4. Is hyperventilation a health hazard?
5. How does bottle-feeding alter a baby's appearance?
6. What are the hazards of enlarged tonsils or being tongue-tied?
7. Does extraction orthodontics lead to poorer health?

## Body Balance

A person with insufficient reserves of either acid or alkaline buffers is a person who is unhealthy. For purposes of this book, an unbalanced pH keeps the body from operating optimally and allows unfriendly bacteria to proliferate. Cavities, gum disease, and most other diseases result from an imbalance in either direction. Most often, the Standard American Diet (SAD) leads to acid waste buildup within cells and more importantly, in the spaces outside of cells, helping to determine what is allowed to enter and exit each cell.

It is beyond the scope of this book to present this complicated, yet highly misunderstood subject in great detail, but it offers those interested in health some direction.

Acidity/alkalinity is primarily a function of dietary imbalances, particularly those resulting from insufficient trace and macro-minerals.

Toxic acid loads can build within cells.[1] [2] The primary acid-binding (alkaline-forming) minerals are: calcium, magnesium, sodium, potassium, iron, and manganese. Alkaline-binding (acid-forming) minerals are: phosphorus, sulfur, copper, silicon, and the halides fluorine, chlorine, bromine, and iodine.

A typical story: One of my clients, a biologist, reported he had endured athlete's foot since his teens – for over 40 years. He had learned to live with it, but recently tried an alkalizing diet. He researched alkalizing foods online and emphasized eating only alkaline-forming foods. He was shocked at how fast his athlete's foot became a memory. I relay his story to other clients who try it, often with the same success.

One lady with a low salivary pH and a similar fungal infection on her toe had already suffered kidney damage from two unsuccessful cycles of drugs her doctor had prescribed to eliminate it. Of course we discussed how the kidney damage only made her body more hospitable to the fungus she was trying to clear, since kidneys help neutralize acids. She jump-started her healing with ozone gas and topical ozonated gel treatments, but understood the fungal infection was opportunistic due to the acid waste build-up in cells her lifestyle had created. She changed her diet; the fungal infection cleared.

I told a friend how I felt unexpectedly different after I added kale and chard to my morning vegetable sauté and changed the vinegar in my salads from distilled to raw apple cider vinegar[3] to raise my slightly low pH. He replied, "I agree. I don't usually notice that foods make me feel one way or another – unless I eat greens for a while. They make me feel better almost immediately." How out of tune with our bodies most of us have become! [Kale rates a perfect 1000 score on the Aggregate Nutrient Density Index (ANDI) adopted by Whole Foods.]**Note:** Though deposits rarely form on my teeth, after adding more greens, they always feel slick and there are zero deposits.

---

1 Complex carbohydrates make more carbonic acid than meats; starches build lactic acid in muscles. We make far more lactic acid when we exercise compared to when we eat, but compensatory mechanisms handle these with ease, *as long as we keep these foods and other general lifestyle habits in balance.* Remember, refined flours and sugars deplete minerals.

2 Robert Walker MA MS DC and Kaye McArthur DDS offer several excellent courses on this. "The Physiologic Aspects of Sleep Disorders and Health," among other things teaches the principals of toxic cell-loading and minerals. "Advanced Occlusal Concepts" teaches one how to measure and address the toxic loads. Exceptional Dental Courses. www.ExceptionalDentalCourses.com. They also teach courses in advanced cranial-sacral work, termed chirodontics.

3 Though an acid, this alkaline- forming vinegar is full of minerals and probiotics.

Acidity/Alkalinity balance is also affected by:

- Hydration/ability to carry minerals (electrolytes) and maintain a proper electrical charge (voltage) – A shocking majority of clients have excessively dry mouths. A person should be able to produce at least 1.5 milliliters of saliva in five minutes if they have not been chewing, eating or drinking anything, 2.5 ml minimum if they have. Many of my clients cannot even produce enough saliva to test. These clients always show a pH less than 5.5. (See Appendix 5-D.)
- Respiration, addressed later
- Protein metabolism imbalance – While meats are notoriously known as acid-forming because meat metabolism results in massive amounts of phosphoric and sulfuric acid waste products, well-functioning kidneys efficiently eliminate them. One can double meat intake and only increase the kidney's workload by about ten percent. Nonetheless, heavy meat intake can load cells with waste products they may have trouble eliminating.
- Nervous system imbalances, often brought on by stress
- Hormonal imbalances (Sex hormones or those hormones deriving from the kidneys, adrenals, thyroid, parathyroid, or the posterior pituitary)
- Kidney function – Kidneys are compensatory as they do their best to excrete or retain acids as needed. Kidneys cause an alkaline/acid imbalance in the body when their ability to excrete or retain acids is compromised.

**Try it:** Salivary pH is a rough measure of the buffering reserves of the body. A healthy saliva pH is 6.8. If that is your typical resting pH (two hours after a snack or meal), test it after a simple carbohydrate challenge dose. It should remain around pH 6.8. (For maximum accuracy, use pHion Diagnostic Test Strips.) You will likely maintain that near-neutral pH if your cells are not carrying a toxic acid load. It indicates you have adequate reserve buffering capacity. In order of importance:

- You have appropriate trace minerals at the cell level
- Macro minerals at the fluid level
- Correct blood balance of carbon dioxide, oxygen, and hemoglobin
- Respiration functions as it should

Respiration as a buffer: Mouth breathers, those using a CPAP machine, and many of the rest of us, hyperventilate. In other words, breathing is too rapid and shallow. The healthy "textbook" nasal breathing rate of an inhale/exhale every five seconds doubles. The result is a serious carbon dioxide ($CO_2$) loss and a poor ratio between carbon dioxide and oxygen. PH and much else suffers because we blow off excessive carbon dioxide ($CO_2$).

**Try it:** Your breathing is normal/healthy only if you have normal tissue oxygenation and carbon dioxide levels in your blood. How can you check it? You should, after five minutes of sitting with good posture in a relaxed state, be able to easily cease breathing for at least 40-60 seconds after an exhalation. At the first strong need to breathe, you should be able to do so comfortably, your first breath being no deeper than your last. Called a Control Pause, Dr. Buteyko developed it as a simple and reliable measure of the carbon dioxide/oxygen blood ratio.

The respiratory rate is set in the brain. One can slowly raise his CP and change the brain's "set point" by practicing Buteyko breathing exercises. There are Buteyko practitioners throughout the world. Dr. Patrick McKeown, an asthmatic for 26 years, no longer exhibits symptoms as a result of this breathing program and has become a tireless advocate of Buteyko breathing methods. I recommend his DVDs and books for those who like to help themselves.

Carbon dioxide influences our health in unimaginable ways:

- $CO_2$ combines with hydrogen ions to make bicarbonate buffer, which guards against alkalosis or acidosis. If this buffer is deficient at the cellular level, our saliva or urine may register as too acidic or too alkaline. Unbalanced conditions favor disease via unfriendly germ populations and heightened blood clotting. Cavities, gum disease and other diseases will be more prevalent.
- If your Control Pause (CP) is twenty seconds or less, you will likely exhibit some of the symptoms in this list. If your CP is between 20 and 40 seconds, symptoms are not apparent, but can quickly express themselves when stressed. These are the people who sometimes must breathe into a paper bag when stressed to raise $CO_2$ levels. When one's CP is in this range, the kidney excretes some of the

bicarbonate buffer, so buffering capacity is limited. A CP of over 40 means this list doesn't apply!

- Alkalinity from low $CO_2$ levels and poor buffering cause nerve and muscle excitability. Muscle tension and ADHD misdiagnosis can result. Those with ADHD not only exhibit muscle excitability, but may be intuitively trying to build blood $CO_2$ levels. Working muscles produce $CO_2$.
- Low $CO_2$ levels constrict arteries, especially in the brain. Low oxygenation from constricted brain arteries can result in headaches, poor concentration and brain fog. Only when carbon dioxide is in the normal range do blood vessels dilate. Constricted arteries and poor oxygenation make the heart, colon, spleen, liver, kidneys, and other organs function suboptimally.
- $CO_2$ helps release oxygen from red blood cells (Bohr effect). Blood may carry sufficient oxygen, but alkaline blood does not allow its release. The less $CO_2$, the less vital organs including the brain are oxygenated. Suboptimal function results. Noticeable symptoms may be breathlessness, dizziness, irritability, obsessiveness, or panic.
- When arteries constrict in the extremities, people experience cold hands and feet.
- $CO_2$ rids us of excess ammonia and urea. Four AM is our body's primary detoxification time. If you often have to get up at 4AM to relieve yourself, you likely have this ammonia-based problem. The body cannot take ammonia to urea without enough $CO_2$, so it irritates the bladder and you have to get up to expel it.
- $CO_2$ prevents smooth muscle spasms. Low carbon dioxide blood levels are an important reason mouth breathers suffer gastric reflux, circulatory problems, disturbed sleep, bedwetting, and asthma. As Dr. McKeown says, "Unless you make the switch to nasal breathing, you will never solve your asthma." [i]

To test the hypothesis of bedwetting as a result of a poor airway, a dentist rapidly expanded the upper jaws of ten mouth breathers who were also bedwetters. He knew an expanded arch would reduce nasal constriction so they could begin to breath through their noses. Bedwetting stopped within a few months for all ten children.[ii]

## Does Beauty Matter?

That our culture values beauty is undeniable:

**Babies:** Attractive babies receive more affection and, and, are more likely to grow up into well-balanced adults.[iii]

**Intelligence:** Attractive people are perceived as being more intelligent. In fact, they actually often are more intelligent, possibly because they receive more attention in schools and elsewhere. They are also more likely to get better jobs, rise to higher positions, and earn more money. [iv]

**Criminals:** An attractive criminal is more likely to receive a shorter sentence from a judge. Unattractive people are more likely to become criminals. Four out of five females committed for aggressive offenses were rated as unattractive.[v] Criminals who improve their appearance with facial surgery are less likely to return to prison.[vi]

**Military:** Handsome cadets achieve higher rank by the time they graduate.[vii]

**Better health:** Surprisingly, beauty often results from a clear airway from birth. Unobstructed breathing brings immeasurable health benefits. Body chemistry changes significantly when one has a compromised airway.

Genetics does not play as large a role in facial development as most of us think.

## Breathing Easy

A clear, wide airway may seem a birthright, but most Americans no longer have one. Most of us have adjusted to and dismissed what seem like minor annoyances.  More likely, we recognize a compromised airway as:

- Sleep disturbances such as sleep apnea; some forms of snoring
- Unbalanced facial features; we are less attractive and functional than we could be.
- Unexplained weight gain
- Early wrinkles around the mouth and nose
- Attention deficit hyperactivity disorder – ADHD
- Depression

- Inflammatory diseases
- Clouded intellect/poor memory
- Frequent ear infections in children
- Poor posture – tilted head, shoulders, and hips with an S-shaped spine
- Forward head posture with sore neck and shoulders
- Mouth breathing
- Bed wetting through early adolescence
- Daytime sleepiness
- TMJ/jaw joint problems; clenching
- Misaligned teeth
- Morning headaches
- Sleepwalking or sleep talking
- Nightmares
- Erectile dysfunction

## Nature's Beauty Code

The Fibonacci Golden Ratio is Nature's Beauty Code. We find the Fibonacci Golden Ratio, this Divine Proportion, (1 to 1.68 0339887 ...[4] ) throughout nature – in birds, insects, flowers, art, architecture … and in faces.

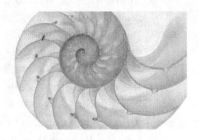

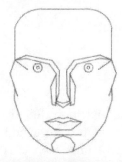

This mask represents a face in harmony with the Golden Ratio. When the overlaid features of this mask match a person's photograph, we perceive the person as attractive.[5] Maybe more importantly, we also can guess they breathe well.

---

4 Two quantities are in the golden ratio if the ratio between the sum of those quantities and the larger one is the same as the ratio between the larger one and the smaller. This is expressed as: $a+b/a = a/b = \Phi$ where phi ($\Phi$) is 1.6180339887.
5 Use this mask in an interactive game with faces we all know: http://www.intmath.com/numbers/math-of-beauty.php. For a fascinating exploration of the Beauty Code of nature, go to: http://www.beautyanalysis.com/index2_mba.htm

## What Affects Growth and Development?

- The choice between breast-feeding or bottle-feeding can affect a baby's future health and appearance as can non-nutritive sucking via pacifiers, finger or arm sucking. These teach babies an incorrect sucking pattern and encourage the tongue to rest on the floor of the mouth. Incorrect oral postures put improper pressures on developing facial bones.
- A clear airway and nasal breathing develop maximum facial attractiveness. Mouth breathers usually develop a poor airway and will have distorted features falling outside the Golden Ratio. The lower third of the face elongates. The angle of the lower jaw increases throughout life such that the lower jaw line becomes less parallel with the floor. This imposes on the airway, it crowds teeth, and often contributes to TMJ problems.
- Swallowing habits and a low resting tongue posture: When resting on the palate, the tongue stimulates stem cells along the palatal midline. This encourages growth into a broad arch resulting in a larger airway, and more room for teeth.
- Enlarged tonsils/adenoids. A child with a deep bite usually has enlarged tonsils and/or adenoids crowding the airway. Their do not develop as "face forward" as they should.
- Tongue-tie: vestigial embryonic tissue under the tongue can lock it down, keeping it from proper function.
- Drugs and diet
- Extraction "Four on the Floor" Orthodontics
- Facial-Skeletal growth abnormalities

## Breast-feeding, Beauty, and Health

Of course baby formula cannot match the nutrition found in mother's milk and can be a significant source of protein allergies. Immunoglobulins and human proteins in breast milk help infants resist allergies. Clear nasal passages allow babies to breath through their noses so their faces develop as they should.

Are there other reasons bottle-feeding prevents babies from maximizing their facial and airway development? In fact, breastfed babies have a far better chance at beauty and health because these infants learn to work their lips, cheeks, and tongue differently. Facial development occurs early, when facial bones are plastic. Genes, skeletal influences, and airway development determine facial shape.[viii]

It takes 1.4 grams of pressure to move teeth or change bone structure. The tongue exerts up to 500 grams of pressure, cheek muscles up to 300 grams. For maximum attractiveness and a lifetime of healthy function, these forces must work properly together. Proper swallowing patterns and an upper tongue rest posture help balance these forces so teeth erupt evenly around the tongue to form a beautiful and functional arch. A wide arch promotes a wide, open airway and room for all teeth.

Breastfeeding and avoiding non-nutritive sucking habits help babies develop good oral posture. The coordination required for an infant to swallow and breathe while breastfeeding is a critical step in learning correct swallow patterns. In a proper swallow, the lips touch lightly. The lower jaw moves slightly upward to touch the upper teeth. The tongue blade lightly moves up and reinforces the good arch form. There is minimal TM/jaw joint compression.[ix] I encourage all readers to go to: http://myoresearch.com/orthodontics/#soft_tissue_dysfunction. Click on "Watch Video" on the right of the page, and then also "More" below that. The video presented shows correct and incorrect swallows. This company, Myofunctional Research Company makes good appliances intended to work in conjunction with orofacial myofunctional therapy to learn correct oral postures.

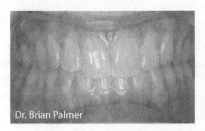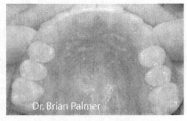

Dr. Brian Palmer          Dr. Brian Palmer

**An adult with a beautiful smile who exclusively breastfed as an infant, nasal breathes, and who never had orthodontics (braces).**

Babies who breastfeed generally keep their tongue on the roof of their mouths, nasal breathe, and develop proper swallowing patterns. They generally have more prominent cheekbones, less constricted sinuses, and a larger eye orbit that allows the eyeball to develop a proper shape. This improves chances of good eyesight. Additionally, they develop far fewer ear infections. Children with deep dental overbites[6] are 2.8 times more likely to have ear tubes placed.[7]

On the other hand, the strong sucking patterns formed with the use of pacifiers, bottles and digits like the thumb create a strong vacuum against the roof of the mouth and at the back of the throat. This can form a very high palatal vault, reduce the width of the arch so teeth are crowded, and constrict the sinuses and airway.

Working in concert to collapse the arch, the cheek muscles suck tightly inward. The amount of distortion relates to the duration and intensity of incorrect oral postures. Switching to a sippy, then real cup as soon as possible shortens the time unequal forces are in play unless the child continues to swallow incorrectly, does not maintain a lip seal, or lets the tongue rest flaccidly on the floor of the mouth.

**Try it:** Make a thick, frozen smoothie, and then try to suck it through a small straw. Notice how hard your lips, tongue, and cheeks work, how much pressure they exert on your teeth and the roof of your mouth.

## Mouth Breathing Leads to Facial Atrophy

In an article published in General Dentistry, Dr. Yosh Jefferson wrote, "Over time, children whose mouth breathing goes untreated may suffer from abnormal facial and dental development, such as long, narrow faces and mouths, gummy smiles, gingivitis (early stage gum disease) and crooked teeth. The poor sleeping habits that result from mouth breathing adversely affect growth and academic performance. Many of these children are misdiagnosed with attention deficit disorder (ADD) and hyperactivity."[x] Mouth breathers usually double their breathing rate. Air volume is higher. The net result is they exhale too much carbon dioxide ($CO_2$). $CO_2$ has many functions in the body. On of its most important is releasing oxygen from blood hemoglobin into tissues. One may have high blood oxygen saturation, but low $CO_2$ levels disallow its release. Tissues are not suffused with the oxygen they need. Hyperactive children are sometimes just trying to build their $CO_2$ blood levels with physical activity, since exercising produces $CO_2$.

---

6 Overbite – a measure of how much top teeth overlap lower teeth when jaws are together. Top teeth overlap the lower by a third in a correct relationship. It is often confused with overjet, which is the horizontal distance between the upper and lower teeth on complete closure.

7 Dental techniques that reshape baby molars to open a deep closed dental overbite, also relieve pressure on the jaw joint by moving the lower jaw bone away from the ears at the jaw joint. (The Functional Orthodontist – 1990.) Removing pacifiers from babies suffering chronic ear infections cures half the chronic infections.

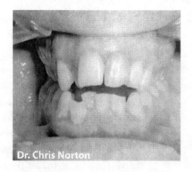

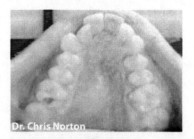

Note the high palatal vault, v-shaped arch, and anterior open bite that can come from a lower tongue rest posture and an active swallow.

Jefferson continues, "Children who mouth breathe typically do not sleep well, causing them to be tired during the day and possibly unable to concentrate on academics. If the child becomes frustrated, he or she may develop behavioral problems. The following images illustrate how mouth breathing can affect facial development.

Left: A six-year-old girl who was a severe mouth breather.
Right: The same girl at age nine, with abnormal facial growth and dental malocclusion as a result of her mouth breathing. Mouth breathing creates a 3D contraction in the jaw. The jaw cross section is smaller as is jaw length. There is less room for teeth and the tongue.

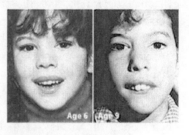

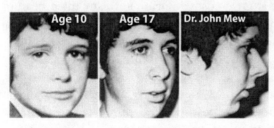

Left images: A young boy who also developed a long face, retruded chin, and dental malocclusion from mouth breathing after allergies set in at age 14.

Practitioners who treat the full face send clients to myofunctional therapists for neuromuscular oral posture repatterning, which includes the tongue resting in the roof of the mouth, a good lip seal, and a passive swallow. They expect this to encourage forward facial growth instead of downward, vertical growth.

Very often, a bottle-fed child or one with a non-nutritive sucking habit develops a lower tongue rest and the "active" swallow introduced earlier.

**Try it:** Place your tongue gently in the roof of your mouth and attempt to breathe through your mouth. It doesn't work well, does it?

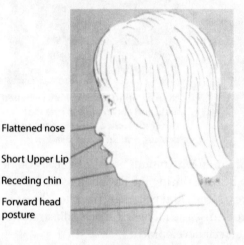

Flattened nose

Short Upper Lip

Receding chin

Forward head posture

**All children who habitually mouth breathe will have misaligned teeth. Their faces appear long and their profiles typically display a flattened nose, short upper lip, receding chin, and a forward head posture. They may have a "gummy smile", one that shows too much gum above the upper teeth.**

In an experiment that illustrates Jefferson's claim, an orthodontist named Harvold placed latex plugs into the noses of young monkeys. Each developed one of three distinctive mouth breathing patterns. All developed the long faces described above. Their faces developed facial disharmonies in three distinctive ways, depending on which of the three patterns they adopted.[8] [xi]

The tilt and forward head posture typical of mouth breathers helps open the airway, as it does in cardio pulmonary resuscitation maneuvers (CPR) but at great cost. Unfortunately, any tilted head or one not aligned with the spine will influence the size, shape and position of all the 29 skull bones, including the jaws. Consider an 8-10 pound bowling ball, weighing about the same as an adult head. When the adult head is tilted, containing mostly water, the fluid flows downhill, pressing on and distorting bones on the down side. The constant tilt also results in poor whole body posture, condemning one to a lifetime of neck and shoulder pain.

Every inch the head moves forward of the shoulders amplifies its weight by ten pounds. If the opening of your ear canal is in line with

---

8 Animals that rhythmically lowered and raised their mandibles with each breath developed a Class I open bite and a skeletal Class I open bite (that is, long faces). Animals that rotated their mandibles in a posterior and inferior direction developed a Class II malocclusion and a skeletal Class II profile. The animals whose mandible maintained an anterior position developed a Class III malocclusion and a skeletal Class III profile.

your spine, your spine supports your ten pound head. If it is three inches forward of your spine, your exhausted muscles must support what feels like forty pounds! This forward head posture contributes to face and neck pain, swallowing difficulties, migraines, pinched nerves, herniated neck discs, and arthritis. Pain causes upregulation of the central nervous system, which can contribute to fibromyalgia, chronic fatigue, and myofascial tender points. The entire gastrointestinal tract can become agitated and result in sluggish peristalsis and evacuation.

A forward head posture can also contribute to high blood pressure, pulse rate, and poor balance. Ninety percent of the brain's energy and output is used to relate the physical body to gravity. Ten percent is dedicated to thinking, metabolism, and healing. Spinal movement contributes ninety percent of the brain's stimulation and nutrition.

A cramped posture also reduces lung capacity by at least thirty percent and keeps one from breathing properly from the diaphragm. Breathing from the lower lungs helps clear them.

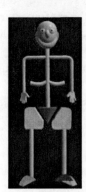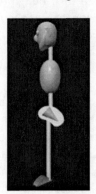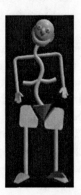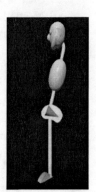

**Developing an open airway, no matter when in life the problem is identified, can grant profound posural benefits. Good posture translates into bodies that move well and feel better for a lifetime. Images: Dr. Chris Norton.**

The tongue at rest should be plastered to the roof of the mouth. The tip should be on the "spot". The spot is about a half inch behind the base of the front teeth. The rest of the tongue should also be in contact with the palate unless speaking or moving food around. The tongue stays there during a swallow. Only the back portion drops down like a dump truck passively emptying its load. There should be no facial muscle movement while swallowing. Mouth breathers cannot maintain this posture and still breathe. Let us turn for a moment to other benefits of keeping the tongue in the roof of the mouth along with a good lip seal.

- A lip seal creates negative pressure within the mouth. When the tongue suctions naturally to the palate, it gently suspends the lower jaw in space. One need not clench to keep the mouth closed.
- A tongue in contact with the midline of the palate during growth and development will stimulate stem cells here to broaden the arch, creating a wide airway and more room for teeth and tongue. The tongue will also be more "toned", thus more compact.
- The tongue is a natural palate expander. It provides push back for pressures exerted by cheek muscles. When up, teeth erupt in a nice, wide pattern around it. Usually a wide arch and shallow palate results.
- When the tongue is up while swallowing, the soft palate rises. This twists the eustachian tubes and changes their internal pressure, keeping them clear while aerating the middle ear.
- When the tongue is up during a correct swallow, it puts pressure on the vomer bone, which in turn nudges the sphenoid bone. Nestled inside the butterfly wings of the sphenoid is the important pituitary gland. A correct swallow "milks" the pituitary of its growth, thyroid, sex, and other hormones.
- When the tongue is up, it completes a crucial meridian circuit.

As mentioned, a highly arched palatal vault reduces the size of the nasal passages. This in turn leads to deviated septums and nasal and sinus congestion. In fact, mouth breathing *causes* congestion: the body senses it is losing too much precious carbon dioxide so it clamps down on the opening it recognizes as its breathing apparatus. Nasal goblet cells produce mucus to narrow nasal passages, never realizing there is a downstream leak!

**Try it!** Buteyko short-term clearing of nasal passages involves walking rapidly while holding one's breath on the exhale until one simply can't hold one's breath any longer. The next inhale, through the nose, should be much clearer. Sometimes it requires a repeat after a two minute rest. The muscle movement raises $CO_2$ levels, which shuts down the nasal goblet cells. Now, keep your lips sealed!

In a downward spiral, frequent upper respiratory tract infections often cause tonsillitis and enlarged adenoids – that further close airways. Many children with constricted airways, especially those due to enlarged adenoids and tonsils, have undiagnosed obstructive sleep apnea (OSA). OSA affects at least 2% of children between ages two to eight. More and more researchers believe there is an association between OSA and

ADHD.[9] Snoring is associated with higher levels of inattention and hyperactivity.[xii] Eighty-one percent of snoring children with ADHD could eliminate it if they could eliminate their habitual snoring.[xiii] Sleep apnea can slow growth and cause behavior and learning problems. IQ scores significantly improve when enlarged tonsils and adenoids are removed and normal sleep patterns return.[xiv]

Mouth breathing exerts other profound negative effects on health and wellbeing. Beyond morphing facial structure and functions, a critical consequence is that it curtails an important way our bodies make nitric oxide (NO). Nitric oxide:

- Has anti-inflammatory effects, for example it improves bacterial clearance in lungs.[xv] Crosstalk between NO and other molecules, cooperatively regulates the fates of unfriendly microorganisms and their hosts.[xvi]
- Improves circulation by dilating blood vessels and facilitating oxygen release to cells.[xvii] Good circulation lowers blood pressure, improves sexual function and nourishes skin. Children who mouth breathe tend to have worse acne and may be prone to eczema and psoriasis. Ineffective oxygen or nitric oxide delivery to cells underlies many diseases.
- Increases alertness by suffusing the brain with oxygen
- Helps regulate blood vessel tone [xviii]
- Increases the amount of oxygen in blood. Low blood oxygenation is associated with high blood pressure, heart attacks, and promotes cancer, diabetes, and other chronic diseases.
- Promotes relaxation and feelings of wellbeing.

Additionally, compared to nasal breathers, mouth breathers have to:

- Process dry, cool air
- Process twice the air
- Process about 180% more allergens, fungi, bacteria, etc.

---

9 Since the ADHD medications Adderall and Ritalin are suspected to cause reduced weight and height, damage the circulatory system, possibly increase risks for cancer and reproductive problems, and may lead to substance abuse, treating children diagnosed with ADHD by changing their breathing patterns could vastly improve their health in many ways. The mouth breathing irritates the tonsils and adenoids, which helps maintain the negative health spiral.

- Function with at least 10% less oxygen
- Function with less brain power
- Suffer more cases of gastric reflux, asthma, circulatory problems, disturbed sleep including apnea, extended bedwetting, and ADHD symptoms
- Suffer more postural problems
- Suffer more diseases and ill health because of an inability to buffer body systems well. Again, the inability to buffer body systems well is easily noticed as bad acne, tooth decay and gum disease.

## Pacifier, Finger, and Arm-Sucking

All sucking habits can change facial structures. Just as the tongue can cause an open bite with an active swallow, so can fingers and other foreign objects. Children who have good opportunity to breastfeed are least likely to develop a sucking habit. The longer a habit continues, the more noticeable the facial changes. Those who continue sucking habits over age four have the greatest changes in facial features.[xix]

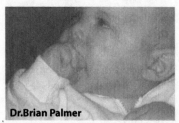
Dr.Brian Palmer

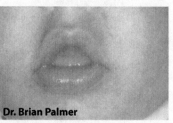
Dr. Brian Palmer

Left: Agressive thumb-sucker at four months.
Right: Lip contour and tongue position of same agressive thumb-sucker with thumb removed. (Four months)

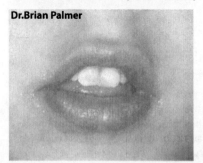
Dr.Brian Palmer

Left: Same patient at 4.5 years of age. Note lip contour and forward position of tongue at rest. This open mouth posture is called "Picard's Bottle Mouth".

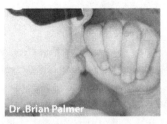

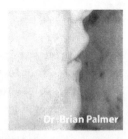

Left: Intense thumb-sucker Right: Retruded chin and elevated upper lip is a result of his thumb-sucking.

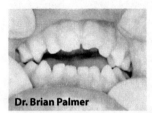

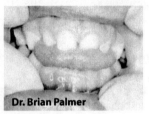

Finger sucking created his open bite (left) and the tongue-thrust upon swallowing (right).

## Tonsils and Adenoids

Enlarged tonsils and adenoids constrict airways and may be the most frequent reason children mouth breath. Immunoglobulins from breast milk protect against allergies that can cause them while today's dairy products may be the biggest allergen culprit. Enlarged tonsils further complicate breathing for those whose facial features are already constricted. As the images below illustrate, there is great variability in airways. Removal of tonsils and adenoids of children misdiagnosed with ADHD improves their behavior, attentiveness, energy levels, performance in school, and growth and development. It can correct nighttime bedwetting. Of course mouth breathing can also *cause* enlarged tonsils!

Repatterning facial muscles through orofacial myofunctional therapy can significantly improve airway opening. Muscles move everything. Good oral posture can increase oral volume just as poor posture can decrease it!

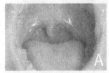

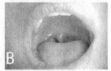

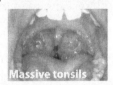

Class I Airway – wide open

Class II Airway – less open

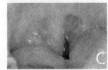

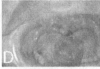

Class III Airway – somewhat closed

Class IV Airway – more closed

A long soft palate (B, D), long skin tag/uvula at the back of the throat (C), a large tongue D, or large tonsils (above), can partially occlude the airway. Images courtesy of Dr. Brian Palmer.

## Tongue-tied

Were you the only person at a party who couldn't tie a knot in a cherry stem in your mouth or do you have trouble licking an ice cream cone? If so, chances are you are what is called tongue-tied. A tongue-tied person is unable to move his tongue freely because the vestigial embryonic tissue fold under the tongue holds it too tightly. It may appear as though the tip of the tongue is heart-shaped when raised, or a depression at the back of the tongue will form, when extended fully out of the mouth. It was once common to help these babies after delivery with a simple tool called a tongue-lifter. Sadly, this practice was discontinued, leaving nearly five percent of the population with difficulty doing normal things. Being tongue-tied:

- Often impedes successful breast-feeding. It can be painful to the mother because it compresses the nipple against the gum pad instead of the tongue. Forming a seal is difficult and the tongue cannot move as it should to express the milk. A similar tissue fold holding the center of the upper lip can also cause a poor seal and breast-feeding problems. All infants with a tongue restriction significant enough to impact breastfeeding show some signs of reflux, colic, wind, gastric distress or all of the above.
- Usually leads to a reverse or active swallow – the tongue thrust causing the collapsed bites discussed above (narrow jaws and anterior open bite). This swallow can put consistent excessive pressure on front teeth – enough to rock them loose.
- Almost always causes development of a narrow, high palate
- Can cause speech impediments
- Can make it difficult to swallow pills and food
- Can lead to digestive problems because it is hard to chew thoroughly or swallow correctly. Often tongue-tied people swallow too much air. Bloating and reflux is common.
- Can cause teeth to separate or rotate
- Causes partial breathing obstructions that can lead to complications like snoring, sleep apnea, and bedwetting into puberty
- Interferes with kissing

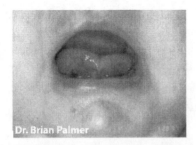
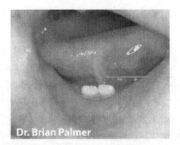

**Left: Tongue-tied three-month-old, weaned because of breast-feeding problems. Note the heart shape the tongue makes when lifted. This is typical of a tied tongue, though not all cases are so obvious.**
**Right: Age 4 months – Note lesion on tissue fold (frenum) caused by teeth.**

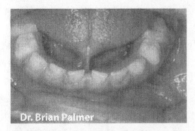
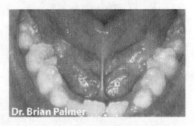

**Left: Same child, age 3: The tissue fold has already caused existing front teeth to rotate. Speech impediments often result.**
**Right: Same child, age 6.5 years**

**Try it:** Place and hold the tip of your tongue into the gum tissue below the lower front teeth. Try to swallow, eat, talk, or kiss with the tongue held here.

## Diet

Many people believe tooth alignment and facial feature formation is all genetically determined. However studies of human skull fossils at the Smithsonian and other leading institutions worldwide show that until 200 years ago, the number of people whose teeth fit together incorrectly was less than one percent. Skulls 200 years old and older also show fully developed, wide dental arches. Therefore today's malocclusions cannot be genetic. One explanation is that baby bottles and pacifiers were introduced about two hundred years ago.

Weston Price, the first President of the American Dental Association, and a well-respected researcher, proposed our diets are to blame. Dr. Price chronicled nutrition's role in the development of poor facial features and tooth misalignment. Specifically, he photographed the drastic facial changes that occurred to people of indigenous cultures occurring within one generation of beginning to barter with westerners. Records show that about ninety percent of the time, these people, used only to their native foods, bartered for sugar and white flour. Within one generation, people whose birthright was perfectly formed dental arches, showed terribly misaligned teeth. Images and a full discussion are available on the Price-Pottinger Nutrition Foundation web site.[10]

## "Four on the Floor" Extraction Orthodontics

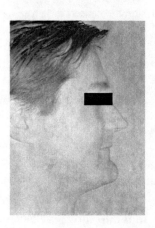

Several generations of orthodontically treated people share a similar profile, often called the silver dollar smile. This man is handsome, but he did not have to have this profile. His chin is too prominent, his nose is somewhat pointed, and he has unremarkable cheekbones. His profile almost looks like an old man with no teeth. This profile arises when dentists extract four teeth prior to orthodontics, and then pull the teeth backwards. (Image: Reed Dana/ Dana Orthodontics)

Many orthodontists now consider this practice does more harm than good. They know it may lead to a nicer smile but a less attractive face. Those who instead help grow attractive faces through early intervention, have clients whose results show more pronounced cheekbones, longer jawbones, wider smiles, and fuller lips. Even better, a clearer airway helps them breathe better. Their heads line up over their spines without the forward head tilt that helps open the airway. Overall posture is better.[11] Sleep apnea is less likely.

Once recognized, these dysfunctions can be treated. Early treatment, while the bones are more plastic, brings the best results.

---

10 http://www.ppnf.org/catalog/ppnf/price.htm.
11 To To view a 60 Minutes (Australian version) story about the negative consequences of extraction orthodontics, go to: http://www.youtube.com/watch?v=VvqndYJRniI.
Also: http://www.youtube.com/watch?v=OAITgloDeAU
And: http://www.youtube.com/watch?v=oKMu38k8SBk&NR=1

## Early Action Parents Can Take

Watch your child for:

- **Flattening of the cheeks or unusual mouth shape**. These conditions almost always worsen. Look for dark circles under the eyes and slumping shoulders.
- **Hanging the mouth open**. This is probably the most important single factor determining facial growth. Open mouth postures cause the face to grow down to such an extent that a child may have trouble closing their lips at all. Once this happens, it is very difficult to correct by means other than by surgery. Try to persuade your child to keep their mouth closed at rest.
- **Adverse Growth**. Downward, vertical facial growth sets the jaw back and restricts throat size. To breathe more easily, the head tilts back. Drop your jaw an inch and you will see why. To restore spinal balance, the neck tilts forward. This unbalances the whole vertebral column. Osteopaths, physiotherapists and chiropractors know this is a common cause of headaches, neck aches, and long-term back trouble. This also contributes to clenching, jaw joint problems, and accompanying headaches. Measure from chin to bottom of the nose while at rest, then with a lip seal. If the difference is more than 3mm, a person continues to remodel the face, jaw joint, and airway.
- **Sucking Habits**. If your child's face does not look quite like other children, seek advice. Sucking habits of any kind, or swallowing with the tongue showing, can also distort the teeth and jaws, and may eventually cause a speech impediment. Remember the only forces that guide teeth into position are the lips, the cheeks, the tongue, and the other teeth. Any faults in these will be reflected by irregularity of the teeth, followed later by facial disfigurement.
- **Spaces**. At the age of five there should be spaces between the front teeth. Their permanent successors, which arrive at about age six, are much larger. If there is insufficient space, they will crowd. It is easier to prevent crowding by creating space than to correct it afterwards.
- **Crowding**. If the lower front teeth are crowded at six years of age, do not adopt a 'wait and see approach'. At the very least, your child may need to improve his mouth posture.

- **Unattractive Eyes.** If the top jaw grows down, the eyes look prominent and the outer corner of the eyelids will sag. Beyond making the child look tired with too much white-of-eye showing, the lower eyelid will develop a ridge rather than slope smoothly into the cheek.
- **Weak Chin.** Check your child's profile to see the position of the chin. If their mouth is open a lot, the chin is likely to be set back and they will have a double chin.
- **Prominent Chin.** Children who fidget or are overactive, may suffer from too much lower jaw growth, even more so if they stick their jaw forward and work it from side to side. Excessive jaw growth can be very difficult to correct when they are older.
- **Excessive Gum.** You will notice the most attractive people do not show a lot of gum when they smile. The more gum that shows, the less attractive the face. If a young child shows a lot of gum, their face is growing downwards.
- **Speech.** The tongue should be in the palate for most sounds. If it protrudes sideways or forwards between the teeth, the teeth are likely to become displaced. A lisp usually indicates the tongue is between the teeth. The lips should come into contact between most syllables. Ask your child to count to five and see how far apart their lips are after the 'five'. If more that 3mm apart, there is a moderate problem; if more than 7mm a severe problem.
- **Eating Habits.** Many children avoid hard foods. This allows their muscles to become weak and can be a principal cause of vertical growth. These habits often develop when a child is first weaned, try to encourage your child to chew unpureed solid foods starting at six months. Read the book, *Baby Led Weaning* and enjoy YouTube videos on the subject.
- **Where should the teeth be?** To measure the correct position of the upper front teeth, put a pencil mark on the most forward point of the nose, and measure from that point to the edge of the upper front teeth. Ideally it should be 28mm at the age of five and increase one mm each year until puberty, when it should be 38 to 42mm for a girl of sixteen, and 40 to 44mm for a boy of seventeen. If it is more than five millimeters over this, there will be some irregularity of the teeth and disfigurement of the face, and if more than eight millimeters the child is certain to grow up with a less attractive face than they should. Know

that upper teeth are almost never too far forward relative to the rest of the face. It is the lower jaw that is too far back that makes the upper teeth appear to be too far forward! (See video links available on www.mouthmattersbook.com.)

- **Allergies.** Allergies, blocked noses, and enlarged tonsils can start soon after birth as a response to tiny dust particles and other pollution, becoming increasingly common. Children born when pollen counts are high tend to have more hay fever.

  House dust is one of the most common allergens. If newborn is exposed to high dust levels, their immature immune system may overreact. If formula-fed, they lack the protective immunoglobulins of mother's milk. Infants can become permanently sensitized, not only to the original agent, but also to other concurrent foreign proteins such as dairy products and gluten. Allergies to these are far more common than they once were. Never leave an infant in a dusty atmosphere. Consider using an ionizer in the home to precipitate allergens to the ground. Vacuum when the child is elsewhere.

Remember, blocked noses lead to open mouth postures. Mouth breathers continue to experience facial changes throughout life. Depending on the extent of mouth breathing, the chin may continue to become more recessive, bringing the soft tissue drape of the cheeks and nose downward. This can pull the cartilage of the nose downwards, making it appear as though there is a bump in the nose where the nose becomes bony. Tilting the head in an unconscious effort to open the airway may mask some of the downward and backward growth occurring. This results in a forehead that slopes backward, but the chin does not appear as recessive.

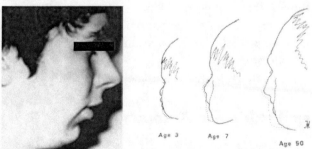

Age 3          Age 7          Age 50

**What will this young man look like in 35 years? How well will he breathe and sleep? (Images courtesy of Dr. Brian Palmer)**

## Sleep Disturbances in Children

As you can see, sleep apnea does happen to children and it has serious repercussions, such as impaired intelligence and nervous system function. The results can be difficulties in concentration, restlessness, behavioral problems, occasional daytime sleepiness and decreased school performance. Children with sleep disturbances are often well below their peers in terms of height and weight.[xx]

Look for:

- Louder breathing at night as opposed to distinct snoring, though there is occasional snoring
- Hyperactivity/ADHD
- Frequent upper airway infections
- Developmental delays
- Poor concentration
- Restless sleep
- Increased need to go to the bathroom at night or bedwetting
- Increased sweating
- Nightmares or night terrors during which time the child seems to awaken, but he or she is not fully awake; sleepwalking, sleep talking, or leg cramps
- Mouth breathing
- Headaches
- Obesity
- Large tonsils
- Chronic runny noses

Watch to see if the shoulders or chest rise and fall during relaxed breathing – they should not. It is the diaphragm that should control breathing, drawing air to the bottom of the lungs. There should be no outward sign audible or otherwise, that someone is breathing when no allergies are present.

Make all efforts to discover and eliminate allergy sources.

## Sleep Disturbances Throughout Life

The primary sleep disturbance dentists treat is obstructive sleep apnea (OSA). Obstructive sleep apnea is any pause of ten seconds or more in breathing during sleep because of a narrow or blocked airway.[12] A loud snort and gasp ends the event as respiration resumes. The pauses allow excessive carbon dioxide build-up in the blood. Blood oxygen levels fall. Severity of sleep apnea is based on the number of events per night and the degree of oxygen desaturation. Those with severe apnea have less than 80 percent oxygen saturation. They also have low levels of NO, and heightened levels inflammatory messengers and clotting factors. White blood cells become sticky.

Low oxygen levels switch on the sympathetic nervous system, that part of the nervous system that clicks into high gear when one's life is at stake. There is a price to pay for constant sympathetic nervous system stimulation. It suppresses the immune system and raises inflammatory markers (TNF and Il-6) and stress hormones. The cortisol released with every event damages blood vessel walls and causes the blood to become sticky. Sticky blood is blood that tends to clot. This partly explains why apnea significantly raises stroke and heart attack risks.

Stress hormones keep the brain aroused, even during sleep. Brain waves are the same as a wakeful person's. A person with apnea may look asleep, but the sleep is non-restorative. Stress also causes blood vessels constriction. This raises blood pressure and can cause morning headaches. Often the heart races. These processes can lead to heart failure. If someone you know is on several blood pressure medications, yet blood pressure is still too high, consider that they likely have obstructive sleep apnea.

Sleep apnea can cause:

- Heavy snoring
- Poor blood sugar control
- Irritability or fatigue
- Mood swings or depression
- Decreased sex drive, loss of intimacy, impotence
- Relationship problems, since it disturbs a partner's sleep
- Excessive daytime sleepiness
- Greatly increased risk of motor vehicle accidents
- Short-term memory loss, intellectual deterioration
- Increased appetite, inability to exercise, rapid weight gain
- Reflux - GERD
- Restless sleep

---

12 Sleep apnea is not the same as primary snoring. Primary snoring may be loud, but there is no change in air flow. Nonetheless, 30-50% of snorers have sleep apnea.

- Severe anxiety
- Dry mouth upon wakening
- Mouth breathing
- Clenching/grinding teeth at night
- Waking up at night in a sweat
- Frequent urination at night
- Morning headaches because blood vessels in the brain are constricted. In the rest of the body, blood vessel constriction reduces the transport of minerals and other nutrients our bodies need to function.
- Death. Sleep apnea takes years off life expectancy. Sixty to eighty percent of strokes are due to apnea.

When asked about the causes of heart attacks, most people would suggest either obesity was a primary factor (obesity raises risks 7.1 times) or high blood pressure (high blood pressure grants 7.8 times the risk). However someone with sleep apnea has 23.3 times the risk of having a heart attack compared to a person without apnea, even after adjusting for age, body mass index, high blood pressure, smoking, and cholesterol levels.[xxi] Sixty-five to eighty percent of patients who have had a stroke have sleep apnea, predominately obstructive sleep apnea.

## Causes of Sleep Apnea

*The tongue can be a six hundred pound tiger in a three foot cage.*

~ Felix K. Liao, D.D.S.~

So, what are the risk factors for obstructive sleep apnea? Of course obesity tops the list. But tooth misalignment ranks at the top, right along with obesity.

We have already seen how mouth breathing, swallowing habits, being tongue-tied, and having a retrusive chin or enlarged adenoids and tonsils changes facial features and constricts the airway. So how does tooth grinding and clenching fit into the scenario?

Those who have flat and elongated facial characteristics, whether from extraction/retraction orthodontics, or whether they simply have a compromised arch form and all that results from it – have lower jaws that reside too far back. This not only causes uncomfortable jaw joint compression, it also makes the lower jaw relax too far backwards into the airway during sleep. The tongue, being tightly attached to the lower jaw at the center of the chin, falls back with the jaw and impinges on the epiglottis. This obstructs the airway.

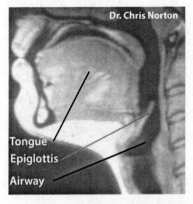

Oddly enough, clenching at night is one way to bring and keep the lower jaw forward to open the airway. It is an adaptive mechanism that pulls the tongue forward and away from the throat. This cutaway image shows how little the tongue must fall back to threaten the breathing by pushing on the epiglottis. Pulling the lower jaw forward is one way emergency responders open the airway to begin cardio-pulmonary resuscitation.

Males with a 17 plus inch neck and females with a 16 plus inch neck have increased risk for sleep apnea. If your profile is similar to this man's, from your chin to the base of your neck, it is likely you have obstructive sleep apnea. It is not just the neck circumference that puts one at risk; it is that it would take very little backward jaw movement during sleep to block the airway.

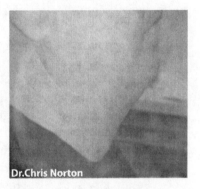

It is tragic OSA is so under-diagnosed because not only do people with OSA spend significantly more time and money on health care than others for at least ten years before they are diagnosed, but as with all chronic diseases, they suffer substantial damage to end organs prior to diagnosis. Ninety-five percent of those with OSA are undiagnosed.

## Diagnosis

Dentists can order formal sleep studies, bill medical insurance for their work, employ home monitoring equipment to screen for sleep apnea, and are in the best position to diagnose sleep apnea. Less expensive alternatives to a formal sleep study are the home study machines that correlate well with those results. Two excellent examples are the Remmers Sleep Recorder and the Ares Unicorder by Watermark Medical, my personal favorite.

For example, the Ares Unicorder measures: oxygen saturation within 0.1%, pulse rate, airflow, snoring, respiratory effort, head position and movement (helps determine the influence of position on the severity of the apnea and is useful in making treatment decisions), sleep and wakeful periods, REM and non-REM sleep, the number of apnea/hypopnea events per hour (during which there is a 4% oxygen desaturation), and the number of respiratory disturbances per hour (during which there is a 1% oxygen desaturation/desaturation event and at least one behavioral arousal indicator).

## Solutions

Who treats sleep apnea? Just about everyone in medicine. The treatment you receive depends on which kind of practitioner you seek.

- Television and the internet can inform you of adjustable beds, pillows, supplements, and prescription medications. Raising the head of the bed is a good partial strategy because the lower jaw will more likely fall down rather than back. Because the tongue is tightly attached, if it slides back, it closes off the airway. Breathe-right strips help open nostrils.
- Chiropractors offer nutrition and adjustments.
- Psychologists offer counseling.
- Pulmonary specialists most often treat sleep. They usually offer the infamous gold standard for treating apnea, the C-Pap machine. This machine is so unwieldy, compliance is extremely low. These are not always titrated correctly. Go to: http://doctorstevenpark.com/. Click on the Borelli interview.
- Ear, Nose, and Throat specialists offer tonsillectomies for younger patients and polysomnograms for mature patients – followed by tonsillectomies, septoplasty, turbinate surgery, hyoid surgery, and a few more surgeries.
- Oral surgeons often remove the skin tag that hangs at the back of the throat, along with other tissue, but it is usually minimally successful. For one thing, it addresses the obstruction too far forward. Remember, blockage most often happens when the tongue falls back into the airway. Other surgeries move the chin forward and sling a particular bone (the hyoid bone) forward in a very messy surgery. Sometimes the jaws are sectioned and moved around.

- General dentists offer non-surgical methods that can treat sleep disordered breathing, including mild to moderate obstructive sleep apnea. Typical devices move the lower jaw forward or act to keep the tongue from falling up and back. These devices are now considered the first treatment for mild to moderate sleep apnea. Teeth almost always shift and over time, the upper jaw may become smaller, but they have helped people avoid the C-Pap for many years.

Most dental devices are based on the same principals as those used in resuscitation and anesthesia. Air passages are cleared of throat structures, so air can flow freely. Currently some physicians are biased against these devices and insurance reimbursements may be insignificant. On the other hand, they are more physiologically compatible, are less invasive, and far less expensive. Because people like them, compliance is better.

Possible side effects are excess salivation and a temporary change in the bite upon awakening. Some will notice a dry mouth in the morning. There can be some jaw joint discomfort. Those who easily gag may not be able to use them. If these appliances are not chosen with care, teeth can over-erupt, causing a permanent change in the bite. Ideally, devices should cover all teeth in an arch, not just the front teeth.

My favorite, the Full Breath Solution device helps hold the tongue off the airway[xxii] and more importantly, causes no facial remodeling compared to the more common "jaw forward positioners" and some nasal C-paps. Learn more at: http://www.cpapalternative.com/. I became an orofacial myofunctional therapist because I recognize myofunctional therapy can greatly enhance all other solutions – the repatterning of orofacial muscles seems essential in many cases.

A few orthodontists can repair the damage of extraction/retraction orthodontics and play a critical role in permanently eliminating OSA by treating a root cause. Reopening these spaces can reverse one's changing appearance, brought on by old-style care. Often, people need orthodontics or jaw surgeries because they never learned to breathe/swallow/chew correctly and lack proper oral posture. Incorrect oral posture is why so many orthodontic cases relapse.

## Prevention is best:

- Try to breastfeed for at least 6-12 months. If you *must* bottle feed, consider Medela Calma bottles; switch to a cup as soon as possible. The La Leche League provides excellent support.

- Avoid pacifiers and baby bottles as much as possible.
- Eliminate tight tissue attachments that anchor the tongue and lips.
- Ensure an upper tongue rest posture, a correct swallowing habit, and a lip seal. All of these habits can influence facial growth throughout one's lifetime.
- Address large tonsils or adenoids.
- Address allergies.
- Evaluate cranial-sacral therapy in conjunction with orofacial myofunctional therapy.
- If you perceive orthodontics is necessary, find a dentist who practices "full face" orthodontics. These practitioners prefer to start around age four to guide growth and develop the face forward, rather than downward. Properly done, the expansion will open the airway and change posture. Proper forward growth gives a greater chance of having enough room for normal wisdom teeth eruption.

These techniques never involve tooth extraction. One approach is to accomplish an arch expansion, followed by wearing a myofunctional training device and/or a Biobloc for one year minimum when myofunctional therapy is not available.

Some appliances train the tongue tip to be in the correct upward position in the roof of the mouth. A built-in trainer tongue guard only allows swallowing when the tongue body is in the correct position. This forces teeth into the correct arch form. The jaw joint no longer compresses. Lip activity decreases and nose breathing establishes. Again, strongly consider adding myofunctional therapy for maximum benefit. The neuromuscular training for lifetime habituation is superior.[13]

As often happens, traditional orthodontics treats symptoms (crooked teeth), not causes. Results are usually unstable; retention is necessary throughout life. A few dentists in the United States work with adults to correct the TMJ/breathing/apnea problems associated with the "extraction and retraction" orthodontics they had the first time around.

13 Find a practitioner trained through the Academy of Orofacial Myofunctional Therapy (AOMT). http://www.myoacademy.com/ For more information see also: http://www.myofunctional-therapy.com/articles.html and http://www.myofunctional-therapy.com/what-is-myofunctional-therapy.html.

It is not within this book's scope to detail solutions, but some guidance is appropriate. Beyond working with an Orofacial Myofunctional Therapist to correct oral postures, practice Buteyko breathing techniques. Buteyko, a Russian doctor who identified the problems caused by low carbon dioxide levels in the body, designed exercises to slow down the breathing rate, thus increasing $CO_2$ levels in blood.[14] Blood saturation of $CO_2$ involves a brain set point, so it is often necessary to learn to reduce hyperventilation with Buteyko breathing techniques. Or you could just become a didgeridoo master![xxiii] I'll let you figure that one out.

Some choose to work with cranio-sacral therapists or functional osteopaths in addition to orthodontics and myofunctional therapy.

The earlier one receives therapy, the more successful and easy it is. The best time to begin therapy is at age two or three. Intervene when you notice a finger habit, allergy shiners under the eyes, enlarged tonsils, mouth breathing, or a low tongue resting posture. Remember:

- At age 4, 60 percent of the facial growth is complete.
- At age 7, 70 percent of facial growth is complete.
- At age 12, 90 percent of craniofacial growth is complete.

Having properly aligned teeth helps them function without breakage for a lifetime.

The discoveries I made while researching this chapter answered a few puzzling questions I have had over the years. I thought I was a nasal breather, but when I took my Control Pause the first time, I came up short. It led to the realization that I often mouth breath! And though slender, I also have apnea. My daughter did only slightly better – until I expressed my surprise because she has had voice training.

Ah! The lights went on. For a few minutes, she breathed from her nose using her strong diaphragm as she has been trained to do. When she repeated the experiment, she hit the target 40 seconds with no effort.

**Try it:** Count how many breaths you normally take per minute. Your maximum should be from 12 - 17. Those trained in the martial arts or yoga often fall in the range of about four to ten breaths per minute.

---

14 To learn more or find resources, visit www.buteyko.com.

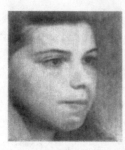
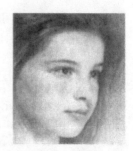

**Left:** This sister had improper oral posture and developed poor facial balance.
**Right:** This sister had proper oral posture and developed good facial balance.
**Images: Brian Palmer**

Kudos to the doctors who have worked their lifetimes to trace the origins of many serious medical conditions, and who work towards their solutions. They graciously donated their time, knowledge, and images to help you become a wise consumer. They are:

- Dr. Brian Palmer (U.S.) and Dr. John Mew (England), researchers/presenters, and primary doctors who developed many of these ideas. Dr. Palmer's web site expands on what you have just read. http://www.brianpalmerdds.com/
- Dr. Chris Norton, McKinney, Texas, (www.fasttraxortho. com) who shared his ideas and power points.
- Dr. William Hang. Dr. Hang's web site has valuable videos to evaluate when you are deciding treatment options. Explore: http://www.facefocused.com/indexb.html. Click on the dropdown menu, "Why Face Focused".
- Dr. Hang guided me to Dr. Brendan Stack, who pioneered treatment of movement disorders such as Tourette's Syndrome with a simple, non-visible dental device. (see it in action at: http://www.tmjstack.com/)
- Dr. Anthony B. Sims similarly treats these disorders with dental orthotics, as well as those with neck and shoulder pain. Dr. Sims studies how dentistry interrelates with many different movement disorders. (http://www.bodymovementdisorders. com. Visit www.mouthmattersbook.com links to these sites and many more.
- Dr. Steven Park, MD. If you are an adult with apnea I strongly recommend you visit the archived experts webinars at: http:// doctorstevenpark.com/expert-interviews. Start with Dr. Joseph Borelli's, his final webinar.

*We inherit mechanisms, not outcomes!*

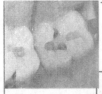

# BEYOND THE DEATH SPIRAL: MODERN DENTISTRY 1908 VS. 1985

*"Accurate decay diagnosis, conservative tooth preparation, and adhesion dentistry can reduce the need for crowns and subsequent root canals by up to eighty percent. When people understand that, they willingly invest in Minimally Invasive, Biomimetic Dentistry."*

**~ Dave Alleman, DDS ~**

## Drill-less Dentistry (1985)

A three-year-old child rests quietly in a dental chair, arms upturned in total relaxation. Back teeth severely rotted, the child's parents have brought him to this clinic because they abhorred the traditional diagnosis/treatment recommended for their child: general anesthetic and unsightly, ill-fitting full stainless steel crowns for his back molars. They had heard of a better way...

The dental team works smoothly in a fifteen-minute, oft repeated choreograph. The assistant maintains eye contact and speaks softly to the child while the dentist behind his microscope silently plies the tools of his trade. Air abrasion powers away most of the tooth decay. A blast of ozone gas to each tooth penetrates deeply to inactivate remaining germ invaders and their toxins. This changes each tooth's internal chemistry to allow rapid remineralization – eventually leading to "petrification" of the lesion. The ozone may also help preserve the pulp's vitality. Next, the dentist paints minerals on prepared tooth surfaces to facilitate the rebuilding. After applying a series of optional resins with today's superior adhesive qualities, a quarter of his mouth is restored!

**Benefits:** A brief, anesthetic-free, relaxed visit for both child and dental team, translates into economical lifetime solutions. Compared with all-too-frequently recommended stainless steel crowns placed while under general anesthetic, natural-colored tooth repairs leave children with higher self-esteem, better function, and pleasant feelings about dental visits.

Welcome to the world of drill-less dentistry!

# Death Spiral (1908)

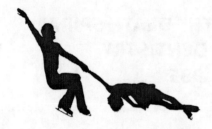

**Death spiral** – noun, (skating term) A dramatic paired skating technique during which, if either partner loses contact with the other, both collapse with possibly dire consequences.

**Death spiral** – noun, (dental term) A destructive dental sequence wherein tooth deterioration is so advanced at time of detection, major repair is necessary – usually using high speed drills to prepare teeth for filling material in designs engineered 100+ years ago. Because this design generally requires breaking tooth sidewalls away from each other, all walls eventually collapse with possible dire consequences.

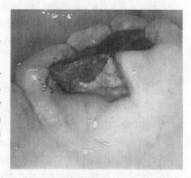

In contrast, the following two images show the rarely seen fragile enamel network that holds teeth together. "Modern" dental techniques usually destroy this webbed network, either with drills or with straight-line lasers. These two, by nature must ignore some of the performance capabilities of the wonderful adhesive resin materials and techniques now available. They never allow the enamel webbing to reveal itself. When intact, the webbing diffuses chewing forces, so teeth hold together. When eliminated, a tooth is doomed to a cycle of breakdown and increasingly complex repair, often ending in death of the tooth and compromised overall health for the owner.

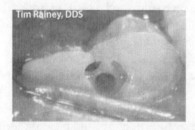

Tim Rainey, DDS

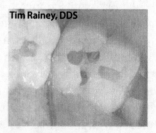

Tim Rainey, DDS

How long does it take research to translate into practice? What does its slow adoption cost you in terms of health and financial reserves?

"Death spiral" is a secret term used by dental professionals who are adverse to the status quo of drilling and filling teeth," write Gutkowski, DiGangi, and Harper in their article, *Economics of the Team Approach: How-to Guide for the Minimally Invasive Dental Practice*. "The tooth enters into a death spiral the first time a drill touches precious enamel. At some point practitioners find their formal education has put them onto the treadmill of repair, restore, and redo until one day it becomes painfully obvious that another filling is not the answer."[i] Cracks lead to failure, infection, re-infection and further failure!

In terms of economic impact on the patient, one of the largest dental insurance providers, Delta Dental, conducted a detailed study on the costs of traditional (drill, fill, and bill mercury/silver/amalgam) fillings with the designs they require. For patients who develop cavities in their molars between ages 7 and 12 and who entered the repair-replacement-repair cycle of traditional dentistry, each tooth required more than $2187 in services by age 79 per initial cavity [2003 dollars]. Lifetime costs increase when a (failing) tooth requires a root canal or extraction and replacement with a prosthetic tooth.[ii]

What about health and "quality of life" costs of broken down or root canal treated teeth? These teeth are generally septic, infected cesspools with which the body's immune system must constantly contend. What happens to the poor when their teeth break down so badly they must shy away from jobs requiring face-to-face contact? One way or the other, drilling into teeth begins a death spiral. This planned obsolescence is no longer necessary or acceptable with the advent of Minimally Invasive Dentistry.

This chapter will illustrate why tooth decay is often diagnosed at the far end of the spectrum and why the predominant filling design used in the United States sets teeth up to fail. This information should no longer be secret. Knowing what follows will help you give true informed consent to whatever dental treatment you choose to receive.

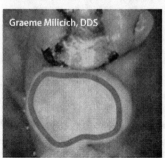
Graeme Milicich, DDS

The elevated rim around the edge of a tooth (overset with a bolded "ring") is like a suspension cable for enamel. It is another stress distribution structure – it transfers occlusal stresses to the root. It too must be preserved whenever possible. Cutting the ridge, as was done on the adjacent tooth, disturbs natural stress relief pathways and concentrates it elsewhere. Future fracturing of the tooth are almost guaranteed. To survive, teeth must be dissected with finesse.

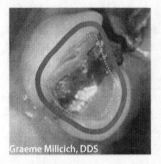
Graeme Milicich, DDS

FLOPPY CUSPS: Once a tooth's stress distribution system (including the peripheral rim – again overset with a bolded ring) is destroyed with a drill following traditional cavity design, it is inevitable the tooth will begin to split just inside the peripheral rim, just as you see in this image. (The dotted line overlies where two kinds of enamel meet – and where enamel delaminates.) You can also see splits developing on the side of the tooth (lower left corner). Eventually, one of the floppy cusps wil break away.

Stripes in this picture represent how a tooth distributes forces placed on it as a person chews or clenches. Increased stripe width shows increased stress. Stress concentration occurs where the fringes are close together.[iii]

Arch architecture, the enamel webbing within molars, and the high organic content of dentin, which makes up the body of a tooth, beautifully distributes chewing stresses to the root.

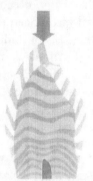
Tim Rainey, DDS

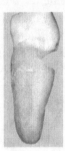

Over time, biting forces cause enough tooth flex and stress concentration at the gum line, that gums recede and "V" shaped tooth pieces break away. Dental professionals used to admonish clients they were scrubbing "back and forth" too hard when they saw these notches. We now know this chipping away is largely the result of clenching. (Refer to Chapter Eleven, "The Nightly Grind.") If you look closely, you can see the fatal fracture developing horizontally across the root just under the notch.
Image: Brian Palmer, DDS

This cross-section shows how traditional filling designs disturb a tooth's natural stress distribution system. The solid line shows another place stresses concentrate – on the enamel shell. The tooth crumbles away in the area represented by the dark void between the filling and the enamel. The wider the filling design, the less force and time it takes to crack a tooth apart.[iv]

An intact tooth can resist 530 pounds of chewing pressure. When a filling preparation removes 1/4 the distance between cusp tips, a tooth resists 333 pounds of pressure; when 1/3 is removed, it withstands only 213 pounds of pressure.

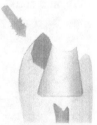
Graeme Milicich DDS

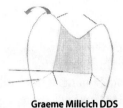
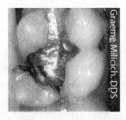
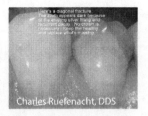

Graeme Milicich DDS

Charles Ruefenacht, DDS

**Above: FLOPPY CUSPS.** Amalgams are never stress-reducing restorations. They are completely incompatible with the crystalline structure of teeth. Just as metal bent back and forth over time will fatigue, so will a tooth's cusps, eventually breaking away at predictable places. The sharp angles created by typical flat bottomed designs concentrate chewing and clenching stresses shown by the dotted lines (left), eventually causing tooth sections to fracture away along that line (center). Additionally, metals expand and contract about a third more than teeth do. This thermal cycling alone causes teeth with this design to fracture. These teeth were set up to fail by design. This traditional design, was originally conceived of in 1879. In 1998, it was declared obsolete.[1]

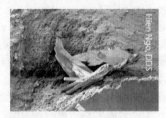
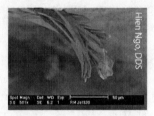

Other damage caused by drilling: Above: Carbide bur edges shatter as they drill through tooth structure and embed in dentin. Below: Scanning electron microscopes show shattered crystalline tooth structure as dental burs touch teeth.

Preparation with a coarse diamond bur initiates cracks in enamel as deep as 84 ± 30µm. Sometimes these cracks propagate.

Dental drills also produce electricity and heat – uncomfortable to a tooth's nerves and the main reason it is necessary to use anesthetic. Heat can also traumatize the pulp.

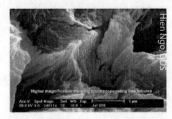
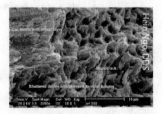

1 Dr. Terry Donovan, Associate Dean and Associate Professor at the Department of Restorative Dentistry at the University of South California made the statement in Auckland, at the Dental Advisory Committee's "A Trilogy In Restorative Dentistry." March, 1998.

## Things Are Rarely What They Seem

"Do I have a cavity?" It would seem an easily answered question, yet most dentists in the United States were not trained to definitively diagnose them – and do not know it. On the other hand, early and appropriate diagnosis is a fundamental standard for those who practice Minimally Invasive Dentistry (MID) correctly. You may not think how the health of your teeth is assessed matters, but as with early detection of any problem, long-term survival and cost savings depend on it.

Traditional dentists use x-rays and a sharp explorer to detect decay in biting surface pits. MID dental professionals call that the "poke and hope" method. They do not rely on these tools because they know they are less reliable than the flip of a coin – correct 25% of the time:

1. 1969, 1987, 1993 – Using a pointed explorer is an unreliable way to diagnose cavities in tooth grooves.[iv] In fact, not only are sharp explorers inaccurate, they "may damage the enamel surface covering early... lesions." [v] Using explorers to detect decay became obsolete in Europe over two decades ago. This has not stopped clinicians in the United States from relying on them to detect end-stage decay.

2. 1996 – Doctors attempting to diagnose decay in tooth fissures using sharp explorers are accurate about 25 percent of the time. Magnification of cross sections from teeth confirmed that 75 percent of the time, seemingly intact enamel surfaces concealed extensive lesions in underlying layers of tooth.[vi]

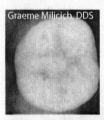

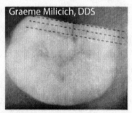

**Left:** A sharp explorer does not stick in the freshly polished grooves of this molar; x-rays show no degeneration.

**Right:** Same molar after air abrasion cleaned out organic material plugging the fissures.

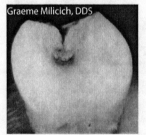

**Left:** To study what can happen in fissures, the tooth above was sectioned in three places, shown by the dotted lines. The image on the left shows the third cross section. Oops!

These kinds of lesions are often sealed to protect seemingly intact surfaces. Improper diagnosis is one reason sealants fail. Graeme Milicich, DDS

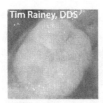

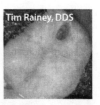

Left: Non-sticky, but visually stained fissure. No signs of decay in x-ray.
Right: The same tooth after air abrasion. Another oops!
Images: Tim Rainey, DDS

3. **1967, 1987** – Additionally, probing restored teeth can be misleading, since a probe may catch in a margin discrepancy that is not in fact [decay].[vii] [This is known as a false positive.]

4. **1967, 1987** – "Probing of root… lesions with a sharp explorer using controlled, modest pressure, may create surface defects that prevent complete remineralization of the lesion." [viii] Based on MID findings since 1987, lesions never completely remineralize anyway. Considering enamel, once the crystalline enamel structure is gone (demineralized), it is gone forever. It may reharden in the presence of fluoride or other minerals, but the now porous structures allow acids to seep through the enamel to continue structural damage in deeper layers. (See point 8.) This is one reason keeping localized plaque off of teeth and a balanced oral pH is important. This is also the first of three ways I introduce, in which decay can happen from the "inside out". Does a focus on remineralizing the outer enamel shell delay diagnosis?

5. **1988** – Decay does not generally show up in x-rays unless it has progressed 2mm to 3mm deep into the softer sub-enamel layer.[ix]

6. **1993** – Typical "check-up" x-rays miss about 23 percent of deep lesions originating in the top surface of molars.

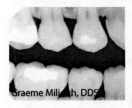

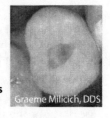

Left: The x-ray reveals no tooth deterioration, yet when the stained fissure was air abraded (right), decay extended nearly to the pulp, the heart of the tooth that keeps it alive and nourished. Furthermore, undiagnosed or late decay diagnosis like this also leads to floppy cusps.

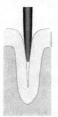

7. **We can always push a probe in hard enough to make it stick.** Depending on explorers to reveal decay sometimes leads to placing fillings in sound surfaces. In these cases, the fissure walls are angled in just such a way as to catch an explorer tip. (Image courtesy of Graeme Milicich, DDS)

**8.** Sectioned teeth examined under microscopes reveal that demineralized or poorly formed enamel, enamel cracks, and other defects in the "protective" enamel surface, allow acids to percolate into subsurface layers. The outer shell of enamel macroscopically appears hard and impermeable, the structural loss is deep within teeth.

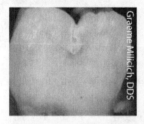 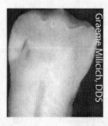 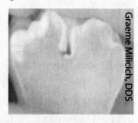

**Left: (The first way teeth decay from the inside out):** Acids seep through porous, cracked, or poorly formed enamel in biting surface fissures. These acids often destroy underlying structure long before traditional techniques detect decay. Left: the fissure is completely closed, yet you can see a triangle of super-white enamel leading into the decaying subsurface layer (dark area). The white wedge represents demineralized (decalcified) enamel. It has no crystalline structure and never will again. This allows acids to percolate into the tooth to erode subsurface layers.

**Center: (The second way teeth decay from the inside out):** Acids have percolated through the super-white demineralized, yet macroscopically intact enamel on the tooth's left side. Note the mineral loss/"decay" in the underlying layer (dentin). Once enamel is porous through to the dentin, the dentin loses minerals. Could hardening enamel with fluoride or other minerals delay diagnosis, allowing for more structural loss?

**Right:** A probe, even if it could enter the fissure, would never detect the crack in the sidewall enamel. X-rays detect nothing.

Complacency about superficial tooth integrity creates a lag in decay identification, allowing an accumulation of undetected decay.

In summary, as MID pioneer Dr. Tim Rainey says, "For anything to be considered within the realm of science, it must be repeatable. If you give ten dentists an explorer and ten patients, the ten dentists cannot agree amongst themselves about where the decay is. Their diagnosis is not repeatable. Further, if they return in a week to examine the same ten patients, they do not agree with their own previous diagnosis. That clearly is not a science!... We know how to fix things but can't agree and are not sure about what it is we should be fixing." [x]

## What About Sealants?

Sealants are still a common dental procedure, but the previous images should give all parties pause. Obviously, without an accurate diagnosis, this practice can hide significant damage for a long time. So, not only is it essential to diagnose fissures carefully before recommending sealants, know only properly placed and maintained sealants placed on mature enamel provide protection. Scanning electron microscope observations of sealant gaps and fractures suggests they fail because their adhesives degrade. Also that gaps and unetched areas may cause failure rates totaling more than 21 per cent after only six months.[xi]

If a sealant is applied to a decalcified area (left image/previous page) or immature enamel, it will not bond properly. A porous tooth allows acids and other fluids to leak under sealants, also causing failure.

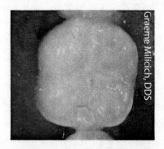 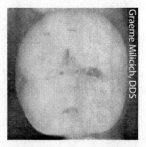

**Left: Twelve-year-old sealant. Right: Sealant was removed, then the area was air abraded and stained with cavity detection dye.**

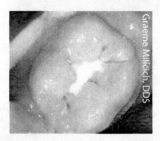 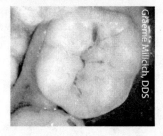

**Left: A sealant was removed from this tooth. Right: Air abrasion and cavity detection dye shows significant decay.**

If you have had sealants placed, frequent, routine check-ups are essential because, as one study says, "*Maintained* sealants provided nearly 100% protection for the tooth over a 15 year period ... As long as the presence of defective fissure enamel is diagnosed accurately and effectively placed, preventive resin restorations are very successful."[xii] [2] This information suggests sealants should not be placed on populations who do not seek or otherwise receive routine care. As stated elsewhere, only half of Americans ever seek dental treatment and of those who do, only half visit routinely.

---

2 Beyond *accurate* diagnosis, MID dentists certified by TIADS use particular techniques and materials for sealants that have proven successful for many years.

Two parting thoughts: Sealant retention is related to each person's incidence of decay. Those patients needing sealant protection most are least likely to have long-term retention.[xiii] Expected rate of sealant loss in permanent molars is 5% – 10% a year.[xiv]

## Minimally Invasive Dentistry (1985)

MID dental professionals are the ultimate preventive specialists. They analyze risk, help clients learn their role in maintaining health, and as we've seen, depend on accurate, early diagnostic techniques. Avoiding the enamel porosity that evolves into hollowed out teeth is a priority. If given the chance, practitioners will diagnose acid conditions and demineralization in its earliest stages and work closely with the client to correct causes. They often perform a saliva analysis including pH, volume, and bacterial DNA signatures, then work with the person to correct imbalances. Good personal oral hygiene, nutrition, oral posture, correcting $CO_2/O_2$ imbalances through breathing exercises, and product counseling are key, as is ozone use.

MID professionals use a stream of high-speed particles to prepare teeth for diagnosis. These particles clear organic plugs from fissures so they can accurately diagnose using new technologies.[3] These technologies aim specific frequencies of light (laser or, more recently, LED) into teeth, then measure the light's reflection and refraction.[4] Some tools accurately detect lesions better than x-rays, even in between teeth.

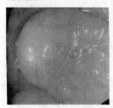 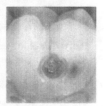

My favorite, the SoProLife's Acteon
Left: A healthy tooth sends a homogeneous green fluorescence signal to a computer screen.
Right: An infected tooth sends a red/dark signal of fluorescence to the screen.

---

3 As researcher Gordon Christianson has said, "In our own research, overt, ongoing dental carious lesions were found under almost all previously placed sealants, with some creating near-pulp exposures. Changes in the sealant technique are desperately needed, including better identification of the presence or lack of caries [decay], [and] much better removal of plaque, stain, and calculus [the organic plug] from occlusal surfaces before sealants." MID dentists know accurate diagnosis is impossible without air abrasion to clear this plug before even attempting to use these new technologies. TIADS-credentialed dentists know how to make sealants work.

4 Kavo, maker of Diagnodent, uses a laser light and is the oldest technology. It measures demineralization only. The Diagnodent does not detect recurring breakdown next to fillings well. LED light technologies are: SoProLife's Acteon,

Early, accurate detection has enormous implications for keeping teeth a lifetime. The sooner problems are noted and addressed, the less invasive treatment can be and the more tooth structure remains to dissipate chewing and clenching forces for a lifetime. MID practitioners use another kind of particle stream to gently remove compromised tooth structure, called air abrasion. Air abrasion is important for several reasons:

1.   Air abrasion is gentle to tooth structure – it doesn't micro-fracture or heat teeth as burs do. Bur wobble initiates tooth cracks. Heat can damage the pulp that keeps teeth vital.

2. Air abrasion is initially selective for compromised tooth structure. In skilled hands, the enamel webbing that dissipates forces can be left intact. Aluminum oxide is the typical currently used air abrasive particle. Bioactive glass (Sylc/NovaMin®) is even more selective for decay.

3. Anesthetic is rarely necessary when warm water is used in parallel with the tiny abrasive particles. A low pressure particle stream is another way the procedure stays comfortable.

4. Smooth air abrasion preps are cleaner. They form superior bonds to dental materials.

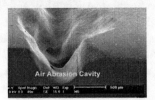 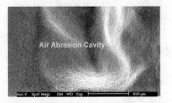

**Air abrasion creates softly contoured filling preparations. The procedure does not create the sharp angles that concentrate forces – the forces shown to predispose teeth to breaking. (Images: University of Ohio.)**

Biomimetic dentists have solutions for teeth that have previously undergone traditional dentistry. These are the teeth whose enamel webbing or rim around the biting surface have already been destroyed and the tooth has broken down as a result.

---

Midwest's Caries I.D., and Airtechniques' Spectra. The principal behind the first two LED technologies is that healthy, affected, and infected enamel all have different optical signatures, so light reflects back differently. Airtechniques' Spectra looks at a byproduct of specific bacteria associated with dental decay. In rebuttal to that concept,  MID inventor/promoter Tim Rainey, DDS says, "We are ... misguided by the misconception that streptococcus mutans [a common oral bacteria implicated in decay] must be present in order to have dental decay. [To do so] makes up criteria for disease and sets up a premise that assumes everyone agrees that without streptococcus mutans, you do not have disease."

## Mimicking Nature: Biomimetic Dentistry

Face it. Most of us have at least a few teeth operating with compromised strength because they received traditional dental therapy. You just read of the late diagnosis typical of traditional dentistry and how dated filling designs cause teeth to break apart. This allows bacterial entry, which can then hollow teeth long before anyone suspects a problem. It can also lead to irreparable fractures and tooth loss or health-compromising root canals.

Dental schools still teach – and dental state board exams still test – traditional, mechanical dentistry. Mechanical dentists drill holes and fill them, or as these repairs fail, cut teeth down to accept full coverage crowns. Is placing these large crowns our only choice?

No! About five percent of dentists have followed the science on these subjects and moved to Minimally Invasive Dentistry and when necessary, biomimetic adhesive dentistry. Biomimetic dentists specialize in helping teeth survive late intervention. They make advantageous use of the advanced ceramic materials and adhesive technology that have been available over the last quarter of a century.

As David Alleman, an early pioneer in biomimetic dentistry explains, biomimetic dentistry treats weak, fractured, and decayed teeth in a way that keeps them strong and seals out bacterial invasion. They employ pre-stressed, pre-fabricated inlays and onlays – and resins. Resin material cannot just be "blobbed" in. Biomimetic dentists rebuild a tooth so its walls are connected from side-to-side, front-to back, and top-to-bottom. The new materials and special techniques allow a tooth to move and flex the way a tooth is supposed to.[5] This eliminates the need for up to 90% of crowns and future root canals.

"Instead of simply filling cavities as though they were potholes, biomimetic dentists ensure the *dental work* will fail in a repairable way, rather than letting teeth fail. Carefully placed repairs last far longer than traditional repairs. Many people most appreciate biomimetic dentistry because these special techniques nearly always eliminate post-treatment discomfort!"

---

5 Forces applied to teeth are similar to those buildings experience during earthquakes. Appropriate engineering and material use mitigate earthquake hazards. Appropriate engineering and material use also mitigate chewing/clenching hazards to teeth compromised by old-style dentistry. An example of earthquake engineering is the mortar-free dry-stack stone construction techniques used by the Incas. Mortar binds stone in walls so they cannot diffuse the pressure vibrations of an earthquake. They fail and crumble. The stones of dry-stack walls can dissipate energy. They shift and resettle without collapsing. MID dentists engineer similarly. They use a fiber reinforcement material that helps prevent fractures and apply resins in careful interlocking layers that dissipate chewing energy accounting for a principle called C-Factor. They also choose resins that expand and contract similarly to the expansion and contraction rate of teeth. They know how to maximize bond strengths."

MID and Biomimetic techniques taken together prevent fracturing of teeth and filling materials without crowns. Aside from systemic toxicity of mercury fillings (amalgams) and the poor repair designs they require,[6] MID dental professionals know there are other reason these fillings are harmful. Fluid-filled zones form underneath mercury fillings.[7] Chewing forces cause a trampoline-like effect as these fillings compress into the voids. Teeth bulge under the intense pressure. This eventually causes small cracks to form on virgin surfaces in between teeth. When plaque remains between teeth, the microclimate here is acidic. As teeth flex during function, these cracks open and shut, pumping acids into the teeth. This eventually causes tooth failure. Similar cracks can develop on teeth with resin (white) fillings not done using biomimetic techniques or materials.

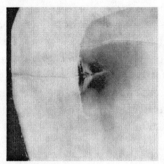

Left: <u>The third way teeth decay from the inside out</u>: Small crack formed on a virgin surface in between teeth due to the "trampoline effect". Deterioration has occurred deep in the sub-enamel layer. The enamel appears intact both in x-rays and to the naked eye. Again, damage can be 3mm deep into the sub-enamel layer before an x-ray can detect it. Sometimes a part of the tooth is so unsupported it breaks away before x-ray detection.

No salivary repair mechanism contributes to the arrest of these subsurface enamel lesions.

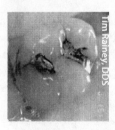

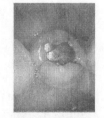

Left and right: Design and material flaws cause teeth to crack. In addition to the obvious cracks, these teeth likely have small cracks in the sides, similar to the above image due to the "trampoline effect".

Late decay diagnosis has the same effect. The loss of so much structure around a fissure allows the tooth to bulge during chewing. Cracks form on the side of the tooth in the same way as mercury fillings do. It is highly likely this tooth also has small cracks on the sides.

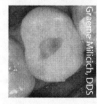

---

6 Just because a dentist has quit using mercury filling materials does not mean they understand MID/Biomimetic dentistry. Most dentists use new materials in old ways.
7 Corrosive alloy by-products from these fillings produce oxides that penetrate decalcified dentin underneath the filling. As the decalcification process proceeds, the metallic ions eventually leave and a "fluid-filled zone" remains.

## Clean Air/Clean Water

Another dirty dental secret: your mouth is not the only place biofilms exist. Biofilms form everywhere there is water. Many dental office water lines are highly contaminated even if the staff uses dispensing bottles with sterilized water and flushes the lines nightly. Recolonization can occur in twenty minutes. Contamination is measured in terms of "colony forming units" or CFUs. The ADA suggests a goal of 200/ml of water. Boil water alerts go out when CFUs exceed 500. Many dental unit lines have between half a million to five million CFUs/ml. Water contamination can occur from either end of the system: the source or the point-of-use. So even if an office uses dispensing bottles as required, they must either ozonate their water or treat it with anti-microbials. I prefer ozonated water because it is alkalizing, it destroys cell wall deficient bacteria, and does not interfere with tissue reconnection, as chlorhexidine can. Dentists must also filter their air source to keep it verifiably oil and contaminant-free. This keeps dental unit air lines from infecting water lines and does not re-contaminate teeth – either with new germs or with oils that contribute to resin filling failure. Clean air/clean water contributes to the quadruple bond strength MID/biomimetic dentists can achieve with their resins.[8] Obviously clean air/clean water also amplifies both surgical and non-surgical dental results.

## Ozone

Ozone is one of the most exciting, versatile tools in the dental toolbox. Not a new idea in medicine, Germans successfully applied ozone to gaseous gangrene wounds during World War I. Used for more than 130 years, oxygen/ozone therapy is the current standard of care in over 20 countries. An inexpensive yet powerful antimicrobial, neither bacteria, nor viruses or fungi develop resistance to it. Ozone is a natural approach to infection control, wound management, and tissue repair. It restores proper oxygen metabolism, increases circulation, and induces a friendly ecology. Oxygen/ozone therapy is fully recognized by the medical community in 14 states.

1. **Do you like the idea of halting or reversing decay?** We know teeth remineralize given the right conditions, but what techniques are predictable? Research shows only unpredictable and less than positive results using chlorhexidine, fluoride, triclosan or other chemical control. What we do know is that teeth are mineral banks – the balance of

---

8 Dentists credentialed by Texas Institute For Advanced Dental Studies, TIADS, must provide verifiably oil and contaminant-free air and water.

minerals into or out of teeth shifts depending on the oral environment. They lose minerals in an acid environment, they gain them in an alkaline environment. Saliva and a tooth's pulp provide all the minerals a tooth needs to stay healthy; we just have to keep the oral environment neutral to mildly alkaline to keep them going in the right direction.

Microbial waste products within teeth create the acid environment (pH 3-3.5) that sustains them and that also dissolves teeth. Ozone gas can penetrate 3 – 5mm into a tooth, killing all the pathogens that have migrated into its miles of tubules *and* neutralizing their erosive waste products.[9] Thus ozone shifts the tooth's internal environment towards a neutral pH. The tooth lesion can then remineralize or *petrify* using minerals primarily from pulp fluids, but also from saliva. Because ozone annihilates both the bugs and their bughouse, it is the only *predictable* way to reverse a decaying lesion.

When ozone is also used selectively in the mouth, friendly microbes begin to predominate. Even when patients do not support therapy with appropriate self-care, it takes months for germ populations to revert to an unfriendly balance. In the meantime, tooth banks are set to receive mineral deposits rather than lose them.

If a person actively seeks health, they support a positive balance by monitoring their oral pH. If saliva consistently tests below 6.8, they detect and address possible causes. Chapter 12 provides a starting point. Taking oral probiotics such as Evora, mechanically removing biofilms daily, and using remineralizing washes and pastes[10] support a permanent terrain change. MID dentists will "gas" a tooth, then paint on Caphasol or its generic to jump start the remineralization process. A 20 nm hydroxyapatite nanoparticle that actually can recrystallize demineralized tooth structure is now available and is introduced in Chapter 16.

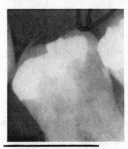
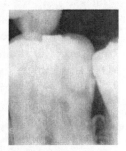

**Left: Deep decay lies near the pulp. Soft tooth material was removed with hand tools and air abrasion, gassed with ozone, then painted with minerals prior to placing a resin filling.**
**Right: Three months later, the pulp is still healthy and the tooth is remineralizing well.**

9 Ozone denatures the protective protein coat that protects germs from pharmaceutical products and the immune system.
10 I encourage my cavity-prone clients to brush every night with straight baking soda, *not* baking soda toothpaste, then use Carifree's baby toothpaste, CTx3 Gel, in the morning. The slightly acidic pH in the morning helps minerals precipitate into the tooth. This children's version omits fluoride.

**Example:** Noted English ozone expert, Professor Lynch and his group showed ozone successfully treats root decay. "The tooth's lesion is exposed to ozone for a period of 40-60 seconds. It is a sort of ozone "hurricane" based on a low ozone concentration... This treatment appears sufficient to kill all microorganisms present." His studies also show the "ozone sterilized dental surface can be quickly (about an hour) remineralized by the calcium phosphate present in saliva, thus becoming hard and resistant to further bacterial attack for at least three months." [xv] Also, important decay-causing germs cannot stick to an ozonated root.

A study by Julian Holmes showed ozone gas application reversed 69 percent of cavities at three months. Repeated applications at three, six, twelve, and eighteen months resulted in 100 percent decay reversal.[xvi]

Usually a MID dentist decides to fill a "pothole" to structurally strengthen the tooth. They know properly used ozone extends the longevity of a dental repair because it increases a resin filling's bond strength to enamel.[11] On the other hand, ozone use without lightly re-air abrading the tooth decreases bond strength.

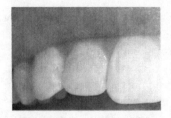

**2. Unhappy with unsightly orthodontic bracket scars? Are you undergoing orthodontic care and want to avoid them?** Acidic oral conditions and poor self-care during orthodontics can leave super-white demineralized lesions that outline where brackets once were. Acids can continue to seep through this de-structured enamel. Ozone therapy can change the structural and optical properties of these lesions. It can also improve the appearance of tetracycline stains. (Mothers who took tetracycline during pregnancy or young children who took this antibiotic while teeth were forming, develop a characteristic brown mottled stain, similar to teeth marking systemic fluoride overdosing.) Ozone treatment during orthodontics is excellent for white spot and decay prevention.[xvii] Make sure bracket bonds are not removed with a drill, which removes precious enamel. Ask your dentist to air polish with Danville's OrthoProphy powder – it is abrasive enough to remove the cement, soft enough not to hurt the enamel.

**3. Are you bothered by cold sores (herpes), oral ulcers, denture sores, or chronic sores at the corners of your mouth?** Ozone gas or ozonated oils

---

11 A glass ionomer base + Ribbond also helps when bonding to dentin or to root surfaces.

will help these heal quickly. Cold sores result from several kinds of herpes viruses that lie dormant within nerve nuclei. When the immune system is stressed, these viruses migrate down the nerve cell and express as "cold sores". Ozone gas not only heals these highly contagious lesions quickly, 65% of the time, they never return! The implications are enormous. Chronic red sores often appear at creased mouth corners. These creases stay moist, therefore welcome fungal proliferation. Ozonated oils can heal these. Be aware these oils can dry the skin; I dilute them. Assure yourself that iron deficiency is not to blame for dry, red areas at mouth corners.

**4. Are your teeth temperature sensitive?** Even in the absence of disease, teeth can be temperature sensitive. As fluids move within tooth tubules, they stimulate the nerves within. Ozone gas applied to root surfaces switches off the painful nerve conduction by clearing the tubules of microbes and their toxins. (See the root canal section below.) This allows minerals to penetrate the tooth deeply to seal it as described in the tooth remineralization section above.

**5. Are you prone to oral yeast infections?** If so, it is likely that is not the only place yeasts thrive. Your body is operating way outside the wellness curve. Address pH issues as best you can including breathing. Ozonated oils can help eradicate oral yeast infections. If you wear a dental prosthetic, have your dentist bag it and gas it with ozone. Alternatively, you may put a thin layer of ozonated oil on the surface for about ten minutes to deactivate the yeast DNA. You must treat your denture and your mouth at the same time so these areas don't re-contaminate each other.

**6. Do you want whiter teeth?** Yellowing teeth arise from many sources. Tea, coffee, smoking, red wine and iron supplements are well-known culprits, but did you know AGEs, inappropriately heated oils (refer to the nutrition chapter) chlorhexidine, antibiotics, anti-fungals, and enzyme inhibitors all form brown-colored pigments? For predictable, fast results with minimal to no sensitivity, a trained dentist can apply a bleach, and then activate them with an ozone gas tray. Ozone breaks down the AGE products bacteria liberally produce into hydroxyl ions.

**7. Do you have implants?** Topically applied ozonated oil improves bone density around implants and the quality of their integration into the jawbone.[xviii] They also help keep tissues around implants healthy. If an implant supports a partial or denture, non-silicone gaskets will degrade more quickly, though most current gaskets are made of silicone.

**8. Have you taken "bone-sparing" drugs like Boniva, Actonel, Aredia and suffered the osteonecrosis discussed in Chapter Seven?** Treating osteonecrosis has been frustrating, at best. Surgery often worsens bone exposure and hyperbaric oxygen therapy is controversial. In a study to learn if ozonated oils could help heal osteonecrosis, the researcher's results were phenomenal. "Complete clinical response with resolution of all the damage was achieved in all patients. Complete response was achieved after three applications of $O_3$ oil in three patients, four applications in four patients and 10 applications in three patients, with a mean recovery time of 27 days."[ixx] There were no adverse effects. Other studies have shown excellent results in two months using ozone gas injections into the wound, weekly nasal and ear insufflation with ozone gas, and daily rinsing at home with ozonated water and ozonated oils and taking the nitric oxide producing supplement called Neo 40. Beyond healing, ozone also takes away the associated pain and stinging of osteonecrosis. Women taking bisphosphonates who must undergo extractions or other dental surgery would greatly benefit from pre- and post-surgical ozone therapy.

**9. Do you suffer from allergies – or acne?** Those with low carbon dioxide saturation often have allergies – and acne. Remember the mouth-breathers from the previous chapter? They blow off too much carbon dioxide. Insufficient carbon dioxide lowers hemoglobin's ability to release oxygen. Deprived of oxygen, cells and organs malfunction.

Ozone is also a biological immune system activator. It upregulates critical antioxidant enzymes like superoxide dismutase (SOD) and reduced glutathione. Allergic-autoimmune diseases such as psoriasis, asthma and rheumatoid arthritis improve. Ozone prevents super infections and stimulates cell proliferation and formation of white blood cells and other healing factors.[12][xx] For these reasons, ozone is also fast becoming a trendy skin rejuvenation adjunct. It benefits those with acne, scarring, or burns.

**10. Gum Disease. Dreaming:** We dream that soon, every client in our practice will have a custom ozone tray. A customized tray forms a seal around the teeth and gums, but leaves a small void around the teeth and surrounding gums. It has an "in" and an "out" port. Ozone suffuses both teeth and gums. These trays allow ozone to saturate all the teeth and gums at the same time. You read about the benefits to teeth and how it modifies the oral environment to make it inhospitable to parasites,

---

12 Fibronectin, collagen III/I, hyaluronic acid, fibroblasts, keratinocytes, and chondroitin sulphate

fungi, and unfriendly bacterial populations. You know microbes enter your circulation via the pockets around your teeth as you go about your daily life. You know "cleaning" procedures create an enormous bacterial shower into your bloodstream.

Now, imagine eliminating that shower by first using either ozone trays or ozonated oil within your pockets. Imagine also having your pockets rinsed with ozonated water as it runs through your hygienist's ultrasonic cleaning tool.

Infected tissues are always acidic. Ozone, being negative, is attracted to the positive charge acidic tissues always give off. Not only does ozone kill the microbes and deactivate their toxic wastes near and within teeth, it alkalizes the chemistry in the gum pockets, painlessly dissolves the bacteria-infested tissue lining the pocket, stimulates a localized immune response that speeds healing time, and powers up fibroblast production so tissues can reconnect to the tooth if necessary.

## Toxic Teeth: What About Root Canals?

Killing virulent germs in inaccessible places is a cornerstone of successful dentistry. MID/Biomimetic dentists are particularly aware of these issues, so it is natural they are early adopters. They know front teeth have at least three miles of microscopic tubules to "sterilize". Tubules are the highway through which nutrient-rich fluids pass from the central pulp to the outer tooth surface to keep teeth nourished and hydrated. As mentioned elsewhere in this text, rendering teeth sterile is a necessary objective of a root canal procedure. It would be the only way to keep a dead structure within a live body without medically challenging the host. Convoluted canals and microscopic tubules have made that task impossible until now.

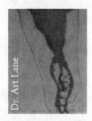
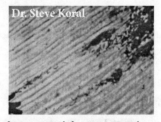

**Left: Difoti transillumination shows partial cross section of a root, demonstrating how convoluted a tooth's main canal can be. Standard root canal therapy hasn't a chance of reaming out, much less appropriately filling and sealing the contents of these canals. Traditional sterilization is equally impossible. Right: High magnification shows bacterial infiltration into dentin's microscopic tubules. Longitudinal view.**

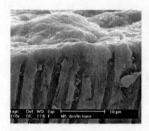

Left: Scanning electron microscope shows a longitudinal view of the miniscule tubules within a tooth's sub-enamel layer. The three miles of tubules in a front tooth have been impossible to sterilize until now.
Right: Cross section of a tooth showing some of the minute tubules radiating out from the central pulp.

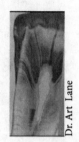

Dr. Art Lane

MID dentists feel if a client insists on saving a tooth at all costs, even if it includes having a root canal, that ozone gas therapy is essential for initially sterilizing the tubules. Ozone gas can permeate these microscopic channels, killing even cystic spirochete forms. [Treponema denticola, a major spirochete implicated in gum disease, is also associated with severely infected tooth pulps. This pathogen has been found in the spleen, heart, and brains of those with root canal infections.[xxi]]

Whether tubules stay that way is the subject of lively debate. Biological dentists suggest that though a root canal treated tooth is sealed at the tip, nothing seals the tubules. Normal fluid flow within live teeth transports nutrients from the blood stream into the tooth's pulp chamber, then through the micro-tubules within the body of the teeth, the enamel, and finally out into the mouth. Sugar intake, among other processes, reverses this fluid flow.[xxii] The reversed flow draws microbial endotoxins into the tooth from the pocket and periodontal ligament. In the same way these miles of tubules in a dead tooth act as a toxic sponge for pathogens and their end products. They incubate within the tooth, their waste products build; both escape to cause serious health threats to the host. This theory is based on the works of doctors Weston Price, George Meinig, Thomas Levy and others. The good news is that early diagnosis and other MID/Biomimetic practices save teeth from the need for root canals. Using ozone gas during even routine repair procedures also helps challenged pulps survive in the first place.

On the other hand, some sincere biological dentists abhor the practice of pulling septic teeth. If a person appears to have no autoimmune medical issues, they offer root canals as an acceptable extraction alternative. They understand sterilizing the tubules with ozone gas before sealing off the pulp chamber(s) as best they can increases chances of success. They reason if a person later develops an autoimmune disease, root canal treated teeth can be extracted, the socket gassed with ozone, and the blood treated with ozone to help reverse any health issues precipitated by toxic teeth. Keep in mind: Once a tooth has undergone a root canal, it lacks the hydrated organic material that helps a tooth stay flexible. Cracks form with just one third the force that would make a hydrated tooth crack.[xxiii]

## Ozone Safety in Medicine

Many people question ozone's safety. Julian Holmes provides an excellent response in his courses, paraphrased as follows:

"The Journal of the American Medical Association and the World Health Organization have abstained from publishing research reporting medical benefits of ozone, possibly because the FDA has taken the stance that ozone is always toxic.

The FDA completed four studies in the 1990s. They did not use medical grade oxygen to generate the ozone and only considered damage to lung tissues. The corona discharge generators they used generate ozone from ambient air instead of pure oxygen.

Further, they evaluated surface tissues. In European circles they know that underneath damaged tissues, living tissues produce huge amounts of protective enzymes.[13] Despite their position on medical ozone, the FDA *does* allow food facilities to ozonate food to fight bacteria.

On the other hand, many international peer reviewed medical journals, have published hundreds of articles reporting benefits of medically used ozone for a range of pathology since the 1990s. They include pre-clinical studies, animal experiments, patient case histories, and placebo-controlled blinded human trials and reviews. All draw conclusions that conflict with the current FDA stance.

Those who live in metropolitan areas breathe an alphabet soup of oxidizing acidic gasses that includes ozone, nitrogen dioxide, carbon monoxide, methane and sulfuric acids. Ozone is a measure of these pollutants, not a pollutant itself. In fact, ozone helps clear the air of these pollutants.

There is no argument this mix is toxic to our respiratory systems. This mix is also not pure ozone. Ozone combines with the nitrogen that comprises the majority of atmospheric air. Nitrogen oxides, especially $NO_2$, are plentiful when one generates ozone from atmospheric air. $NO_2$

---

13 Superoxide dismutase, glutathione peroxidase, catalase, and reductase

*is* toxic. Further, $NO_2$ easily combines with water to form nitric acid (HNO3), an aggressive protein destroyer. This explains why moist lungs are particularly at risk from ozone generated from atmospheric air.

In 2000, the prestigious Scripps institute designed a study to see if typical ozone autohemotherapy administration negatively impacted red blood cell enzyme integrity, since there were some concerns that using ozone in this way could cause the cell membranes and their metabolites to degenerate.[xxiv][xxv] They found zero impact by ozone, and encouraged further clinical trials.[xxvi] Studies all over the world excluding the United States confirm this. It seems blood is resistant to ozone's oxidative powers when administered in concentrations less than 42μg/ml. On the other hand, pathogenic organisms in the body die off when subjected to ozone."

Some worry about ozone's oxidation potential in the body. In mammals, ozone makes the antioxidant enzyme system far more efficient. Cells respond to the beneficial oxidative stress of ozone by increasing their production of protective enzymes like superoxide dismutase.

Scripps Institute researchers also discovered that atherosclerotic arteries produce ozone as a by-product of inflammation. [xxvii]

Respiratory tract ozone toxicity cannot be extrapolated to blood because of the huge anatomical, biochemical and metabolic dissimilarities between the two. Respiratory mucosa has a very weak buffering and antioxidant capacity.

Pure ozone in the low concentrations and dose times used in medicine seem not to threaten lungs. New evidence suggests ozone up to about 400 ppm initiates a "preconditioning" response and is not dangerous.

We all know there are problems with how the FDA is run and therefore, how it makes decisions. They would have you believe there is a gold standard for pharmaceutical safety. However in their own 1978 report:

- 1.5 million people were hospitalized by a pharmaceutical side effect
- 140,000 died from prescription drug use

Compare that to a 1980 German Medical Society Report regarding ozone therapy:

- 5.6 million ozone treatments carried out
- 40 cases of side effects (.000007%)… operator generated
- no deaths from ozone ever reported.

Ozone's medical/dental uses are grandfathered in the United States. The medical community determines standards of care for ozone, its purity, and its uses. Frank Shallenberger, MD, president of the American Academy of Ozonetherapy (AAOT), is also a founding member of the International Scientific Committee on Ozonotherapy (ISCO3), whose purpose was to standardize scientifically acceptable ozone practice. The resulting "Madrid Protocol" was signed by the AAOT, and European, and Latin American ozone societies. A key point is that ozone generators meet EU standards to assure the public the ozone product is pure/medical grade. Refer to Appendix IX.

## Other Ozone Uses

Ozone is the third most powerful oxidizer after fluorine and persulfate. It oxidizes at dramatically lower concentration than chlorine and with none of the toxic side effects of chlorine or fluorine. One molecule of ozone equals between 3,000 to 10,000 molecules of chlorine in oxidizing power; it kills pathogenic organisms 3,500 times faster![xxviii]

This is one reason some public and private water treatment systems have converted to ozone. They use it to inactivate parasites, bacteria, and other pathogens, control odor, and to oxidize heavy metals, rendering them safer. **Note:** Ozone converts a naturally occurring element in water, bromide, into its cancer-causing cousin, bromate. Dentists ozonate only distilled water.

Veterinarians use ozone for:
- animal infections/infestations
- operatory odors/surface/water supply sterilization
- wound management
- peritoneal and rectal insufflation

Doctors use ozone for:
- instrument sterilization
- bacterial, fungal, and viral elimination
- lower inflammatory mediators
- major and minor autohemotherapy
- trauma and wound management including damaged ligaments and joints
- pain control; it switches off nerve propagation
- tissue regeneration and healing
- dermatology
- non-healing diabetic sores and ulcerations

Industry uses it for:
- produce and poultry sanitation
- surface sanitation
- bottle and canning sanitation (just as it uses fluoride, but again, without the toxic side effects)
- fish farmers use it to keep fungae at bay and to suppress odors
- odor control in general
- electronic pcb manufacture
- soft drink manufacturing
- bleaching paper and textiles

Hotels and homes use ozone for:
- removal of unwanted odors like fish and cigarettes
- ice manufacture, showers
- handwashing
- food prep
- extended food products life

Public buildings use ozone to:
- sterilize conditioned air
- sterilize unoccupied rooms and spaces
- reduce air-born infections like SARS, tuberculosis, and influenza
- disinfect water supplies and prevent diseases like leagionella

## The Second Millennium

*"Before biomimetic dentistry I used to be a serial pulp killer."*

**~Dr. Pascal Magne ~**

The University of Geneva no longer teaches 100-year-old dentistry. No full crowns, no pins, no posts, no flat-bottomed, sharply angled filling preparations. They teach only Minimally Invasive and Biomimetic dentistry.

In a 2006 article in the Journal of the California Dental Association, Dr. Richard Kao wrote, "Although the concept of evidence-based dentistry appears fundamentally simple and reasonable, clinicians have been slow to implement it... Perhaps as little as eight percent of dental care is justified by peer-reviewed, published and appropriately analyzed dental research." Again, when people know they can avoid of eighty percent of future restorations by visiting doctors who use advanced techniques, they willingly invest.

The faster research clarifies how our bodies function within our changing environment, the further away we operate from a scientific basis. It is safe to say that many practitioners in all professions don't keep up. Others are afraid to think beyond what they learned in school; they are comfortable or afraid to try new things, but weighing new research and acting on it is what defines a professional. None of us will ever know everything. We will not always be right. We must make our best treatment decisions based on current knowledge.

Dentistry has come far. Towards the end of World War I, the U.S. army had to lower its admission standards for army recruits. Early in the war, recruits had to have at least six sets of opposing teeth. By the end of the war, that standard was lowered to fill the army. We owe much to dentistry. In fact, all dental professionals put themselves at great daily health risk. Those who maintain the old ways are at highest risk. We should appreciate all they do for us. But we can and must do better.

Up until now decay has been:

- poorly diagnosed
- has involved tooth amputation with drills
- have put children at risk for brain dysfunction if they undergo multiple episodes of general anesthesia
- has been poorly accepted by the public
- has been poorly executed
- so that the average lifetime of a filling is low...
- resulting in spiraling costs from ever larger and more complicated restorations...
- often followed by either root canals or extractions, themselves a health risk.

We can do better. Today's dentistry, based on the best science, is fast, pain-free, and affordable.

*"The days of "drill and fill" are numbered. Dental drills have had their day. They belong to another era."*
~ Julian Holmes ~

*"The biggest impediment to new learning is old learning."*
~ Albert Einstein ~

Note to dentists concerned about the safety of air abrasion, but interested in it:

- Some dentists worry about compromised lung function as they age should they use abrasive particles. Generally these aware dentists are the same ones who wear respiratory masks for mercury filling removal. Three pertinent points: particle size, shape, and reactivity are what matter. Anything with a ratio of 3/1 in the range of around 5 microns or less can enter and injure lungs. Particles larger than 5 microns never reach lung alveoli; lung cilia beat them out or they are trapped by nasal passageways. The particles used in air abrasion dentistry range from 15 to about 80 microns. Further, manufacturing processes for dental abrasives produce an amorphous shape rather than a crystalline shape. It is the crystalline shape that often has a "J" hook on it, by which means particles could lock into lung tissues – should a particle be small enough to ever reach them.

- Some dentists are concerned the particles contain aluminum, however aluminum oxide is completely inert. The aluminum is so tightly bound that, in the rare instance aluminum oxide is found in nature, it is extracted using one of the strongest acids available, hydrofluoric acid. The acid melts everything around it, but leaves the aluminum oxide (corundum) completely unscathed. See Appendix XII for more information.

- Order an aluminum oxide product low in titanium dioxide. CrystalMark has one with .02%, the lowest I've found. (http://www.crystalmarkdental.com/about.html) Pure aluminum oxide is white by nature. Iron particles impart a brown color to some brands, but do increase abrasivity, thus they cut faster.

- Air abrasion units are available that use a parallel water spray to keep particles from becoming airborne. Alternative units are highly efficient and use much less powder. If dentists are concerned, they might consider what happens when they grind on "feldsparic" or standard porcelain crown material. That produces a *cloud* of dust particles less than 5 microns, much of which is $Al_2O_3$!

Profound thanks to Dr. Tim Rainey, principal architect of Minimally Invasive Dentistry, and the biomimetic dentists Dave Alleman, Pascal Magne, and Simon Delaperi for generously sharing their work.

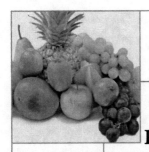

# 14

# FOOD AS MEDICINE

*"If we're not willing to settle for junk living, we certainly shouldn't settle for junk food."*

~ **Sally Edwards** ~

**Explore:**
1. How do American food policies, laws, and farm subsidy programs threaten our health and our freedom to make certain healthy food choices?
2. How does diet fuel inflammation?
3. How does your body manage and store energy via fats and simple carbohydrates?
4. What should you know about saturated fats, omega 3 and 6 fats, trans fats, the modern oil industry, and labeling?
5. Corn fed *what*?
6. Which foods suppress inflammation?
7. CoQ10. Who needs it?
8. Sugars, leptin, insulin and AGEing
9. Fructose metabolism and when to worry about cholesterol levels
10. Sugar addictions and rewiring the brain
11. Celiac disease/gluten intolerance, malnutrition, and nutrient absorption

## Love Your Body, Love Your Life!

Our circulatory systems carry nutrients and toxins to each cell. Because these come from what we eat, breathe, and slather onto our skin, each cell reflects the lifestyle choices we make. Every aspect of our diets influences how we age and whether we fight or succumb to disease. Inflammation is affected by how and when we eat refined carbohydrates, fiber, and various types and amounts of fats, antioxidants, and other nutrients. Foods also influence cancer risks, osteoporosis and help mitigate damage from smoking.

Ultimately, we must be able to absorb nutrients from the foods we eat. Many of us no longer produce sufficient intestinal enzymes to properly break down foods. Others have skewed the balance between beneficial and harmful gut bacteria through poor eating habits. Still others have an undiagnosed autoimmune disease, Celiac Disease, and are unaware that they suffer malnutrition from malabsorption.

Clients diagnosed with one or more degenerative diseases and who are working to improve their health report they experience a cascade of beneficial effects – increased energy, focus and happiness – as they reinvent themselves and their lifestyles. They are amazed at how easy and self-reinforcing these effects are. Degenerative changes stole their health so slowly that early symptoms went unnoticed. They had lost the ability to "listen" to their own bodies, but as health improved, they felt energized and empowered. Dr. Oz – cardiothoracic surgeon, author, and talk show host – calls this phenomenon a "resetting of our brains and bodies." We reset our blood chemistry by what we eat, how we live, and how we think about ourselves, and our place in the world.

As research unveils immune system secrets, we learn what keeps body systems strong. The condition of your mouth absolutely matters, but what you put into it matters more! Depending on what it is and how it is grown, processed, transported, stored, and prepared, food can be powerfully inflammatory or powerfully healing.

It is clear Americans' health is held hostage by the vast changes in food production and delivery that have evolved over the last fifty years. As Dr. Chilton – inflammatory disease expert and author – says, "We are all feeding from a poisoned trough."[i] Highly industrialized agribusinesses produce petroleum-based, genetically modified monoculture crops. Their livestock feeds on commodities grown this way. These foods sabotage our health, pollinator honeybee health, the health of our soils, and our individual and national financial health.

There are alternatives to our current system that can satisfy the market at lower costs in all areas. Small organic farms are successful. The foods from these farms are superior when they are not GMO Round-Up Ready and grown in soil alive with micronutrients and minerals. These soils are built by crop rotation, planting cover crops, incorporating compost, adding minerals, and implementing other organic strategies. The nutrition of the produce and animals raised on these farms reflects the rich, alive soils.

Argentina and Brazil successfully experiment with large-scale solar-based agriculture and rotating commodity crops and livestock. These methods are a return to the farming and soil conservation practices that were successful for thousands of years.

If we seek health, we must care about what we eat and how it arrives at our table. We must care about the laws that govern seeds, food production, distribution, and retailing under the guise of food safety.[1] American consumers and small farmers must fight for the freedom to discuss and publicize their concerns about food production and safety concerns without threat of prohibitively expensive lawsuits.[ii iii] We must demand changes in food policy, especially regarding the products our government chooses to subsidize, if we want our food supply to underpin and complement our health.

If we do not, it may be that only the wealthiest, most motivated, and most informed citizens will be able to stay optimally healthy. Those who understand the dangers of what we have allowed to happen to our food supply know that eating sustainably grown local organic food is key to health. We must work to help our local biodynamic farmers stay viable under proposed food policy and law. With every food purchase, we either vote for change or the status quo. If you buy good food, you choose to invest in lifelong health; if you buy cheap food, you choose to invest in the health care system instead. Make no mistake, this choice will bankrupt the U.S. It is not sustainable.

Regulatory organic food definitions and labeling are not what they should be;[2] in fact, organic regulations continue to be diluted. Until our food production and delivery models change, we must make careful lifestyle choices.[3]

---

1 Bills continuously lay siege to food freedom. Monsanto has patents on many crop seeds and aggressively sues farmers whose non-GMO crops have been contaminated by the inevitable pollen drift from nearby GMO crops. Today, after hundreds of farmers have been sued for patent infringement after Monsanto's patented seeds were found growing where they weren't supposed to, we know how ridiculous such assertions are. Monsanto patent protections also keep farmers from saving seed from current crops to use in future growing seasons. Further, Monsanto has genetically modified some seeds to be sterile, traits that can be passed on to seeds of nearby crops. The repercussions of this may be more disastrous to a region than their patented Roundup-Ready seeds.
2 For instance, crops grown organically and labeled as such, are allowed to be fumigated post-harvest with sulfuryl fluoride, a complex particularly damaging to human health.
3 This critical subject is beyond this book's scope. Learn more about the origins of your food from The Omnivore's Dilemma: A Natural History of Four Meals (Michael Pollan New York: Penguin Books, 2007). Food, Inc., a follow-up movie also introduces the subject. (Food, Inc. Theater viewing. Directed by Robert Kenner. 2009; Los Angeles: Magnolia Home Entertainment.)

## You Are What You Eat

Luxurious hair, radiant skin, and strong nails are products of a healthy, nutrient-filled diet. "Your skin is the fingerprint of what is going on inside your body, and all skin conditions, from psoriasis to acne to aging, are the manifestations of your body's internal needs, including its nutritional needs," points out Georgiana Donadio, PhD, DC, MSc, founder and director of the National Institute of Whole Health in Boston.[iv] The cells of your body repair and replace themselves daily with the foods you eat. Youthful, supple tissues require cellular building blocks like omega-3 fatty acids, niacin, and vitamin E.

Nowhere is that more true than in your mouth. Oral soft tissue cells recycle about every three to seven days, seven times faster than many other tissues, so they require a lot of care and feeding to be healthy. Gums are fed by default. If they are unhealthy, how are the rest of your tissues? If you want to be healthy, start by healing from the inside out.

Defining excellent nutrition is a challenge, yet likely the most critical key in the fight to keep or regain your health. Refer to Appendix X to review immune system support strategies. Remember, it is best to consume vitamins and minerals in whole, natural foods, rather than the fractionated, isolated forms found in supplements.

Foods are inflammatory or anti-inflammatory based on antioxidant value, glycemic index, mineral content (determines if a food is acid- or alkaline-forming) and essential fatty acid ratios between omega-3 fatty acids (like EPA and DHA) and omega-6 fatty acids (like GLA, DGLA and arachidonic acid). The first three are introduced elsewhere in this book, but neither fat oxidation nor fat ratios have been discussed until now. For optimal health and vitality, do not overlook them.

Though detailed fat oxidation and fatty acid profiles are beyond the scope of this book, I must introduce them because fats, particularly saturated fats, have an undeserved poor reputation. It is an absurd notion that all fats are bad for us. We unknowingly choose the wrong ones. Fats are critical to health, but you must understand them in order to benefit from them.

- Saturated fats slow food digestion; they keep you feeling full longer and increase contact time with digestive enzymes so one can extract and absorb tightly-bound minerals, like calcium.
- Fats are a critical internal component of each cell and cell membrane. They comprise roughly half of every cell membrane in your body,

including your brain. Saturated fats keep these membranes stiff, yet flexible. Cell membranes regulate what enters and exits each cell, including nutrients, allergens, toxins, and viruses. What those fats are and whether they oxidize or not makes a tremendous difference in how cells function – or don't function.

- Fats are building blocks for the inflammatory and anti-inflammatory hormones called prostaglandins. The kinds of fats you consume influence how much overall inflammation you will suffer.
- Fats comprise a major part of the protective sheaths around nerves (myelin) and nearly half the dry weight of our brains. The kinds of fats we eat predict brain function.
- Fats carry minerals, vitamins A, D, E, and K and convert carotenes to vitamin A. Without fats your body will not absorb these nutrients. Therefore it is wise to include fats with every meal.
- Butyric acid in animal fats and plant oils help prevent cancer.
- Saturated palmitic and stearic acids normalize cholesterol levels.

Saturated fats, are so important our bodies have the ability to manufacture them. Coconut oil is a good example of a wrongfully maligned saturated fat. Pacific Island populations have almost no heart disease yet thirty to sixty percent of their total caloric intake comes from fully saturated coconut oil.[v][vi] In fact, studies show these populations have excellent vascular health. Another benefit is that our bodies convert coconut's lauric acid into monolaurin. Monolaurin is anti-viral, anti-bacterial and anti-protozoan. Coconut oil has more lauric acid than any other food. Capric acid, another coconut fatty acid, is also antimicrobial.

Essential fatty acids (EFAs) are like vitamins. We must obtain them from our diets because our bodies cannot make them. When we consume alpha-linolenic acid, an omega-3 fatty acid found in flax, leafy green vegetables, walnuts, perilla and linseed oils, we can convert about 10 percent of it into the anti-inflammatory fatty acids EPA and DHA. We consume EPA and DHA in other foods, too. EPA is in fish liver oils and fish eggs. DHA is in human milk, organic egg yolks, fish liver oils, fish eggs, and organ meats.

## The Billion Dollar Highway

Omega-6 fatty acids are more complicated. Corn, soy, cottonseed and safflower oils are rich in alpha-linoleic acid (not to be confused with the anti-inflammatory omega-3 fatty acid, alpha-linolenic acid).

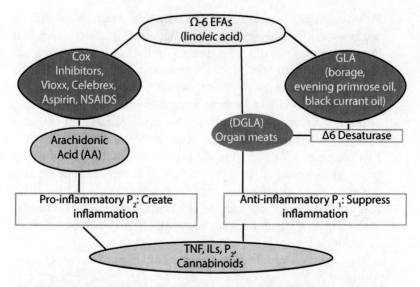

**The Billion Dollar Highway.** Omega-6 fatty acids tend to follow the inflammatory pathway on the left branch of the above chart. This pathway converts omega-6 fatty acids into Arachadonic Acid, a pro-inflammatory molecule that recruits other inflammatory molecules. Ibuprofens like Advil and Motrin, Celebrex, aspirin, and other anti-inflammatory drugs work by interrupting this pathway.
Some omega-6s suppress inflammation. Borage, black currant oil, evening primrose oil (EPO), and the DGLA found in liver and other organ meats are examples. When available, they can divert some of the Ω-6s into anti-inflammatory compounds.

Linoleic acid gives rise to two branches of fatty acids. One produces pro-inflammatory prostaglandins, the $P_2$ series, while the other branch produces *anti*-inflammatory prostaglandins, the $P_1$ series. The $P_2$ pro-inflammatory series is derived from arachidonic acid (AA).

Pharmaceuticals like Vioxx and Celebrex as well as less powerful NSAIDs like ibuprofen and aspirin reduce inflammation by interrupting the AA inflammatory pathway, though not without occasional, unfortunate side effects as we learned when Vioxx was removed from the market. AA breakdown products are also a problem. They create overproduction of an inflammatory mediator, TGF-alpha1, found in fibrotic diseases like liver fibrosis, atherosclerosis and Crohn's disease. This overproduction may also feed colon tumor-promoting events.[vii]

Our bodies do convert a small amount of the omega-6 alpha-linoleic acid we eat into the anti-inflammatory $P_1$ series of prostaglandins. We can also consume these anti-inflammatory essential fatty acids directly. The anti-inflammatory $P_1$ series include GLA, derived from borage, black currant oil, and evening primrose oil, and DGLA, found in liver and other organ meats. An enzyme, called delta-6 desaturase, rapidly coverts GLA to DGLA. In doing so, it limits the conversion of GLA to inflammatory AAs. While we need some omega-6 fatty acids, unbalanced levels raise the incidences of blood clotting, allergies, asthma, cancer risks, and all the inflammation-based diseases.

According to Undurti Das, in an article, "Can Essential Fatty Acids Reduce the Burden of Disease(s)?" those with the inflammatory diseases of heart disease, diabetes, pre-diabetes, psoriasis, Alzheimer's disease, schizophrenia, depression, cancer, and high blood pressure have significantly low blood and tissues levels of the anti-inflammatory fatty acids GLA, EPA, and DHA compared to normal. [viii]

These compounds have important anti-inflammatory actions by themselves, and they give rise to biologically active compounds that help to suppress inflammation, such as the lipoxins, resolvins, and protectins mentioned elsewhere in this book. Researchers successfully use them to improve gum disease treatment outcomes. These fatty acids and their metabolites relax blood vessel walls, decrease clotting, help cell membranes remain fluid, enhance Nitric Oxide production, regulate DNA's telomere length, and suppress inflammatory mediators like TNF-alpha, IL-IBeta, IL-6, and prostaglandin E2 ($PGE_2$), the prostaglandin that softens the cervix and causes the uterine contractions of labor. $PGE_2$ also promotes bone loss. TNF-alpha is the inflammatory molecule that increases fever, shock, and blood vessel permeability.

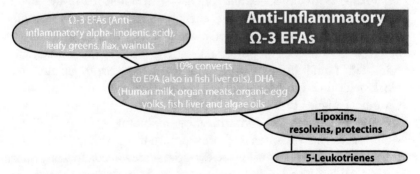

The omega-3 fatty acid, DHA, helps maintain optimal levels of the "feel-good" brain chemicals serotonin and dopamine and ensures proper nerve signaling. Omega-3 fatty acids promote bone strength when diets also include low levels of boron.[ix] Deficiencies in omega-

3s can compromise blood flow to the brain,[x][xi] compromise the blood-brain barrier,[xii] and decrease Brain Derived Neurotropic Factor (BDNF) levels.[xiii] The compound BDNF helps make our brains and nervous systems function. People whose diets are rich in omega-3 fatty acids may also be happier! [xiv][xv]

We need saturated fats to store and use omega-3 fatty acids. All omega-3 and -6 oils are polyunsaturated oils that are vulnerable to oxidation. If you supplement, make sure your diet is rich in the antioxidants found in fruits and vegetables. Five hundred mg of vitamin E per day (in both the gamma and alpha forms of the E vitamin, tocopherol), encapsulated together within an omega-3 supplement protect the omega-3 fatty acids from oxidizing within the capsules, as well as within the blood stream and in cell membranes. You'll read more about this in a moment.

Humans evolved on a diet of evenly balanced omega-3s and omega-6s in a more or less one-to-one ratio. Current American diets are typically 20 or 25-to-1 in favor of omega-6s, found especially in corn, soy, the oils of soy, corn, cottonseed and safflower, and in the meat and eggs of animals fed these products. An exaggerated presence of omega-6 fatty acids leads to an exaggerated production of arachidonic acid (AA), the precursor for pro-inflammatory mediators. Arachidonic acids are also precursors for the cannabinoids referred to in the diabetes chapter. Cannabinoids trigger hunger and impede insulin's ability to move sugar from the blood stream into fat, muscle and liver cells – a classic symptom of pre-diabetes, and the definition of insulin resistance.

Finally, both omega-3 and omega-6 metabolic pathways begin with processes that require the enzyme delta-6 desaturase. A diet overburdened with omega-6 fatty acids will consume this enzyme before it is available for processing omega-3 pathways. Incidentally, trans fats found in margarine, shortening, and hydrogenated fats block delta-6 desaturase, as do some viruses like the one that causes Chronic Fatigue. Excessive alcohol and sugars inhibit its function. Delta-6 desaturase works with magnesium, biotin, vitamin E, zinc, B vitamins and protein, often in short supply in those with inflammation. Certainly omega-6 fatty acids are essential – they make up a large part of the total brain and over 15 percent of body lipids. But if you live in America, you can be sure you are getting more of these than you need. The pharmaceutical industry makes billions of dollars a year from the sale of anti-inflammatory drugs. Doesn't it make sense to simply eat less inflammatory omega-6 fatty acids in the first place?

## You are What They Eat – You've Got Corn!

Corn forms the basis of the U.S. food supply. It is used as animal feed, sweetener, thickener, filler, and gum base. It is also eaten as bread, cereal, and popcorn. Corn is pro-inflammatory with its 32 to 1 omega-6 to omega-3 ratio.

### ESSENTIAL FATTY ACID RATIOS OF SELECTED FOODS [xvi]

| FOOD | Omega-6 EFA/ mg | Omega-3 EFA/ mg | Omega-6/ Omega-3 Ratio |
|------|------|------|------|
| Corn | 1996.0 | 62.0 | 32/1 |
| Rice, brown | 603.0 | 27.3 | 22/1 |
| Wheat | 886.0 | 45.6 | 19/1 |
| Barley | 1838.0 | 202.0 | 9/1 |
| Raw soybeans | 18,459 | 2473 | 7.46/1 |
| Broccoli, raw | 15.5 | 19.1 | .81/1 |
| Broccoli, cooked | 143.0 | 333.0 | .43/1 |

Have you ever puzzled about the vacillating reputation of eggs? First we hear they are good for you, then bad, and now good again. The secret as to whether eggs are healthful or not lies in what the animal that laid them ate. Just as grains and many oils are high in omega-6s, so are industrial agribusiness's grain-fed animals and their offshoot products. Grain-fed beef and chickens and their eggs have a ratio of 20 plus to 1, whereas grass-fed/pasture-raised animals generally have a ratio of about 4 to 1. Remember that when media stories tell you animal fats are bad for you. Inadvertently, they are referring to fats from corn-fattened animals.

In an amusing twist, The New York Times published a story, "Greening the Herds: A New Diet to Cap Gas," that describes how a cow's diet affects global warming. It states that if cows follow EFA guidelines – if they eat the alfalfa and flaxseed their bodies were designed to digest rather than the corn and soy most are fed now and cannot digest – they belch less and produce about 18 percent less methane. According to the article, methane is a "potent heat-trapping gas (twenty times that of carbon dioxide) that has been linked to climate change." The article also notes that when the cows eat correctly, their "coats are shinier, and their breath is sweet." [xvii] I think we humans would enjoy equivalent benefits!

Another point the story made is that when cows eat what they are supposed to, their stomachs do not develop erosive holes that allow their stomachs to leak their contents into their abdomens, which in turn causes life threatening cases of peritonitis. Feedlot cattle are fed corn because it adds weight fast. Hummm...

The health problems they suffer from eating this erosive diet is the reason they need heavy doses of antibiotics. Feedlots are deemed highly toxic. The heavy antibiotic concentrations and the ammonia and hydrogen sulfide gas emissions from the millions of pounds of feces feedlot cows produce, are part of the reason. Currently, factory farms do not have to report the neurotoxic emissions of these two gasses.

Salmon are highly touted for their omega-3 content, but the same nutritional concerns about beef apply to salmon and other meat products. Farm-raised Atlantic salmon floods your body with about 150 mg/serving of omega-6s compared to 1 to 3mg/serving found in wild salmon populations.[xviii] The media never specifies this when they advise you to eat salmon. Grass-fed animals are higher in omega-3s and lower in omega-6s and saturated fat.

Just as notable, the modern vegetable oil industry is skewed towards omega-6 fatty acids. The following table is derived from the USDA's National Nutrient Database for Standard Reference.[ixx] It illustrates why one must analyze omega-6 intake as well as boost omega-3s with fish oils, flax, and other sources in an effort to achieve balance between fatty acids.

| OIL/Tablespoon | Omega-6 | Omega-3 | Ratio (rounded) |
|---|---|---|---|
| Canola, low erucic acid rapeseed oil | 2, 610 mg | 1279 mg | 2/1 |
| Walnut oil | 7,141 mg | 1,404 mg | 5/1 |
| Soybean oil | 109,921 mg | 14,800 mg | 7.43/1 |
| Oil, wheat germ | 7,398 mg | 923 mg | 8/1 |
| Butter from non-pasture-raised cows | 382 mg | 44 mg | 8.5/1 |
| Canola oil, partially hydrogenated | 1,693 mg | 202 mg | 8.5/1 |
| Olive oil | 1,318 mg | 103 mg | 13/1 |
| Corn oil | 7,224 mg | 157 mg | 46/1 |
| Coconut oil (97% saturated) | 243 mg | 0 mg | 243/0 |
| Grapeseed oil | 151,708 mg | 218 mg | 696/1 |
| Sunflower oil | 3,905 mg | 5 mg | 781/1 |
| Safflower oil, oleic | 1,937 mg | 0 mg | 1,937/1 |
| Almond oil | 2,349 mg | 0 mg | 2349/1 |
| Peanut oil | 4,231 mg | 0 mg | 4231/1 |
| Safflower oil, linoleic | 10,073 mg | 0 mg | 10,073/0 |

An analysis of this table reveals that EFA ratios are only part of the story when considering what mix of dietary oils to use. If you want to avoid heart disease and reduce inflammation, also consider fat stability. Once again, politics and business interests have skewed what the general public "knows" about fats. In a nutshell, consumers have been taught that a diet high in fat, especially saturated fats, leads to high cholesterol levels and thus heart disease. A diet containing naturally saturated oils, such as tropical oils (coconut and palm oils) is more favorable than a diet filled with unnaturally saturated, hydrogenated, or trans, oils and highly refined, oxidized polyunsaturated oils. Consumers have been given confusing information about the difference between the two, much like the information about inflammatory saturated fats derived from unnaturally corn-fed animals being confused with fats from grass-fattened animals.

It is worthwhile to note that statin drugs (Lipitor, Crestor, etc.) reduce cholesterol numbers throughout the body without regard to function. Besides being an important precursor of all the hormones that direct cellular function, cholesterols also aid the formation and function of the junctions between nerves, called synapses.[xx] The reduction of cholesterol in brain synapses may explain why those on statin drugs often suffer confusion, forgetfulness, and other cerebral dysfunctions.

Think for a moment:

- Is it likely our circulatory systems can only be healthy if we consume the highly refined, polyunsaturated oils derived from vegetables of low oil content that have only recently entered the food supply?
- Did the advent of these highly refined oils coincide with the meteoric rise we've seen in heart disease in Western countries?
- Why is it that Japanese and Mediterranean people with cholesterol levels similar to Americans have far less mortality from heart disease?[xxi]
- What about the French? French diets are rich in butter, cream, and other saturated fats. Their cholesterol levels are higher than those in all other European nations, yet they have low rates of heart disease.

We need saturated fats. Saturated fatty acids are stable. They do not oxidize. They do not turn rancid. This fact has enormous ramifications. Inflammation is one cause of aging. Oxidation is another.

## Commentary on Fats and Oils

All oils and fats are hydrocarbons. Chains of carbons are linked together with varying numbers of hydrogen attached to them. Saturated fats have the maximum possible number of hydrogen atoms bonded to each carbon. Monounsaturated fats lack one pair of hydrogen atoms in each fatty acid chain. Polyunsaturated oils lack several pairs of hydrogen atoms. Oxidation, or free radical damage, occurs where hydrogen pairs are missing.

Saturated Fatty Acid

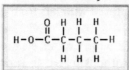

**Building Blocks of Fat**

Mono-unsaturated Fatty Acid

Poly-unsaturated Fatty Acid

All saturated fats are not created equal. First, all fats are a mix of saturated, monounsaturated and polyunsaturated fats. The predominant type of fat is what determines how a fat or oil is labeled. Hydrogenated fats are polyunsaturated fats to which hydrogen atoms are artificially added to carbons to stabilize them. This protects them from oxidation and gives them the consistency and qualities associated with naturally occurring saturated fats and tropical oils. Complete saturation makes polyunsaturates too rigid, thus impractical and inedible. Partial hydrogenation converts polyunsaturated fats into trans fats. The safe limit for artificial trans fat intake is zero.

Trans fats:

- Clog arteries. They morph LDL/HDL cholesterol carrier ratios. LDL carriers carry cholesterol *to* arteries to repair damage. HDL carriers carry cholesterols *away* from arteries back to the liver for recycling or degradation and excretion.
- Contribute to cancer, autoimmune problems, diabetes, poor brain function, and obesity.
- Deplete omega-3s and hinder their utilization. When trans fats substitute for natural fats in the brain and the sheaths that protect our nerves, they alter their function.
- Are difficult for our bodies to break down and excrete.
- Fats constitute about 50 percent of all cell membranes. When a person has a diet that includes trans fats, these unnatural trans fats replace about 20 percent of the natural fats. This causes the membranes to weaken and distort. They admit compounds they shouldn't into cells. When cell membranes no longer function as they should, the immune system may not recognize the membrane and may attack them, which leads to autoimmune dysfunction.

Many processed foods advertise they are trans fat free, hoping to infer a healthy product. Often the label numbers are deceptively manipulated. If there is less than 0.5 gram of trans fat per serving, labels can advertise their product as trans fat free. The fact that people easily consume more than one miniscule serving of a "trans fat free" product without realizing it, invalidates the claim.

Also, these products often use a mixture of polyunsaturated and inedible fully hydrogenated oils to create the desired texture. Technically, they are not trans fats, but they are unhealthy.

Many of the vegetables and grains from which oils are extracted have low oil content. The oil content of corn, for instance, is about 2.8 percent. The modern oil industry uses high temperature, high pressure, and the toxic solvent, hexane, to extract oil from most seeds and grains. Heat causes oils to oxidize, or turn rancid. Most oils are subsequently bleached, de-gummed, and deodorized to mask their rancidity. Since oxidation is a principal player in inflammatory aging, it should be clear the EFA ratios in the chart do not tell the whole story. Depending on how listed oils are refined, most of them are garbage to your body. They are already highly oxidized when you buy them. They also may contain hexane residues.

Since fats are critical to every cell, and oxidation damages cell structures, people whose diets are rich in highly refined polyunsaturated vegetable oils suffer excessive oxidative damage. The fats available to make up cell membranes and other structures are pre-oxidized by oil processors, or they are susceptible to oxidation within the bloodstream or once they integrate within the cell. The mitochondrial energy furnaces and DNA found in each cell are particularly susceptible to oxidation. Energy generation within each cell declines as oxidative damage to mitochondria accumulates. Damage to and lack of mitochondria is significantly related to aging and diseases like diabetes.

High levels of antioxidants are required to prevent oxidative damage to cellular structures. It is one reason supplemental CoQ10 becomes more necessary as we age. This is because CoQ10 recycles the potent antioxidant vitamins C and E, yet we produce less and less of it as we age. Note that statin drugs and red rice yeast that lower cholesterol also lower natural CoQ10 production, so supplementation with the ubiquinol form of CoQ10 is essential.

Because canola oil is presented as a heart-healthy oil, it deserves mention. Canola oil may have a great omega-3/omega-6 ratio, but during the deodorizing process, nearly five percent of the omega-3s morph into trans fats. If manufacturers manipulate labeling numbers via serving size, canola oil can still be advertised as being trans fat free. During processing, heat oxidizes susceptible omega-3 chains in all oils, so a high fraction of canola oil is already oxidized when you buy it.

You may be unaware that more than half of all rapeseed from which canola oil is derived has been genetically modified and heavily treated with pesticides, as are corn and soybean crops. In fact, pesticides enter our bodies most often through oils. Partially hydrogenated canola oil is preferentially used in many processed foods because it increases shelf life and gives fried food the crunchy texture consumers seek. Heart healthy? I don't think so.

*Unprocessed* canola oil has its problems, too. Vitamin E deficiencies, a decrease in blood platelet counts, and an increase in blood platelet size have been reported. Interestingly, these deficiencies reverse when combined with a diet that includes saturated fats.[xxii] Saturated fats help the body to convert omega-3s into the important EPA and DHA forms of omega-3s. Unfortunately, many people who use canola oil have bought into the notion that all saturated fats are bad and no longer consume the saturated fats that would protect them.

Do your own research and reconsider what mix of oils you choose to consume. Take a long look at saturated, thus stable palm and coconut oils as a part of a healthy diet. They have abundant benefits and rarely cause the rise in cholesterol so often ascribed to them. After all, it is polyunsaturated fats in vegetable and seed oils that encourage blood clot formation by increasing platelet stickiness. In fact, coconut oil helps promote normal platelet function. The medium-chain fats in coconut oil are considered so nutritious they are used in baby formulas, in hospitals to feed the critically ill, those being tube fed, and those with digestive problems. Unrefined red palm oil has a prominent place in my home kitchen.

Recognize that oil processing, storage, and cooking techniques matter because heat and air oxidize oils. Use only oils that have been extracted with stone, hydraulic, or cold pressing techniques, preferably in that order. Mechanical pressing can heat oils to 190° Fahrenheit, while the deodorizing process subjects them to much higher temperatures. Pay attention to an oil's smoking point when you cook, too. When oils smoke or discolor, it means they have oxidized and created both airborne and solid carcinogens, which are toxic when inhaled or ingested. Refined oils also lose taste and nutrition. Unrefined oils, rich in taste, aroma, and nutrients, are more susceptible to oxidation, depending on how saturated they are. Buy small amounts and store unrefined oils (including omega-3 supplements) carefully. Match the oil to the task: cook with them as little as possible, If a recipe requires high heat, choose oils with high smoking points. Be sensible about the amounts of fats you consume because they are all calorie dense.

If you want to know more about oils, begin with a web article, "Tripping Lightly Down the Prostaglandin Pathways,"[xxiii] by Dr. Mary Enig and Sally Fallon. In this article, they review the roles of healthy traditional fats in balanced diets and how they influence the complicated feedback loops of pro-inflammatory and anti-inflammatory prostaglandins, compared to the rancid, processed vegetable oils, such as corn, canola, and soy oils. They also co-authored several books about fat, such as, *Eat Fat, Lose Fat: Lose Weight and Feel Great with the Delicious, Science-Based Coconut Diet.*

*New Good Food* by Margaret Wittenberg,[xxiv] is an excellent source of information about oils, their health benefits, uses, and smoking points. She reviews the fatty acid profiles of meats, eggs, seeds, nuts, and dairy products.

People who understand fats can experience significant healing. Their diets often mimic the diets of those from the Greek island of Crete in the 1950's. These Greeks had the lowest rates of heart disease in the world at the time, despite the fact that their diet was not particularly low fat. In fact, 37 percent of the Cretin diet came from fat calories, some from saturated fats, most from monounsaturated fats rich in ALA (alpha-linolenic fatty acid) and omega-3s.

The food program currently referred to as the "Mediterranean Diet" follows the same principles and is largely plant-based. Every meal includes foods high in antioxidant value because one cannot store these mostly water-soluble nutrients. Meat, oil, and dairy products are chosen with care. Ideally, the Mediterranean diet includes many wild greens grown in selenium-rich soils and an abundance of herbs, walnuts, dried figs, flaxseeds, sardines, and wild salmon. Meat and dairy come from true pasture-raised, foraging animals. This program avoids processed foods so one can control the amount and types of ingested fats. People following this program take omega-3 supplements[4] or eat fish known to be high in omega-3s, and incorporate a small amount of pesticide-free, saturated fat with every meal. This is because, as has been previously discussed, many nutrients are fat soluble, so cannot be absorbed without fats. These fats also make you feel full faster so you stop eating when your body gets what it needs.

If ever there was an inspiring example of how "changing the terrain" of a body can heal it, the following example shows it. A man much like the rancher described in the stroke chapter, experienced significant healing after following much of the advice offered in this book. In reviewing his chart before I met him I noted his X-rays showed only about 2 mm of bone anchoring his teeth. Adult tooth roots average 12 mm in length. His roots were heavily encrusted with hard black deposits and likely reflected the crusty stiffness of his arteries. Not surprisingly, I learned he had suffered a heart attack two years prior to his dental visit.

Backed by twenty-five years of experience and knowledge, I was prepared to explain how he clearly had a predisposition for inflammatory diseases; that his mouth, which harbored its own inflammatory disease, was a septic reservoir of toxins that fed his

---

4 Oils should be bioavailable and fresh. Look at the certificate of analysis (COA) to be sure oxidation numbers are low. Be sure Anisidine and peroxide values are both listed and comparatively low. Also assess purity. You want arsenic, cadmium, mercury, lead, PCB, dioxin and furan contamination to be as low as possible.

other diseases. I thought removing his teeth might improve his overall health, but his case reminded me that sometimes I am the student. Even before his "cleaning," the negligible tissues supporting his teeth showed no signs of inflammation. During my conversation with him, I learned his heart attack had prompted him to begin following the diet strategies I recommend. Therefore the tightening of his teeth in his sockets and the lack of tissue inflammation were no surprise. Preliminary research shows strong evidence to support that balancing fatty acids, reducing simple carbohydrates, and avoiding unhealthy oils can counter genetic susceptibilities that predispose some people to inflammatory diseases.

If you suffer from inflammation, consider taking pancreatic enzyme supplements.[5] Eat anthocyanin-rich foods, known to suppress inflammation. These foods are a deep red, blue, or purple color. Beets, red peppers, eggplant, oranges, and berries are great examples. An important antioxidant, alpha lipoic acid (ALA), also reduces inflammation. Additionally, it enhances insulin sensitivity, chelates heavy metals, and assists in recycling vitamin C, E, CoQ10, and glutathione, described below. You may want to explore the various essential oils and herbal and green teas[6] that reduce inflammation. For example, Oolong teas can cut triglyceride levels and lower A1c levels; [xxv] green teas can lower arthritis risk and black teas suppress the Cox-2 enzyme that triggers inflammation via the same pathway as Vioxx did and Celebrex does. Again, the emerging field of epigenetics illuminates the critical role nutrition plays in modulating inflammation. As Hippocrates said, "Let food be your medicine and medicine be your food."

## Glutathione/GSH

Glutathione levels are deficient in many inflammatory disease states. Glutathione (GSH) is so protective of our wellbeing that every human cell can synthesize it from three amino acids (L-cysteine, L-glutamic acid and glycine). Glutathione scavenges and metabolizes cholesterols, helps synthesize DNA, and helps dampen carbohydrate cravings for some. (Leafy green vegetables and apple cider vinegar also cut cravings.)

---

5 Stress, antacids, an unhealthy diet or a lack of pancreatic enzymes often lead to incomplete protein breakdown during digestion. These poorly digested proteins can result in constipation or diarrhea, bloating, gas, food allergies, and inflammation when chronic, inflammatory breakdown overrides healing.

6 Green teas lose their antioxidant powers quickly. Drink fresh organic tea steeped in tepid water.

However GSH's most important functions are commonly remembered with the acronym "AIDE":

**A**ntioxidant – Every cell of the body needs glutathione to reduce oxidative stress to its valuable mitochondria, the "energy furnace" for each cell. Since it takes two molecules of glutathione to escort one atom of mercury and other heavy metals out of the body, many people are glutathione deficient, resulting in mitochondrial damage from glutathione depletion. GSH also recycles the antioxidant vitamins C and E and supports their function.

**I**nflammation reducer – GSH regulates immune function in multiple ways including the production of inflammatory mediators and the various prostaglandins that suppress inflammation.

**D**etoxifier – GSH binds directly to toxins, preparing them for elimination. As mentioned, GSH chelates heavy metals like mercury, and binds to cancer-causing agents and other toxins like molds and the mycotoxins found in some alcoholic beverages. Most toxins are fat soluble and thus become stored in fat cells. In order to eliminate them, they must be made to become water soluble. Some people lack the enzyme that helps match glutathione to toxins. Enhancing glutathione levels increases one's chances of toxin elimination.

**E**nergizer - High energy levels require a healthy heart. Because of its relentless beating, heart cells are prone to oxidative stress. GSH provides the antioxidants to reduce the stress. GSH also aides DNA production and repair and scavenges and metabolizes cholesterol. There are strong correlations between low glutathione levels, atherosclerosis, and heart attack recurrence.

High energy also requires optimal brain function, orchestrated by neurotransmitters. Without sufficient antioxidants or the brain chemical serotonin,[7] the brain may decide it is unsafe to produce the excitatory "feel good" brain chemicals, dopamine and norepinephrine. Low levels of these energizing brain compounds partially define aging and diseases like chronic fatigue syndrome.

Aging, aluminum from many vaccines, and some diseases create an inability to produce glutathione efficiently. Poorly controlled diabetics have runaway oxidation and are unable to form glutathione well. Those

---

7 Reducing stress gently raises serotonin levels. Exercise, meditation, and reducing the stress of chronic low-grade infections like gum disease, toxins, poor sleep patterns, and poor diet also raise serotonin levels.

with Parkinson's disease are poor detoxifiers and often have low GSH levels in the liver and the dopamine-producing regions of the brain. They are particularly susceptible to pesticide exposure and respond well to GSH-boosting. Oxidative stress is a major driver of AIDS progression. Pro-inflammatory compounds such as TNF, help activate the virus. Maintaining high GSH levels and good gum disease control is therefore critical for those with HIV/AIDS. GSH also boosts cytotoxic T-cells and lymphocytes.

Those with asthma, hepatitis, cancers, Alzheimer's, respiratory diseases, malnutrition, physical stress, and again, heart disease, often experience sub-optimal level GSH levels as well. A toxic metabolite of acetaminophen depletes glutathione, so if you pop Tylenol or other acetaminophens frequently, you likely need to boost GSH levels.

Glutathione made within body cells is generally more effective than consuming supplemental forms, which are destroyed by digestion. However consuming high levels of glutathione precursors does boost cellular glutathione levels. Cysteine is the amino acid that usually limits GSH production. Cysteine is rarely found in foods, though it is found in whey protein in the form of glutamine and glutamylcysteine.

You must be aware that whey protein *isolates* do not contain glutamine and glutamylcysteine because they are found in fat globules. Isolates have been stripped of their beneficial fats, vitamins, and minerals. Also lost from the fats are the phospholipids, phosphatidylserine, and conjugated linoleic acid (CLA), which grant additional immunological value. Stripped of their minerals, the isolates are also acid-forming. Whey proteins alkalize.

High quality matters in other ways. Proteins from milk that is overheated and treated with acids during processing, morph the protein's shape into what is called a D isomer, a form not recognized by the body and which causes damage as it accumulates in muscles, bones, and the brain. D isomer protein accumulation in the brain is linked to Parkinson's and Alzheimer's. This method of processing also releases free cysteine, degrading its bioavailability.

Poor manufacturing processes also make cheap whey protein products insoluble in water. As with low grade cooking oils, unhealthy chemicals make the product more palatable. Whey proteins should be derived from organic, unpasteurized milk from, grass-fed cows, and should be cold processed. Treat your high quality whey protein with respect at home. Do not heat it or slip it into blenderized drinks. Stir or shake gently!

Other excellent sources of the fragile cysteine precursor molecule are pea or brown rice protein, Immunocal® and silymarin from milk thistle. Many people take the glutathione precursor, N-acetylcysteine (NAC) to help boost glutathione levels. For many reasons, it is less useful than these other products.

Diabetics need special help because they have difficulties producing GSH even when cysteine is abundant. For these people liposomal glutathione[8] may be an answer. The fatty exterior made from the same material as cell membranes allows it to bypass the digestive tract to enter the blood stream. The lipid exterior also protects the water-soluble interior that keeps glutathione in its active state. Don't overlook transdermal methods. Lifewave patches may also raise levels.

Diabetics should also know that alpha lipoic acid (ALA) recycles glutathione. In fact, it may be a diabetic's most effective supplement for boosting glutathione levels. ALA is also another important antioxidant. It reduces inflammation, enhances insulin sensitivity, chelates heavy metals, and assists in recycling vitamin C, E, and CoQ10.

Maintain good digestive tract flora and a high fiber diet when detoxing or chelating with glutathione or any other agent to prevent reabsorption of toxins.

## Our Sweet Lifestyle!  From Simple to Complex

Much has been said about nutrition throughout these pages. A review of sugars and a foray into the related subject of energy and fat metabolism might help tie these ideas together.

In dental school, sugars were a narrowly viewed, elementary subject. Can you believe the following picture represents what I was taught there?

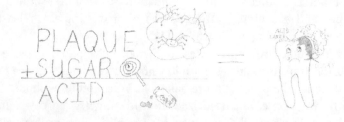

PLAQUE
+SUGAR
ACID

---

8 RediSorb by Complementary Prescriptions is one example.

We are obviously worlds away from this simple concept, just as we are worlds away from those simpler days. Certainly, the equation above still stands. But just as our lives are more complex than those of our parents, our understanding of the science behind our choices is more complex. You know simple sugars feed the germs that cause tooth decay and undermine your health in insidious and destructive ways far beyond their calorie count. In fact, sugars contribute to all the inflammatory diseases, tooth decay, and "brain fog."

You may know all this and still find it difficult to juggle the demands on your time with good nutrition. In America, most of us are in overdrive all the time. If your family mimics mine, it careens from school or work to countless activities, often tempted by the call of convenience foods. We try to lead financially secure, activity-rich lives, but at what cost?

I suspect most adults know we trade our family's health for expediency. Learning about and implementing good nutritional strategies seem the least of our priorities. Therefore we are at the mercy of the American food chain, from government-subsidized agribusiness to the final food products we vote for with our dollars. Unfortunately, our votes are often cast in favor of highly processed foods that cut our precious lives short.

Since this book was first published, there is a burgeoning awareness that environment and lifestyle choices trump genetics when it comes to overall health. We are starting to understand our beleaguered immune systems simply reflect our life's imbalances.

To review, uncontrolled gum disease and other inflammatory diseases contribute to and are symptoms of impaired immune function. An immune system in chronic overdrive contributes to osteoporosis, diabetes, atherosclerosis and related circulatory system damage, and the number of pre-term deliveries. Other diseases related to the immune system are cancers, chronic fatigue syndrome, neurological problems, multiple chemical sensitivities, allergies, and hormonal disturbances.

We reap enormous payoffs when we strengthen rather than depress our immune systems. Doing so can delay for years many diseases to which we are genetically prone. A diabetic client of mine is an example. A gifted, hardworking man of 35, he has worn an insulin pump for years. He avoids simple carbohydrates and fanatically follows healthy lifestyle guidelines. When he was diagnosed with diabetes, his doctor suggested his extremely stressful job had probably tripped the early expression of his disease. Had he not had such a demanding job, he was told, the disease likely would not have appeared for another fifteen years or more, if ever.

Chapter Five highlighted the ways sugar challenges our immune systems through glycation, oxidation, and skewed hormonal sensitivities. The resulting inflammation damages soft tissues and slows healing.

High sugar and other simple carbohydrate loads exert other effects:

- **Sugar overtaxes adrenal glands.** The destruction of adrenal glands may be the most significant challenge a person faces as they try to overcome health problems. Through the adrenal hormones cortisol and DHEA, the precursor to human sex hormones, the adrenal glands influence most body functions. They influence bone and connective tissue turnover rates, memory and learning, nerve conductivity, sleep, mood, muscle integrity, glucose balance, pro- and anti-inflammatory states, protein turnover, the integrity of the mucosal lining of organs, and the capacity of the liver to process toxins like pesticides and heavy metals. The adrenal hormones also control blood pressure and mineral balance. If you want to restore health, you must restore adrenal function. Chapter Fifteen addresses this subject further.

- **Excessive sugar consumption depletes two critical minerals: zinc and chromium.** Zinc is a component of the insulin molecule that moves sugar out of the blood stream. Zinc combats cold and flu viruses. It helps wounds heal and supports the immune and reproductive systems, especially the prostate. Zinc also supports liver function. Chromium activates insulin and changes cell membranes to allow sugars to move into cells.

- **Sugar contributes to osteoporosis because it causes magnesium excretion.** Calcium requires magnesium for it to be utilized and absorbed. Magnesium also activates most of the enzymes that turn sugar and fat into energy (the Krebs cycle/ATP formation/storage that occurs in each cell's mitochondria). Magnesium deficiencies reduce bone mass and increase skeletal fragility.[xxvi] Magnesium deficiencies are common in those whose diets rely on processed foods.

- **AGE products** from excessive sugars accumulate in bone collagen and weaken its structure, which makes bones less resilient.
- **Depressed phosphorus levels contribute to having an acidic system,** that is, having inadequate buffering capacity at the cellular level. Refined carbohydrates, alcohol, and caffeine depress phosphorus levels and increase blood acidity. One way our bodies neutralize acidic conditions is to extract alkalizing calcium from bone. Much of it becomes free calcium that deposits in unwanted places like kidneys and blood vessel walls – and dental plaques. Often, taking a good quality phosphorus supplements decreases hard deposits on teeth.
- **Another side effect of an acidic system is a chronically inflamed gut.** First, an acidic system unbalances microorganism ecologies, as you've learned. Yeast (candida) infections especially proliferate when one has high sugar intake and/or leaky gut syndrome from a chronically inflamed gut. These people are often insulin resistant.

  Blood vessels in the gut become porous and leaky when inflamed just as blood vessels in the gums do. Undigested proteins and peptides spill out of the intestines into places they do not belong. The body recognizes these as "foreign," and, voila, food allergies are born.
- **Simple carbohydrates negate the positive effects of probiotics.** Found in fermented foods, probiotics are the proper "friendly bacteria" flora human digestive systems require. Sugars wipe out the beneficial bacteria that populate the digestive tract, leaving a niche in which harmful bacteria thrive. A crucial part of the immune system depends on these beneficial bacteria. Some produce vitamins. Others help our bodies distinguish between disease-causing germs and non-harmful antigens. When the beneficial ratio of good/bad bacteria is imbalanced, the immune system can overreact to non-harmful antigens by creating allergies. Friendly bacteria also help produce the antibodies required to fight the pathogens that enter our bodies.
- **Even small amounts of sugar seriously impede the infection-fighting function of white blood cells for hours.**

- **High sugar intake impedes memory** by decreasing the brain compound BDNF (brain-derived neurotrophic factor). BDNF is a "memory food." We need BDNF in order to store long-term memories. BDNF supports existing nerves, stimulates the growth of new ones, enhances neurotransmission, and supports normal brain structure. Stress, inflammation, and poor diet decrease BDNF levels. Conditions associated with low levels of BDNF are depression, schizophrenia, obsessive-compulsive disorder, dementia, and Alzheimer's.

  Exercise and a diet rich in omega-3s and few simple carbohydrates raise levels. Depressed people have low levels of BDNF. If you take an omega-3 supplement like fish oil, be sure your diet is rich in antioxidants because, though they are important, omega-3s can oxidize and thus become damaging. Coconut oil does not oxidize and raises BDNF levels.

## From Complex to Simple

As our human genetic code evolved, food was scarce. Our ancestors' energy derived from the complex carbohydrates found in fibrous foods; access to simple sugars was rare. Complex carbohydrates like fiber and cellulose are more difficult to digest and provide low energy. To survive, our forebears' bodies were programmed to maximize all high-energy foods they found. Once discovered, body systems signaled them to devour rare concentrated carbohydrates like honey. Those who survived passed on their strong cravings. Our genes still carry these cravings for fatty and simple sugary foods.

Sugar was prohibitively expensive for all but the wealthiest people during most of human history. Only as European countries expanded into the New World and enslaved various populations to grow and harvest labor-intensive sugar cane did sugar prices begin to decline enough to become more affordable for the middle classes. Still, in the early 1700s, individual intake in England was estimated to be about a teaspoon a day, or four pounds a year.

I often ask clients to guess the average amount of sugar consumed per American per year. Rarely does anyone come close to the correct answer.

Cost and availability no longer limit sugar consumption. Best estimates suggest Americans consume an average of 154 pounds of sugar a year. That is a sharp increase from 2001 when the USDA estimated American's total sugar consumption was roughly 105 pounds a year.[9] Corn sweeteners made up 55 percent of the total in that year. It is certainly higher now. By 2003, corn sweetener consumption alone rose to 79 pounds per person – an increase of more than ten pounds per year in just two years![xxvii] These are averages, of course. Currently, teenagers tend to consume far more sodas than adults. But consulting the numbers, I must assume many keep this habit into adulthood.

Our bodies evolved to process sugars as a part of complex carbohydrates. This means that for eons they dealt only with sugars that were slowly released into the blood stream. When we eat sugar as part of a complex carbohydrate, we feel full quickly. But who feels full after drinking fruit juice or a soda with many times the sugar content? In fact, American sodas (and almost all prepackaged foods, from whole grain breads to pasta sauces) sabotage us with cheap, high fructose corn syrup (HFCS). Unfortunately, we produce less leptin when we ingest fructose. Leptin signals our brains that we are full, so we stop eating. Less leptin means less signaling, so we continue eating.

Other than not signalling fullness, what else happens when a person drinks a 12-ounce can of soda? Blood normally contains about a teaspoon of circulating sugar, so when a person suddenly dumps 11+ teaspoons of high fructose corn syrup into their blood stream, insulin must rapidly transfer it to other organs and tissues to avoid damage. That is, if the pancreas still makes insulin. Insulin production is a primary job. In fact, the pancreas usually stores limited insulin amounts in order to respond to sugar jolts. But what happens when blood sugar loads exceed what stored insulin can remove? It takes time for the pancreas to churn out more insulin, so the person that has drunk a 12-ounce can of soda operates with high levels of damaging blood sugar until production catches up. Imagine what happens to a person's body when they take a walk on the wild side and drink a Big Gulp that packs 800 calories and about 53 teaspoons of high fructose corn syrup?

---

9 An article in the October 2006 issue of the *Harvard Health Letter*, entitled "Sugar and Obesity: High Calorie Drinks to Blame?" suggests that between soda, specialty coffee drinks, alcoholic beverages, and smoothies, beverages for a typical American can account for about 450 calories or a fourth of our daily calories. This has doubled over the last thirty years. It suggests that people who forgo sweet drinks could lose roughly 29 pounds over the course of a year.

## Organ Damage and Rapid Aging

Let us review some key points from the diabetes chapter. The pancreas must go into overdrive to keep insulin production in line with simple carbohydrate consumption. Eventually the pancreas begins to burn out. Fat, muscle and liver cells become less responsive to insulin and eventually, if one has the gene for it as many do, the person becomes a diabetic. Unregulated diabetics suffer significant kidney, eye, blood vessel, and nerve damage because sugar levels are often excessive. Nerve damage might first be noticed as numbness in the arms and legs, slower reflexes, and general weakness. Diabetes also leads to high blood pressure.

The longer sugar freely circulates in the blood, the more time it has to bind irrevocably to proteins, fats, and red blood cells. This is true whether a person is diabetic or not. Doctors call the resulting complex, tightly cross-linked, and rigidly bound molecules advanced glycation end products or AGEs. AGEs cause organs and tissues to degenerate. As a matter of fact, much of the damage diabetics suffer is due to these AGEs, though they accumulate throughout life and age everyone.

## Obesity

When we overindulge in simple carbohydrates, our bodies make new fat cells. At first, the liver converts sugars into glycogen for delivery into muscle cells to be used as fuel. When muscle cells have what they need, the liver stores a small amount. The rest is converted into triglycerides and stored within fat cells. When current fat cells bulge with fats, the body makes new fat cells. Most people let their bodies balloon by making new fat cells as necessary. Most people think they will deal with their few extra pounds later. But no matter how hard they try, many of those pounds refuse to budge. This is because fat cells are around forever, once formed. We can only reduce the amount of stored fat in each cell by half. Not knowing why they cannot lose their last few pounds of fat, this may be what drives people to consider liposuction.[10]

---

10 Liposuction only gets rid of fat immediately under the skin. It address aesthetic issues, but does not change blood pressure, blood sugar, or cholesterol levels. Those benefits are only experienced as one loses deep abdominal fat and fat from muscles including the heart muscle, the liver and so on. It is deep abdominal fat that releases the molecules of inflammation discussed previously: IL-6 and TNF-alpha. These molecules are also involved in the dangerous dissolution of the plaques in our blood vessels that lead to blood vessel blockage by clots or debris.

## The Immune System, Sex Hormones, and Osteoporosis

Eating or drinking a few teaspoons of sugar causes a large part of our body's defense system to limp along at less than 50 percent capacity for hours. As stated earlier, overeating refined carbohydrates also stresses the adrenal glands. The adrenals control sex hormones, stress hormones,[11] blood pressure and mineral balance, so mineral balances are skewed this way also. People who drink over two liters of liquid calories in soda per day tend to have dangerously low levels of potassium. Muscle weakness and cramps as well as an irregular heartbeat can result. Many doctors are sure acids, particularly the phosphoric acid in sodas, cause osteoporosis. Corn syrup in them is known to be a contributor. Sugars in general lower a body's buffering capacity – commonly understood as having an acidic body chemistry. Meager buffering abilities require calcium release from bones to keep blood at the pH require to sustain life (pH 7.35 – 7.45).

## Beer Without the Buzz: Fructose Metabolism

If you lay aside for a moment, the issue of genetically engineered crops and possible contamination of high fructose corn syrup (HFCS) with mercury, our bodies process table sugar (sucrose) and HFCS almost the same way because their chemical structures are nearly identical. They are both roughly half fructose and half glucose. Sucrose is fifty percent glucose, fifty percent fructose. HFCS is 42 percent glucose, 55 percent fructose.

Glucose in moderation is not a problem. It is what our bodies were designed to run on. The body in normal metabolism can use eighty percent of glucose. Fructose is the common denominator that makes table sugar and HFCS equally toxic.

It is the context and dosage that matter. Neither pure fructose nor sugar was ever meant to be dissociated from the fiber and nutrients with which they naturally occur. The high fiber content of fruits and sugar cane for instance discourages excessive consumption, slows fructose entry into the bloodstream, and helps moderate negative metabolic effects. Also, the nutrients and enzymes in foods that contain fructose help metabolize it. To reiterate, whole foods, including their fiber, are perfect nutrition packets.

---

11 Adrenaline and cortisol

Dr. Robert Lustig, a pediatric metabolic specialist from the University of Southern California says fructose, whether from sucrose or HFCS, is metabolized exactly like ethanol alcohol with but one exception – where each is metabolized. Your brain metabolizes your favorite whiskey so you fully experience its toxicity. It is your liver that must process nearly three-fourths of your favorite fruit juice, soda, or other fructose-loaded beverage – into ethanol – so you never feel the damage. Dr. Lustig points out that fructose causes eight out of the twelve problems excessive alcohol consumption is known for: liver dysfunction, heart problems, high blood pressure, improper fat metabolism, inflammation of the pancreas, obesity, fetal alcohol syndrome, and addiction.[xxviii] He says:

- Uric acid, from fructose metabolism increases blood pressure – and contributes to gout. Gout may be a major sign one is insulin resistant.
- Thirty percent of fructose ends up as fat, not glucose. He points to a study of medical students who ingested high amounts of fructose for six days. In that six-day period, their triglyceride levels doubled. Fat-making increased by more than five times, and the number of free fatty acids in the blood (FFAs) also doubled, causing a doubling of insulin resistance. As you have learned, insulin resistance is an early warning sign of diabetes development.
- Some of the fat does not exit the liver, so it contributes to a fatty liver – a kind of hepatitis.
- Dr. Lustig reasserts that fructose keeps your brain from sensing leptin (leptin resistance), so you overeat and likely make more fat. Again, leptin works through the brain's hypothalamus, therefore it also influences other functions as well. Some of these are the stress response through the adrenal glands, bone growth, thyroid function, the sympathetic nervous system, and reproductive behavior.
- Fructose metabolism contributes to insulin resistance in the liver. In this case, the pancreas has to work harder to pump out more insulin. High insulin leads to higher blood pressure. High insulin also leads leptin resistance, further fat making, and other metabolic problems.
- Fructose makes seven times more AGEs than glucose.

- The sugars that make it into the liver go through phosphorylation. This process quickly depletes phosphate from the body.
- Cells use sugar to generate energy called ATP. As ATP breaks down, it degrades into the waste product, uric acid. Uric acid causes gout. It also contributes to high blood pressure because it blocks nitric oxide (NO) in the blood vessels. NO decreases blood pressure.

## When to Worry about Your Cholesterol Levels

Perhaps more critical than all the above: after all the metabolic passes fructose makes through the body, roughly 60 percent exit as LDLs, the reason so many doctors pass out statin prescriptions, such as Lipitor and Crestor. And these are not just any LDLs. Remember there are two kinds of LDLS: LDLs and VLDLs. LDLs are "floaters," roughly composed of 10 percent triglycerides, 45 percent cholesterol, and 25 percent protein. The emulsifying outer shell that allows the internal fat to mix with liquid blood makes up the other 20 percent of the complex. LDLs are too buoyant to pass through the lining of blood vessel walls to cause the damage of atherosclerosis.

Conversely VLDLs are the very low density LDLs that can burrow into your circulatory system. They carry 55-65 percent triglycerides and 10-15 percent cholesterol. The five to ten percent protein content is lower than that of LDLs. Because most tests do not yet differentiate the ratio of LDLs to VLDLs (two that do are available at www.healthylife labs.com and directlabs.com.), Dr. Lustig contends a more accurate assessment of heart disease risk is the triglyceride to HDL ratio. If your triglycerides are low and HDLs high, you have a high fraction of large, buoyant LDLs. High triglycerides and low HDLs signal a problem. Dietary fat raises large, buoyant LDLs; sugars raise VLDL numbers!

Glucose metabolism does not move you to type 2 diabetes, obesity, and heart disease. Fructose metabolism does.

I sometimes remind my young clients that theirs is the first generation whose lifespan will be shorter than that of their parents. Generally speaking, this is because their parents' generation was far more active growing up than they are. Junk foods were not as readily available to them during their formative years. Most American children eat highly processed food at almost every meal. Our environment is also more toxic. I remind these young clients that they are the only ones who can make courageous choices and find the power within themselves to live long and healthy lives.

I know many of my generation know better than to eat the way they do. We might not have known the facts when we were establishing our habits, but dawning concerns about our wrecked health and wrecked environment deserve our full attention. Unfortunately, many bad habits are entrenched. Sugar addictions are well established and no longer look to us like the true addictions they are. We are stressed. We think our children will not listen to our guidance about food and its relationship to their health. We do not have time to prepare healthy meals. It may be too late for many in my generation because the damage is likely done, but our children deserve better guidance and choices.

## Sugar: An Unrecognized American Addiction

Sugar addictions are strong addictions, and once people know how detrimental they are to human health, they ask about less damaging substitutes. Are artificial sugars any better than the real thing? This is a great question. My first response however, is that if you have to ask that question – if you are already strategizing a new game plan similar to your old unhealthy game plan, you are likely addicted to sugars and the answer is not to find a substitute, but to change your body chemistry so you do not crave sweets and simple carbohydrates.

First, it helps to know humans are fighting biology – a strong, preprogrammed urge that evolved eons ago. It is also important to know that ancient mechanisms fail us in today's world, since financial constraints and availability currently do not limit sugar consumption. Culturally, Americans are biased towards sugary treats.

When a person is really hungry, what is usually the first thing he or she reaches for to provide satisfaction and energy? Most Americans crave something sweet. What if a person reaches for a liquid sugar source – a high fructose corn syrup soda, fruit juice, sport drink, energy drink, vitamin water or latte? Since most sugary drinks do not signal fullness – even a calorie-laden Big Gulp – that person would still feel hungry after they had finished one.

Sugar cravings follow several addiction pathways. Sugars stimulate the pleasure centers of the brain by releasing high levels of dopamine, a powerfully addictive "feel good" brain chemical. "Dopamine produces anticipatory pleasure – it initiates food seeking," says Dr. Bart Hoebel, a noted researcher from Princeton University, who has spent decades studying addiction pathways. In a recent study published in the Journal of Nutrition, rats that had elevated brain dopamine levels because they binged on sugars for a month, developed fewer dopamine receptors and more opioid receptors,[12] just as mice addicted to cocaine and heroin do. Together, these receptors create a motivation and reward system.

When their sugar supply was suddenly denied, the rats suffered all the classical signs of withdrawal, including teeth chattering and intense anxiety. When sugar was reintroduced, these rats worked harder to obtain it, and consumed more than they previously had. Also, in the absence of sugar, these rats more frequently turned to alcohol.[xxix] As many studies before it have, this study shows that sugar mimics the behavioral and neurochemical changes in the brain that abused substances like alcohol, heroin and cocaine produce. Sugar is an addiction. It is a reaction to hunger or a need to artificially trigger pleasure.

Sugar addicts can be born or made. Many people are biologically programmed to be true sugar addicts, but do not realize a chemical explanation for their sugar sensitivity exists. For these people, sugar rules their lives – they experience intense volatility in their emotions, energy levels, and feelings of self worth. Sugar sensitive people are often depressed. They know sugars elevate their mood. Sugar addicts are those born with a heightened sensitivity to carbohydrates and chronically low levels of the brain neurotransmitters serotonin and beta-endorphins. These neurotransmitters are called opioids because their action in the brain mimics morphine.

Serotonin is responsible for feelings of wellbeing and for curbing impulsive behavior. When a person has low levels, he or she is usually depressed and lacks willpower. The drugs Paxil, Effexor, Prozac, and Zoloft elevate mood by elevating serotonin levels. Beta-endorphins stimulate confidence and euphoria. Sugar, alcohol, heroin, and morphine all activate beta-endorphin release. Beta-endorphins have many times the potency of morphine.

Many people lose their cravings and find energy by consuming raw foods, especially green smoothies. Some people worry about oxalates found in greens. Do your homework, but I always include broccoli, brussel sprouts, and kale. (See: http://www.whfoods.com/genpage.php?tname=foodspice&dbid=38.)

---

12 Opioids are neurotransmitters, such as beta-endorphins and serotonin, which work by binding to opioid receptors throughout the central nervous system and in the gut. They mimic morphine's actions.

To answer the initial question, I believe artificial sweeteners are more damaging than table sugar. Research abounds on this subject.

## Rewiring the Brain

Knowing what we know about epigenetics – how tags turn gene expression off and on, and how these changes are then passed on to at least two subsequent generations – it is interesting to note that children and grandchildren of alcoholics are often born with low beta-endorphin transmitter and receptor levels. People with low levels of beta-endorphins and serotonin are predisposed to two closely associated syndromes: alcoholism and sugar addiction. The good news is that lifestyle changes can manipulate these neurotransmitters and their receptors. When and how a person sleeps, exercises, eats, drinks, and copes with stress can rewire the brain.

Women should be particularly careful to manage these factors when estrogen levels are low just before menstruation because this is when beta-endorphins are at their lowest.

If you hate the thought of breakfast, are often exhausted and moody, crave sweets, and berate yourself for not having the power to avoid them despite the fact that you know they are killing you, you should know you can readjust your body chemistry so you can begin to heal and change your life. There is no "one size fits all" when it comes to nutritional needs. Everyone is unique and responds differently to the same foods. As we commonly say, "One man's food is another man's poison."

Whether you were born with a predisposition towards simple carbohydrate cravings or you eased into it over a lifetime of over-indulging, you can reset your body chemistry. It is important to include high quality proteins and vegetables at every meal. Proteins are key to reducing sugar cravings. Proteins are made from amino acids.

The amino acids, L-Tyrosine and L-Phenylalanine, boost levels of the brain chemicals dopamine and norepinephrine. These neurotransmitters increase energy and focus. The amino acid tryptophan, or 5-Hydroxy Tryptophan (5HTP), is a precursor for the neurotransmitter, serotonin. Tryptophan relieves insomnia, depression, and anxiety. It also helps you feel full. Serotonin helps you relax. The amino acid glutamine dampens carbohydrate cravings. A good source for all of these amino acids is complete whey proteins, discussed in the "Glutathione" section above.

One of my daughters was able to tame her lifelong sugar addiction by stirring two scoops of whey protein into her morning glass of water for two weeks. Though concerned at the outset about how it would feel to give up something she had always enjoyed, she was palpably amazed at the end of the experiment; and she was relieved at how easy it was. More than anything, she was relieved to be free!

If you are worried about quitting something that brings you great pleasure and comfort, remember that your body compensates. As John Yudkin, M.D., author of the book, *Sweet and Dangerous* says, "When you have become used to taking very little sugar in your foods and drinks, you will notice that all your foods have a wide range of interesting flavors you have forgotten." [xxx] Many clients have told me they notice this and enjoy healthy foods so much more than they ever did before.

Some people rely on gamma-amino butyric acid, or GABA, to curb appetite and sugar cravings. GABA is an important inhibitory neurotransmitter in the brain that signals fullness. It reduces brain excitability and is often effective in treating obsessive–compulsive disorder. This supplement induces relaxation. Green tea can boost GABA levels.

Dr. Amen, a clinical neuroscientist, psychiatrist, and brain-imaging expert, works extensively with people trying to regain control of their weight and their lives. Through studying brain scans, he has learned there are six types of brain activity patterns that lead to weight management difficulty. His ground-breaking book, "Change Your Brain, Change Your Body," [xxxi] offers further guidance about how to reduce cravings depending on personal neurochemistry.

For those not yet committed to total health, I will return to the original question about sugar substitutes. I know I have reviewed enough literature about artificial sweeteners to convince me to avoid them. A comprehensive book, "Sweet Deception: Why Splenda®, NutraSweet®, and the FDA May Be Hazardous to Your Health," [xxxii] succinctly summarizes what I learned from extensive reading. Its author, Dr. Mercola, reviews sugar toxicity and addiction pathways. He also assesses artificial sugars, alcohol sugars, and alternative sweeteners like stevia, honey, and agave nectar. He reviews the politics of the FDA approval process in great detail.

If I were to use a substitute, I would choose stevia, a South American herb with a long safety track record. It is two to three hundred times sweeter than sugar, has almost no calories and little effect on blood sugar levels. It is found only on the nutritional supplement aisle because the FDA has not approved stevia's use as a sweetener, presumably to protect the artificial sweetener manufacturers, according to Dr. Mercola. Avoid agave syrup, which is often relabeled high fructose corn syrup.

If you do choose to use artificial sweeteners, know that the contents of the familiar packets are not what they pretend to be. The familiar .5 and 1.0-gram packets of powdered artificial sugar contain more than 90 percent sugar in the form sucrose, dextrose, or maltodextrin as bulking agents. Splenda No Calorie Sweetener® is actually 99 percent sugar. Manufacturers again manipulate serving sizes to write off calories. The labeling laws allow a "no calorie" label if the serving size contains less than five calories. In Splenda's case, each packet contains four calories. I expect diabetics are as unaware of this manipulation as are most other Americans.

## Nutrient Absorption

Sometimes we eat right but still do not absorb nutrients. Often we do not properly synthesize what we need. For instance, as we age, our bodies make less of the antioxidant CoQ10, less intrinsic factor (a compound secreted by the digestive system that helps us extract vitamin B-12 from animal products), less digestive and pancreatic enzymes, and less hydrochloric acid to help us break down foods. Increasingly, Americans are diagnosed with gluten intolerance or outright celiac disease. It gets more and better play in the media all the time. This is good because celiac disease is basically a disease of malnutrition.

## Celiac Disease

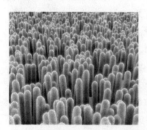
A celiac disease (CD) diagnosis was once rare, but its prevalence has climbed. The Celiac Disease Foundation estimates that 1 in every 133 Americans has it. Other credible sources suggest one percent of Americans suffer it,[xxix] especially those of English, Italian, Scandinavian, or Irish descent.

CD is an autoimmune disease caused by a strong immune response to gluten, a component of most grains.[13] This response happens as the

---

13 Today's hybridized and genetically modified wheats contain between 30-50 per-

bristle-like filaments that profusely line the small intestines (villi) try to absorb nutrients. When a person with CD eats gluten in any form, antibodies in the blood attack the gluten to destroy it. As the villi absorb the gluten, they are also attacked. The villi are slowly destroyed along with the body's ability to absorb nutrients. The resulting malnutrition affects every system. As damage progresses, it can become life threatening.

CD is linked to specific genetic markers.[14] Almost all people with CD have these markers, whereas less than half of those without CD have them. One is not born with the disease, but with a genetic tendency to develop it; stress, pregnancy, viruses, and other chance occurrences can activate it. The disease is usually active for over a decade before enough symptoms surface to cause a person to seek diagnosis. Diagnosis often occurs during a person's middle to late forties. And as with diabetes and early heart disease, bodies suffer damage from ignored symptoms and misdiagnoses.

Because malnutrition appears as myriad symptoms, CD is easily misdiagnosed, leading to needless suffering. Worse, the longer one suffers before diagnosis, the more likely that person will develop another autoimmune disease like rheumatoid arthritis, type 1 diabetes, lupus, thyroid disease (Hashimoto's and Graves' disease), Sjögren's syndrome, or microscopic colitis. Cancers of the lymph glands, kidney disease, seizures, nerve problems and osteoporosis are some other risks of long-standing, unmanaged CD.

If you suffer any or several of the symptoms listed below that are not easily explained, consider the possibility that you have either celiac disease or gluten intolerance:

- Intestinal tract discomfort is a classic symptom, although it does not always surface. A sufferer might experience cramping, bloating, excessive gas, or poor water regulation leading to either diarrhea or constipation.

---

cent gluten. Barley and triticale (a recent cross between rye and wheat) also contain significant amounts of gluten. Ancient wheats like kamut, spelt, and rye, have less gluten and contain more protein, minerals, and fatty acids. Rice, corn, millet, ragi and tiff are ancient grains that do not contain gluten. Oats, Buckwheat, amaranth, soy, cassava, arrowroot, flax, Indian rice grass, quinoa, wild rice, sorghum, bean and other legume flours, yucca, tapioca, or potato flours do not cause problems for most with celiac.

14 HLA–DQ2 and HLA–DQ8

- A constantly dry mouth might be a symptom.
- Anemias (due to nutrient deficiencies)
- Weight loss in spite of a normal or excessive appetite
- Conversely, weight gain can be a symptom.
- Other chameleon-like symptoms might be bone or joint pain
- Lactose intolerance
- Low energy
- Infertility in either gender
- Recurrent miscarriages
- Elevated liver enzymes
- Depression
- Tooth enamel defects
- Low bone density
- Recurring painful oral ulcers occur in about 25 percent of those with unmanaged CD. A beefy-red, smooth tongue signals a lack of adequate iron or B-complex vitamin absorption.

Most links between celiac disease and oral health are not clearly established, but because it is a disease of malnutrition, oral structures are not spared. To see why this disease is hard to diagnose, one simply has to look at some deficiencies created from nutrient malabsorption.

CD is thought to precede some cases of type 1 diabetes. Sometimes a person's immune system turns against itself and destroys the pancreatic cells that make insulin, which leads to diabetes. When gluten is avoided after a CD diagnosis, this response ceases.

Because of its higher prevalence in Europe, several countries conduct routine screenings for CD. Positive results lead to either a small bowel biopsy or the newer capsule endoscopy[15] for a definitive diagnosis. As with diabetes and other diseases, early diagnosis and intervention increases success economically. Screening is still rare in America.

## Gluten Intolerance

Gluten intolerance, while not as severe a diagnosis as celiac disease, can still be debilitating. There are many degrees of intolerance to

---

15 Capsule endoscopy involves swallowing a tiny encapsulated digital camera. As it traverses the GI tract, digestion is visually monitored.

gluten, but best success comes from gluten avoidance, as one might expect. Diagnosing gluten intolerance is not as straightforward as it may seem. Traditional blood tests for gluten sensitivities only look at one component of gluten to determine if one is sensitive, alpha gliadin. There are other components of gluten that make one intolerant. If a person is not intolerant to the alpha gliadin component, they will test negative on most tests.

A home test from Cyrex Labs[16] identifies twelve wheat components that promote inflammatory responses that lead to allergies, celiac disease, and other autoimmune diseases in some people. The test includes a free celiac disease test to rule out the disease. It also looks for gluten's potential to cause addictive behaviors in each person. Specific enzymes in the gut break gluten down into opioids that promote addictive behaviors. Opioids are a major reason for the spike in ADD/ADHD, depression, anxiety and other neurological dysfunctions. Since opioids are addictive, if you start a gluten free program, you may well have major withdrawal symptoms. Discuss test results with your physician so you can learn how to support brain function to minimize withdrawal symptoms.[xxxiii]

## Malnutrition Manifestations

- **Calcium:** Calcium builds strong teeth and bones. Vitamin D is the body's main calcium regulator and is crucial for calcium absorption. Compromised absorption can create tooth enamel deficiencies as well as osteopenia or osteoporosis. Calcium deficiencies also prompt exhaustion, since muscles need calcium to contract. Dentally, periodontal disease intensifies when osteopenia or osteoporosis weaken jawbones. Oral tissues need calcium and phosphate to stay intact. Many CD sufferers concurrently have lactose intolerance, which exacerbates low calcium levels.

- **Vitamin D:** Vitamin D was misclassified as a vitamin. It is really a steroidal hormone that regulates about 2,000 to 3,000 genes. Vitamin D affects not genes themselves, but tags that turn genes on and off, what is termed epigenetics. Almost all

---

16 To order gluten associated home test kits, go to True Health Labs at: http://www.truehealthlabs.com/categories/Cyrex-Gluten-Testing/.

of what we know about vitamin D has been learned in the last decade. Most adults need 5000 units per day. Vitamin D is found in organ meats. We get about 250 to 300 IU per day from fortified foods so most adults are deficient. There are associations between low vitamin D levels and rheumatoid arthritis, multiple sclerosis, type 1 diabetes, high blood pressure, obesity, preeclampsia, asthma, cystic fibrosis, migraines, psoriasis, eczema, insomnia, hearing loss, gum disease, macular degeneration, myopia, seizures, fertility, and autism. The majority of pregnant women are vitamin D deficient. Vitamin D is also a potent antibiotic many times more potent than the ones usually prescribed. It helps create 200 to 300 antimicrobial protein peptides in the human body. For short-term acute infection therapy, one can take as much of 50,000 units for three days. Further, there are strong associations between low levels of vitamin D and cancer, especially of breast, colon, prostate, and lung cancer.

The best way to get vitamin D is through sunshine. Many sunscreens filter out the UVB rays that create protective vitamin $D_3$ in the skin, but not the UVA rays that cause cancer. UVA rays deactivate vitamin $D_3$ in your skin. Since vitamin D helps fight skin cancer, skin cancer risks increase rather than decrease if you use UVB filtering sunscreen. These increased cancer risks do not include elevated risks from absorbing the toxins that are a part of most sunscreen formulas.

Glass also selectively transmits UVA rays while it filters out UVB rays. The best time to convert sunlight into $D_3$ is at noon when UVB rays are the strongest and UVA rays the weakest. Sunburns increase cancer risks, but tans do not. Stop exposure when your skin starts to turn pink. Any more will cause photo aging without conferring extra benefits. Do not wash the D from your skin with soap. The longer you leave it, the more you will absorb.

**Note:** As mentioned in the osteoporosis chapter/Marshall protocol, vitamin D presents us with a paradox: It may be that "optimal" vitamin D levels are really optimal only for healthy people. For those with autoimmune diseases, surfacing research muddies the conversation. Also, excessive vitamin D reduces magnesium absorption.

- **Magnesium:** According to the National Institute of Health, "Magnesium is used in more than 300 biochemical reactions. It helps maintain normal muscle and nerve function, keeps heart rhythm steady, supports a healthy immune system, and keeps bones strong. Magnesium also helps regulate blood sugar levels, promotes normal blood pressure, and is involved in energy metabolism and protein synthesis. There is increasing interest in magnesium's role in preventing and managing disorders such as hypertension, cardiovascular disease, and diabetes." [xxxiv] Magnesium can help slow noise-related hearing loss and can reduce ringing and buzzing in the ears.

  Since an excessive influx of calcium ions can cause nerve death, a balanced calcium/magnesium intake ratio can provide protection. In pre-agrarian days when humans evolved, calcium to magnesium intake was about 1:1. Diets today usually reflect a skewed ratio. In dairy products it is about 12:1. As magnesium and calcium compete for absorption in the gut, modern diets are often deficient in magnesium. High sugar intake depletes magnesium for instance. Inadequate magnesium intake impairs absorption of vitamin D, calcium, and phosphorus. If you supplement with these vitamins, be sure you also supplement with magnesium.

  Try to avoid magnesium stearate. First, magnesium stearate is an excipient with no nutritive value. It is a filler, carrier, and adds anti-caking properties. Stearates are most commonly produced by hydrogenating cottonseed oil. They are pre-oxidized and contain heavy pesticide residues. Those made with organic palm oils would be a better choice. Stearates can coat every particle in a supplement, which may lead to compromised nutrient absorption. Magnesium stearate may suppress the immune system's T-cells.[xxxv] A rule of thumb when buying vitamins in general is to buy only veggie caps. Magnesium stearate is a particular hallmark of shellacked, hard-shelled vitamins, which often exit the digestive tract completely intact. Preferred forms: magnesium citrate, picolate, or magnesium L-lactate dihydrate; better yet, eat dark leafy green foods!

- **B$_{12}$ or Cobalamin:** B$_{12}$ is known as the "energy vitamin." It boosts energy at the cellular level and optimizes mental abilities by maintaining various nerve and brain cell functions. For most people, just knowing deficiencies are associated with brain atrophy[xxxvi] is reason enough to pay attention, but B$_{12}$ also maintains the fatty sheathes around nerves. If these degrade, mental and physical abilities likewise suffer. B$_{12}$ helps produce melatonin, the "sleep hormone" and the body's ubiquitous antioxidant. Along with folic acid (B$_9$), B$_{12}$ regulates red blood cell formation and helps your body use iron and other nutrients. This is why pernicious anemia is associated with CD: oxygen-carrying red blood cell levels drop because B$_{12}$ is not absorbed, which results in exhaustion. B$_{12}$ also provides immune system support, increases cellular longevity (think anti-aging), and helps make the adrenal hormones that partially regulate metabolism, blood chemistry, and a host of other functions.

  Those without the absorption problems of CD often still suffer deficiencies. B$_{12}$ is a huge molecule, so the stomach secretes intrinsic factor, which binds to the large B$_{12}$ vitamin to enable its absorption. After age 50, one's body makes less intrinsic factor. Aging and frequent antacids or anti-ulcer drug use also inhibits absorption because B$_{12}$ requires stomach acids for its release from foods. Vegans and vegetarians often lack B$_{12}$ because it is found mainly in animal food proteins like meat and eggs. If supplementing, note only humans can only use the form cyanocobalamin. The B$_{12}$ in multivitamins create B$_{12}$ analogues as they react with copper, iron and vitamin C. Not only are they unusable in this form, they keep you from absorbing forms you *can* use. *Take B vitamins separately from other supplements.* If you are over 50, have CD or poor GI health from other causes, consider sublingual (under-the-tongue) sprays or drops that bypass the need for intrinsic factor and digestion.

- **B$_9$ (Folate or folic acid):** The list of complications resulting from any vitamin B complex deficiency is long and serious. For instance, if a mother is folate-deficient during the earliest phase of pregnancy, possible if she has been on birth control pills which deplete folate, her baby has an increased risk of developing a neural tube defect (NTD). NTD results in a malformation of the brain and spinal cord. In addition to celiac disease, about a fourth of our population has a gene mutation that causes difficulty with folate metabolism. Women with this genetic mutation are 2.5 times more likely to have a child with Down syndrome. This mutation is also tied to inflammatory bowel disease, colon cancer, oral clefts and high levels of homocysteine.[xxvii] High homocysteine levels are associated with cardiovascular disease and stroke risk. Homocysteine eats tiny pits in arterial walls. The repair requires LDLs to transport cholesterol to the area. This leads to the plaque formation and artery hardening described in Chapter Three. Homocysteine interferes with clotting and oxidizes bad cholesterol (VLDLs). Many doctors recommend B complex to reduce atherosclerosis.

Low folate levels also lead to congenital heart defects, obstructions of the urinary tract, limb deficiencies, pre-term deliveries and slow fetal development. Insufficient folate weakens and breaks chromosomes and turns off tumor-suppressing genes, so insufficient folate is also associated with increased risk of various cancers.[xxxviii] Folate is the $B_9$ form found naturally in dark green leafy vegetables, citrus fruits, beans, etc. Folic acid is the synthetic vitamin our bodies may actually absorb more easily that the folate form found in foods. Excess $B_9$ can mask a $B_{12}$ deficiency.

Oral symptoms of B complex deficiencies vary, but often include an inflammation of the tongue, sometimes accompanied by a deep fiery red or magenta color. Other times, the tongue will be smooth and dry. Soreness and burning can accompany these changes.

Supplementation exceeding 1,000 micrograms per day in the form of folic acid could trigger symptoms of a vitamin $B_{12}$ deficiency, such as anemia and nerve damage. While anemia can be corrected, nerve damage cannot. Take vitamin B as a complex separate from other vitamins or under the advice of your doctor.

- **Vitamin K:** Vitamin $K_1$ is necessary for clot or scab formation. Without it, hemorrhaging risks increase. People with stroke risk should be aware of this since careful control of blood viscosity is a preventive goal for their condition. Vitamin $K_2$ directs calcium deposition in the body. It directs it away from blood vessel walls, where it contributes to atherosclerosis, and to bones. If one's diet is deficient in fats, this fat soluble vitamin may not be well absorbed.

- **Iron:** Iron deficiency anemia is common in those with CD. Iron carries and delivers oxygen throughout the body. It is but one reason CD might express as exhaustion. The tongue can look and feel as it does with pernicious anemia.

- **Fats:** Fats are used throughout the body. They help transport molecules across cell membranes and function as structural components of cell membranes. They are necessary for energy reserves. They are a component of and help synthesize and store other vitamins and hormones. The normal human brain is comprised of about seventy percent fat. A lack of fat absorption could lead to a range of symptoms, including nervous system disorders. This is because fat is a component in the protective sheathes around nerves. Avoid trans fats and oils heated above their smoking point.

The only treatment known for CD is avoidance of all gluten. This is a severe restriction, but as with diabetes, this particular lifestyle change involves a learning curve and a brain and body chemical reset. Celiacs must avoid all grains classified as wheats (spelt, triticale, and often, kamut) as well as rye and barley. Some allowed grains are rice, soy, millet, cassava, arrowroot, corn, flax, Indian rice grass, amaranth, quinoa, sago, seeds, buckwheat, wild rice, sorghum, bean and other legume flours, yucca, tapioca, or potato flours.

Since the FDA's Food Allergen Labeling and Consumer Protection Act of 2004 became effective on January 1, 2006, consumers have some help in appropriately identifying this protein allergen. Still, take care to look for gluten-free labels. Consulting the ingredient list is insufficient. As with peanut allergens, many factories producing ostensibly gluten-free products also make products containing wheat. Similarly, there is sometimes contamination between grains out in the fields during harvest time. It is possible traces of wheat might still exist even if gluten is not labeled as a product ingredient. Discovering hidden sources of wheat products is part of the learning curve as they are often used in preservatives, stabilizers and thickeners, adhesives on stamps and envelopes, baking powder, various drugs, vitamins, and texture enhancers. In fact, wheat products are found in most processed foods, lipstick, gum, and toothpaste. Tom's of Maine and The Natural Dentist manufacture gluten-free hygiene products.

During the healing process, taking supplements to compensate for poor nutrient absorption helps. The fat soluble vitamins A, D, E, and K, plus vitamin C, zinc, calcium, magnesium, omega-3 fatty acids and the antioxidants that protect them, and probiotics are often recommended. Anti-bacterial and anti-inflammatory herbs like goldenseal, echinacea, and turmeric may speed recovery.

## ANNE

I worked with Anne for many years to try to identify the variables that kept her gums unhealthy. Though a young woman, her complicated health history included several autoimmune factors. Her home care was consistently better than most, but her gums never reflected the health we wanted for her.

At a wellness appointment several years ago, her gums finally showed remarkable improvement. I searched for clues to explain her improved health. We began discussing immune system factors. She was used to my querying and knew a change she had made might be pertinent. She said she was told when a child that she had inherited celiac disease from her grandmother. At that time she had not wanted to accept it and restrict her diet. But with increasing maturity and yet another trip to the hospital, she decided she needed to accept and address this genetic disease. She bought, among other books, a copy of: *A Personal Touch On... Celiac Disease (The #1 Misdiagnosed Intestinal Disorder)* [xxxix] to inspire her. This book is a compilation of essays people wrote about their journey toward discovering and living with celiac disease.

Anne said she is making the necessary dietary changes. Her improved sense of wellbeing fuels her strength to make the required adjustments. Her motto has become, "Change is how you think about reality." Instead of focusing on the loss of certain favorite foods, she is thrilled to be reclaiming her health.

## Innocent Until Proven Guilty:
## Allergies and Engineered Proteins

When your immune system registers proteins as foreign, that is an allergy.

- Between 1997-2002, the number of children with peanut allergies doubled, according to the CDC.
- The CDC also reports a 265 percent increase in doctor-mandated hospitalizations due to food reactions.
- One in seventeen children now has a food allergy.

What foreign proteins are in our foods that were not there before? Milk allergies are the most common food allergy. In 1990s, synthetic growth hormones were engineered and introduced into the food supply without any human trials. Governments around the world, excepting the U. S. banned these proteins – guilty until proven innocent. Of course these growth hormones benefitted the dairy industry, but at what cost?

Just as in feedlots, the cows became unhealthy. They required antibiotics to treat their abundant cases of ovarian cysts, skin disorders, and mastitis. The U.S. government took the stance that these foreign proteins were considered benign until proven dangerous and allowed them. These growth hormones elevate human hormones related to breast, prostate, and colon cancers. Compared to the rest of the world, Americans have elevated levels of these hormones – and correspondingly elevated rates of these diseases compared to other countries. We know one out of eight American women has breast cancer, yet only a tenth of these cases are attributed to genes; most cases are environmentally triggered.

In 1996, new proteins were engineered into soy to handle increasing doses of week killer. Soy, mainly used to fatten livestock, is also a top eight food allergen. No other country allows GMO engineered soy.

In the late 1990s, the EPA had to register some corn as an insecticide because the DNA of the kernels was engineered to repel pests.

National corporations formulate their products differently to meet consumer demand in other countries. Nonetheless, they continue to be profitable, so it can be done. Vote with your pocketbook when you buy food. And vote to abandon the agricultural subsidies that force many people to make short-term economic choices that cost them dearly in the long term as health inevitably fails.

Mouth breathers must consider these foods or other allergens, when seeking solutions. See Chapter 12.

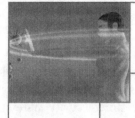

# 15

## IMMUNE SYSTEM SUPPORT
## ARE YOU READY?

*"Our belief system creates our reality."*

**~ Gary Null, Ph. D. in human nutrition and public health science ~**

**Explore:**
1. Easy, energizing immune system support strategies.
2. The ongoing controversy over the oral use of mercury; a fresh look at mercury toxicity.

    a) Personal safety. Are your teeth smoking? How much vapor do mercury fillings release as teeth function?

    b) Environmental concerns. It is not just about you any more.

## Simple Solutions Avert Serious Consequences

"All gum disease and cavities are preventable."

It was a brilliant lecture opener. In the silence before the speaker continued, the audience of hygienists mentally raced through its knowledge and experience base to match what we observed in practice with what we had just heard. Did our practical observations match the speaker's assertion?

The speaker continued by asking if anyone had suffered decay since becoming health professionals. No one raised a hand.

Then she asked if anyone had gum disease. Again, there were no positive responses.

In that moment, we got it. Hygienists understand prevention. We believe in it. We do it.

Why would anyone be casual about their own oral health if they understand the critical link between it, degenerative diseases, and immune system dysfunction? We all make simple, everyday choices that either boost or challenge our body's full-time security system. Challenging the immune system instead of supporting it causes our health balance to tip towards disease. Being healthy is fun, but it takes commitment.

## Heredity and Epigenetics
## Shifting From Destiny To Responsibility and Hope

The Human Genome Project identified all the genes in human DNA and sequenced the three billion chemical base pairs that make up these genes. It was to be the definitive "Book of Life", but it was just the first chapter. The emerging field of epigenetics studies how our dynamic environment sculpts our genes, and thus our health. There are tags that turn genes on and off; they control which genes are expressed. This is why encoded diseases are not always inevitable, why risk is not destiny.

Identical twins with identical genes can have very different health profiles. DNA strands from young identical twins show nearly identical gene expression when superimposed. As the twins age, the same DNA strands may show virtually no similarities in gene expression.[i] Our environments and the choices we make, especially at key times during development, influence the tags that switch genes on and off.

These changes are passed on to future generations. Therefore what epigenetics seems to tell us is that we are ethically charged with the task of protecting our genes. It also gives us hope that we can alter our destinies. The health and longevity we desire for ourselves and our offspring requires us to master our lifestyles. It gives us a moral imperative to clean up our internal and external environments. We can no longer mistreat our fragile ecosystem or ourselves. Our health is tied to both. We can no longer think of our lifestyles as "our way of life." We are awakening to the fact that our current way of life is not sustainable on any level. We can think of this awakening as an opportunity to remake our world and ourselves. In fact, our bodies are a reflection of our external world.

Complementary medicine encourages health by using the body's own internal healing mechanisms and systems. Nutrition, exercise, mental outlook, and toxin avoidance are important cornerstones.

Generally speaking, complementary medicine promotes disease resistance.

Individually, professionally, and collectively, we must incorporate expanded prevention practices into our lives. We must also understand how politics and money impact our health and the information we rely on to maintain it. What are our sources for that information? Is it from talk show hosts and other popular media outlets? Does advertising money influence them? Does advertising influence you?

And what about Pharma's influences on our trusted doctors? Their influences begin early. Harvard Medical school student, Matt Zerden, began what became a full-blown movement to tighten up conflict-of-interest policies at Harvard between medical professors, their duties to their students, and their financial ties to pharmaceutical companies. It began when a pharmacology professor, while teaching the benefits of statin drugs, was queried by a student concerned about their side effects. This professor derided the student for asking. Mr. Zerden investigated and discovered the professor was a consultant for eight pharmaceutical companies, five of whom produce statin drugs. As Kirsten Austad, one movement leader said, "We are being indoctrinated into a field of medicine that is becoming more and more commercialized. Before coming here, I had no idea how much influence companies had on medical education. It is something that's purposely meant to be under the table, providing information under the guise of education when that information is also presented for marketing purposes."

As Duff Wilson reported in The New York Times, about 1600 medical school professors and lecturers report financial interests related to their teaching, research, or clinical care.[ii] Big Pharma's reach into the FDA and what we know about health is deep and broad. We would do well to question the motives backing our belief systems.

Limited awareness, time, and resources hamper conventional medicine, whose focus is to fight localized symptoms of disease, not underlying causes. We cannot maintain health through management and repair of localized disease.

Alternative medicine practitioners and their non-pharmaceutical treatments are usually less expensive than conventional doctor's fees and pharmaceutical drugs. Again, conventional medicine attacks late stage disease with crisis intervention. Complementary medicine focuses on disease prevention and a whole body approach. Clearly, conventional medicine cannot work alone.

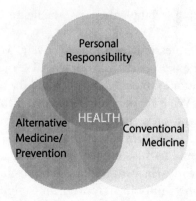

## Stress and Cortisol

Stress is the number one enemy of our immune systems because stress raises cortisol and adrenaline levels. The human stress response, orchestrated by cortisol and adrenaline, once helped us survive immediate life-or-death threats. This response immediately spikes blood pressure and heart rate to provide oxygen to muscles for fight-or-flight. It raises blood sugar levels to feed muscles. Insulin levels also rise. Tissue damage accelerates while tissue repair stops. Reproductive abilities shut down. Brain chemistry changes.

Stress keeps stem cells from keeping pace with the body's need to repair damage caused by age, toxins, or inflammation. In excess, cortisol results in low levels of the sex hormones testosterone, progesterone, and DHEA.[1] High cortisol levels lead to abdominal fat accumulation, sleep disorders, depression, fatigue, poor concentration and poor memory. They create anxiety, mood swings, and sugar cravings.

Stress sabotages digestion by decreasing enzyme activity and blood flow to the gut. Digestive capabilities dwindle, which can lead to food allergies, constipation, bloating, poor nutrient absorption, irritable bowel syndrome (IBS), pain and an inflamed gut lining. A chronically inflamed gut is biologically similar to chronically inflamed gums – the blood vessels that feed both are no longer fine filters, but leaky sieves. In the gut, a compromised intestinal lining allows incompletely digested food particles, wastes, bacteria, fungi, and their toxins to enter the bloodstream. These toxins are not normally released into the

---

1 DHEA is a steroidal hormone that supports the sex hormones, increases lean muscle tissue, burns stored body fat, balances blood sugar, improves memory and supports immune function.

bloodstream. They are usually excreted. The liver can get backed up trying to detoxify these excessive wastes. It is during times of high stress that parasites, bacteria or yeast pathogens can gain a firm foothold in a person's body, though it may be years before symptoms develop.

Stress leads to epigenetic changes, specifically to heart disease, cancers, diabetes, and other diseases. Stress shortens telomeres. Telomeres are protective caps on the ends of DNA strands that keep them from unraveling, fusing with other DNA strands, or rearranging themselves. These abnormalities can lead to cancer. Telomeres shorten every time a cell divides. This limits cells to a fixed number of duplications before they die. This is one way poor lifestyle choices can speed cellular damage, thus aging. For instance, weight gain and insulin resistance correlate with faster telomere shortening.[iii] Like an immune system in constant overdrive, the stress response has life threatening consequences.

There are three kinds of stress that spike cortisol levels:

1.  Emotional stress. Emotional stress is influenced by one's perception of life events, not the life events themselves. Release unresolved emotional issues. Learn how to improve your general outlook, focus on what is important, and develop everyday coping skills.
2.  Dietary stress. Consuming excess sugars and grains leads to unstable blood sugars, which affect cortisol rhythms.
3.  Inflammatory stress. Untreated inflammatory conditions such as gum disease raise cortisol levels.[v]

## Enzymes

Your body contains from 80 to 100 trillion cells, all with a different structure and function, but basically the same chemistry. Twenty thousand enzymes within our body's cells carry on about 100,000 chemical reactions each second. They could be called the master chemists of the cell. Cells do not work well when enzymes are unavailable or improperly synthesized. Beyond proper cell function, enzymes help kill pathogens and break down collagen to dissolve blood clots.

Many people work to maximize their enzymes. Forty percent of their diet is raw food, they avoid microwaved food, and their diets include plenty of probiotics and fermented foods to restore gut microbiota. Why are amino acid supplements, neurotransmitters, probiotics, cleanses, parasite detoxes, and so on, not enough?

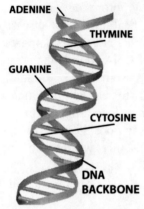

ADENINE

THYMINE

GUANINE

CYTOSINE

DNA BACKBONE

Let us examine how enzymes are made and how their production can go wrong. Inside the nucleus are 46 chromosomes, each with 30,000 to 40,000 genes. Each gene contains about seventeen inches of wound DNA. There are four sugar bases that must combine specifically to form twenty amino acids. (See image.). These in turn must line up in specific ways to produce the 20,000 enzymes. In biology, function follows form. If an enzyme form twists out of shape because the sugar bases line up incorrectly, it loses function. Disease follows when there are too many "misspellings".

Oxidative stress messes up this "spelling", forcing the genetic code to make the wrong enzyme. These chemical reactions are one of the biggest problems caused by free radical oxidation.

Vitamins are co-enzymes; minerals are co-factors. You don't want too many minerals or they become enzyme inhibitors. For example fluoride is a major enzyme inhibitor (and creates acid-forming wastes in tissues that must be buffered). Enzyme biologists were the first to oppose city water fluoridation. But if you do not get enough enzymes, you die. You must consume 27 chemical elements in the proper amounts found in the cell. You have to consume 45 nutrients in their proper amounts: carbohydrates, fats, proteins, 18 vitamins, 19 minerals and pure water. This is easiest if you get most of your nutrients from food. Again, I must mention an alkaline diet and nasal breathing to maintain health. The pH of a normal human cell ranges between 7.35 – 7.45. Enzyme development is affected below 7.3. If pH drops below 7.3, enzymes do not survive.

Taking protease enzymes can boost health. Proteolytic (protease) enzymes break down fibrotic scar tissue, which over time creates so much restriction and strain on our organs they no longer function well. When there aren't sufficient proteolytic enzymes in the blood stream, protease enzymes can also help free red blood cells that get stuck in and amongst fibrin. They break down proteins, support circulation, and are natural anti-oxidants. Protease enzymes also make glutathione.

## Probiotics

After enzymes, your gut's ecosystem determines much of how your immune system functions. Liberally enjoy unpasteurized fermented foods like natto, miso, kefir, and sauerkraut to help repopulate your gut with good bacteria destroyed by antacids, sugars, and other processed foods. While fermented foods deliver many times the beneficial bacteria of supplements at a fraction of the cost, probiotic supplements can help, especially after taking antibiotics or straying from a healthy diet.

Take quality supplements with fiber so they last long enough to survive until they reach the intestines. Prebiotic, high fiber foods like bananas, whole grains, greens, tomatoes, onions, legumes, and garlic are important because they help probiotic bacteria survive long enough to gain a foothold in your gut. Yogurt can have many beneficial bacteria, but if you are using it to replace good bacteria destroyed by refined carbohydrates, it makes no sense to add sugar. Unpasteurized kefir contains friendly bacterial strains as well as beneficial yeasts. These yeasts likewise maintain balance. They control and eliminate pathogenic yeasts because these small molecules can penetrate the intestinal lining where unhealthy bacteria and yeasts reside. The probiotics in kefir also help digest the food you eat. Beyond improved food digestion and assimilation, probiotics influence genes' disease-fighting capabilities. They may even help lower blood pressure! Once again, avoid GMO soy.

For a partial listing of where to obtain raw milk from which to make healthful kefir, go to: http://realmilk.com/where.html.

For those who drink milk, the raw milk movement is gaining ground despite governmental crack-downs citing safety concerns. Pasteurization transforms fats and denatures healthful proteins and enzymes. The process also creates AGEs. Sloppy mass production of milk requires pasteurization, no doubt about it. Raw milk producers must follow stringent practices to keep their milk safe.

**Note:** Fermented soy increases isoflavone availability, and decreases the negative effects of phytic acid found in nonfermented soy products such as tofu, soy milk, nuts, baby formula, and other processed foods. Phytic acid binds to nutrients and thus, hinders their absorption. Nattokinase, found in natto, has an enzyme produced in the fermentation process that has a powerful ability to dissolve blood clots and seems to dissolve the amyloid plaques in the brain associated with Alzheimer's. (Fibrin, a component of blood clots, is a key indicator of whole-body inflammation.)

Bacterial colonizers must be matched to the site of the desired benefit. Yogurt may contain live cultures such as acidophilus that improves digestion, strengthens your immune system and helps maintain vaginal and urinary tract health, but if you want to rebalance oral microorganisms, you will have longer-lasting results if you supplement with Evora lozenges. These may particularly help those who have trouble regulating their oral acid-base balance – elderly people on multiple drugs, the institutionalized, those with excessive areas of root surface exposure, those with a documented high caries incidence, and patients who have physical and dexterity limitations.

## Alpha Lipoic Acid (ALA)

The more energy generators (mitochondria) you have within each cell and the more alpha lipoic acid (ALA) you have available, the more body fat you will burn. ALA increases the number of mitochondria within each cell and is also a critical coenzyme that helps the mitochondria generate energy. This antioxidant also recycles other antioxidants – vitamins C and E. ALA is known to lower blood sugar levels; diabetics use it to treat nerve damage. ALA also elevates the glutathione levels you read about in the last chapter. Since ALA is both water and fat soluble, it can move into all parts of a cell to neutralize free radicals. Vitamin C, on the other hand, is limited to the watery parts of cells because it is soluble only in water, while vitamin E is only fat soluble. ALA is particularly good at crossing the blood-brain barrier to reduce oxidative stress in the brain.

ALA further regulates immune cells, called T-cells and provides protection against the toxins arsenic, cadmium, and mercury. It may bind to other metals like iron, copper and zinc. It may be beneficial to include a B complex supplement in a regimen containing alpha lipoic acid. The preferred form is R-alpha lipoic acid in conjunction with methylated resveratrol and quercetin, which extends the life of resveratrol. [Example: Xymogen's: ALAmax CR Take two tablets 30 minutes before breakfast and 1 tablet 30 minutes before dinner. You may take this with Xymogen's Resveratin. Take one 2 X per day. Many people take ALA in conjunction with Acetyl L-Carnitine. Together they are known to boost the immune system even in HIV patients.]

Incidentally, mercury fillings and pink-colored removable dental appliances and partials contain and release cadmium. Many people request clear colored appliances to avoid this toxin.

## Immune Boosting Strategies That Restore Health

1. **Stress-Reduction Strategies: breathing.** Learn to breathe. How many times did you breathe in as you read the last page? How shallow or erratic were your breaths? Did only your chest rise? Most of us do not inhale or exhale regularly and have no idea how to breathe using our diaphragms. Unlike children who breathe naturally, we ignore this vital rejuvenator.

   Inhale deeply through your nose. Feel your stomach rise, then your chest. Count slowly to four, then slowly release through your nose, letting chest air release first. Repeat three to ten times. How do you feel? Did your shoulders drop? Did you feel your heart rate drop? By breathing using your diaphragm, you slow your respiration rate. By breathing through your nose, you created nitric oxide (NO), a transient gas that relaxes blood vessels and soothes the vagus nerve. Exercise also creates NO. In fact, NO is what Viagra, that famous blue pill, delivers.

   Nitric oxide is created in the upper nasal passages during nasal breathing. It acts as a fuel injector for your body by increasing the number of cellular mitochondria and fueling them with oxygen. It dilates blood vessels, which lowers blood pressure and improves blood flow.[v] NO improves oxygen delivery to all tissues. In fact, nitric oxide has been shown to increase oxygen exchange efficiency and increase blood oxygen by 18%, while improving the lungs' ability to absorb it.[vi]

   Beyond improved sexual function, NO provides better circulation, improved skin nourishment, increased alertness by suffusing the brain with oxygen, and promotes relaxation and feelings of wellbeing. Even a few short periods of slow, deep nasal/diaphragm breathing during the day enhances body and mind. Develop a strong diaphragm. Many people lack the diaphragmatic strength and breathing coordination to intentionally breathe deeply without hyperventilating. This important meditation practice is integrated into martial art and yoga forms. Practitioners typically reduce their breathing rate to between four to ten breaths a minute.

Deep, diaphragmatic breathing also plays into your blood's critical acid/base balance and is often overlooked. To review, the more rapidly you breath, the more carbon dioxide you blow off. Less is available to combine with hydrogen ions to make bicarbonate buffer. It may be possible to create an awareness of breathing patterns during waking hours, but what happens when you sleep? Sleep apnea may be as under-diagnosed as gum disease, especially as ballooning waistlines restrict the diaphragm, leading to rapid, shallow breathing. Because gum disease, heart disease, a tendency towards acidity, and sleep apnea are highly correlated and dental solutions are available, there is a growing movement to train dental professionals to understand, recognize and refer for diagnosis those people they suspect have sleep apnea. Once diagnosed, dentists can work with other specialists to design therapy.

As introduced in Chapter Twelve, many people, especially mouth breathers, are hyperventilated and need to raise carbon dioxide levels in their blood. Carbon dioxide is what allows oxygen release into tissues and is how your body rids itself of ammonia and urea. If nature routinely calls at 4 AM, a primary detoxification time, you likely have an ammonia-based problem. Your body can't transform ammonia to urea, so it irritates your bladder.

If you feel powerless at work, but cannot quit your job, find another place where you feel more in control. Find a way to offer compassion and nurturing to others. These behaviors increase levels of the enzyme telomerase, whose sole function is to repair damage to telomeres.

Many people release blocked emotions by a process called tapping – the Emotional Freedom Technique (EFT), or Meridian Tapping Technique (MTT).

A recent study showed that the more the stress hormone cortisol is produced in the body, the more the destructive protein-destroying enzyme collagenase is produced in the gums. The effect was dose-dependent. The logical conclusion was that more gum disease occurred during times of psycho-social stress.[viii] A literature review indicated 57 percent of the studies showed a positive relationship between gum diseases and stress, anxiety, depression, and loneliness.[ix]

Dr. Preston Miller, president of the American Association of Periodontists said, "Individuals with high stress levels tend to increase their bad habits, which can be harmful to periodontal health. They are less attentive to their oral hygiene and may increase their use of nicotine, alcohol or drugs. Patients should seek healthy ways to relieve stress through exercise, balanced eating, plenty of sleep and maintaining a positive mental attitude." (If you have apnea, you also produce excessive cortisol, releasing the collagenase that causes gum disease.)

It is clear that far more than gum disease is at stake during periods of stress and depression.

2. **Limit or eliminate processed carbohydrate (grain and sugar) intake** to amounts your body was programmed to handle. If you overindulge, consider probiotics taken with fiber. I particularly like natto, apple cider vinegar, and kefir, taken for their myriad other beneficial properties. If you must supplement, choose with care. Non-pasteurized fermented foods are the preferred way to reinstitute proper digestive health. Since much of your immune system depends on a positive balance of healthy gut bacteria, it would be a mistake to overlook ways to maintain that balance.

   When beneficial bacteria are destroyed, bad bacteria multiply quickly to fill the void. This wrecks the bacterial balance in your gut. Prebiotic, high fiber foods like bananas, whole grains, greens, tomatoes, onions, legumes, and garlic are important because they help probiotic bacteria survive long enough to gain a foothold in your gut.

3. **Reduce high AGE foods in your diet.** When grilling, use acidic marinades such as lemon juice and vinegar. Trim fat before cooking and the browned or charred portions of cooked meats and cheeses after cooking. Limit grilled, fried, and broiled foods. The higher the heat used, the more AGEs are created. Emphasize "wet" cooking methods such as stewing, boiling, braising, steaming, and crock-pot cooking. Cooking with water prevents sugars from combining with proteins to form AGEs. Limit processed foods including dairy, which are often pasteurized at high temperatures to kill germs.

Fructose sugars found in fruits and high fructose corn syrup (think sodas) are particularly susceptible to forming AGEs. Glutathione is an antioxidant that may help protect white blood cells, nervous system cells, retinal cells, and may help LDLs not oxidize. L-Carnosine, guava, and Yerba maté tea can help prevent LDLs from transforming into AGEs. Alpha lipoic acid. Vitamin $B_1$, in the form of benfotiamine, may block AGE formation after eating AGE-promoting foods.

4. **Enjoy foods that boost immune system function.** About ninety percent of the food Americans buy is processed and contributes to poor health. If you want to be healthy, you have to spend some time in the kitchen. Eat foods rich in carotenoids, bioflavenoids, zinc,[2] magnesium, curcumin, turmeric, selenium,[3] vitamins C, E,[4] and B complex, quality fish or krill oils, oils high in EPA, and pro- and prebiotics. Enjoy liberal amounts of organic mushrooms, seeds, and nuts. If you are deficient in vitamin D, spend some time outside or take a good $D_3$ supplement. If you must supplement with vitamin C, make sure to buy a buffered form, not an ascorbic acid form. Decrease mercury and other heavy metal sources. Know your iron levels. High iron levels impair immune system function.

5. **Avoid refined salts.** Autoimmune diseases like multiple sclerosis, psoriasis, rheumatoid arthritis, and ankylosing spondylitis are linked to an overproduction of a specialized immune T-cell called Th17. Refined salts seem to make these T-cells more aggressive, so more likely to assault the host. Use like Celtic or Himalayan sea salt instead.

6. **Explore the power of essential oils.** Essential oils are preventive medicine at its most delightful! The use of hundreds of

---

2 Take zinc separately from copper. Taken together, they create a shower of free radicals. (Interesting – mercury amalgam fillings contain both.)

3 Selenium fights viral infections.

4 Vitamin E is an antioxidant that reduces synthesis of the inflammatory molecule called $PGE_2$ and reduces IL-6 production. Wu D, et al. "Age-associated increase in $PGE_2$ synthesis and COX activity in murine macrophages is reversed by vitamin E." *Cell Physiology* 1998;275(3):C661-C668.

plant oil essences as medicine dates back thousands of years. Ancient writings tell us they played a daily role in the lives of Egyptian, Chinese, and Middle Eastern peoples. Being fat soluble, they can enter cell walls throughout the body within 20 minutes of application. Various pure, therapeutic-grade oils are known to be antibacterial, anti-fungal, anti-viral, and anti-cancerous. When diffused, they can purify the air.

Individual oils contain between 200 and 800 chemical constituents, all with different properties. Many of them are used for aromatherapy. Some, such as frankincense, cedarwood, Melissa, and sandalwood, can change your mood in predictable ways because they contain high levels of sesquiterpenes. Sesquiterpenes cross the blood-brain barrier, the membrane present between the blood vessels and the brain that protect the brain and central nervous system from damaging substances.

These oils can stimulate the pineal and pituitary glands, and the limbic system of the brain. The ability to cross the blood-brain barrier is the key to why certain essential oils high in antioxidants can have an effect on diseases that originate in the brain like Alzheimer's, Parkinson's, Multiple Sclerosis, and Lou Gehrig's disease. They can also carry their antioxidant powers deep into the delicate cells of the inner ear to prevent or reverse some cases of ringing in the ears, known as tinnitus.

I routinely use oregano, cinnamon, clove, rosewood, peppermint, frankincense, lemon, hyssop, wormwood, myrrh, and eucalyptus oils. My favorite is a blend called "Thieves" which contains clove, cinnamon, lemon, rosemary, and eucalyptus oils. It is reportedly 99.96 percent effective at killing airborne bacteria. Thyme, oregano, mint, cinnamon, sage, and clove oils have also been shown to be extremely effective at killing airborne bacteria.[xi] A 2009 study demonstrated that a blend of thyme white, lemon, lemongrass and cinnamon essential oils[xii] inhibited bacterial and yeast strains, including MRSA and five other Staphylococcus strains, four Streptococcus strains, and three Candida strains, including a drug-resistant strain of yeast, Candida krusei. For those looking for a safe underarm deodorant, Waleda makes an effective aluminum-free product based on essential oils.

There are multiple ways to use essential oils: orally, applied to skin, or diffused throughout a living environment. As with ozone, a principal reason for using these oils is that they kill viruses and bacteria without allowing them to mutate, unlike antibiotics. Educate yourself on the proper use of essential oils, and enjoy the results!

7.  **Use it or lose it.** Exercise is a powerful tool. Fifty percent of Americans get no exercise. Only 25 percent exercise as much as they should. Losses in muscle mass or strength can be due to hormonal changes, sedentary lifestyles, oxidative damage, fat infiltration into muscles, inflammation and insulin resistance. Exercise can change much of that through improving blood chemistry.

    Exercise increases the number of energy generators in each cell (mitochondria); this profoundly influences how you process energy and how energetic you feel. A doctor can tell by looking at your red blood cells if you exercise. If you do, you have a lot of hemoglobin that can carry oxygen. Exercise removes wastes from the cell, changes hormone balance, stabilizes insulin levels, and improves digestion, circulation, mental and physical agility, blood pressure, oxygen transport, liver function, metabolism, sleep patterns, reaction time, mood, and sexuality.[5]

    Exercise reduces stress, depression, breast cancer risk, heart attack, and osteoporosis. Exercise curbs emotional eating. When you exercise, muscular contractions pump lymph throughout your body. The lymphatic system is integral to immune system function. Unlike the heart that pumps blood through the circulatory system, the immune

---

5 A review of the many ways exercise enhances sexuality is found an article, "Sexual Desirability and Sexual Performance: Does Exercise and Fitness Really Matter?" A summary of their review of the scientific literature: "Exercise frequency and physical fitness enhance attractiveness and increase energy levels, both of which make people feel better about themselves. Those who exercise are more likely to experience a greater level of satisfaction and a positive perception of self. Moreover, those who feel better about themselves may perceive they are more sexually desirable and may perform better sexually. The majority of individuals who are regularly physically active are healthier, and perhaps healthier individuals may be more willing and able to have sex." (Electronic Journal of Human Sexuality, Volume 7, October 5, 2004.http://www.ejhs.org/volume7/fitness.html (Accessed October 10, 2009)

system has no pump. It depends on muscular contractions to pump lymph. A regular exercise routine creates improved discipline and self-esteem. Finally, exercise sculpts your body. You may not lose a lot of weight, but fat pounds convert to muscle. Exercise until you feel energized, but not exhausted. Enjoying a massage after exercising is a pleasurable way to augment lymph movement.

8.  **Be alert to everyday toxicity exposure.** We gravitate to organic foods when we consider limiting toxins, but beyond pesticides and herbicides on and in foods, lawns, gardens, and houses, consider other types of products that contain absorbable chemicals. These include lotions, cosmetics, aerosol-delivered products, aromatic products used to freshen living spaces, soaps, toothpastes, paints, deodorants, etc. There are websites that rate ingredients in thousands of products against definitive toxicity and regulatory databases. The most popular and extensive site is Skin Deep, the Environmental Working Group's cosmetic safety database. To help break down bacteria and pesticides on produce, if you don't have ozone gas available, consider soaking your food in a solution of ¼ cup of conventional 3% peroxide in a gallon of water or 1 teaspoon of pure bleach to a sink-full of water for five minutes. Diluted bleach is not toxic. Our own bodies make sodium chlorite (bleach) to kill invaders.

9.  **Drink "pure" water.** Try to bathe in filtered water. Realize whatever is flushed into the city water supply is in your water – hormones, heavy metals, cleaners, solvents, medical wastes, and prescription drugs. Chlorine reacts with organic materials in water to form trihalomethanes and other compounds far more toxic than chlorine itself. Defining high quality drinking water is difficult enough. Obtaining it is far more difficult – and expensive. Some use reverse osmosis (RO) filtration to remove chlorine, fluorine, and other toxins, but it also removes important minerals. RO-filtered water is also acidic and lacks the electrical charge that can help reduce free radicals and pull out positively charged heavy metals and other acid wastes stored in cells. Minerals can be added back to water, then run through an ionizer, a complicated routine

and resource intense. Distilled water has similar problems, though these may be your best option. See: http://www. phionbalance.com/pH-Balancing-The-Body-Blog.    Spring water delivered in glass bottles is a nuisance, but if you can manage the heavy glass bottles, it may be a great option.

10. **Sleep promotes balance.** Adults consistently require seven to nine hours daily. Teens need nine hours.
   - A Pennsylvania State University study showed a 60 percent increase in inflammatory proteins, like the inflammatory marker CRP, in subjects who slept only six hours a night for a week.
   - Other studies show chronic sleep deprivation substantially increases heart attack and stroke risk.
   - Hormones produced during sleep regulate appetite, thus lean/fat body mass ratios.[6] If you sleep less than seven hours each night, you likely carry more body fat.
   - Just one sleepless night can increase insulin resistance.
   - If you sleep eight hours a night, your risk of colds melts.[xii]
   - Regenerative processes occur during sleep cycles. Sleep enhances physical and mental tasks. Serotonin, produced during sleep (and enhanced by omega-3 fatty acid intake and drugs like Prozac and other SSRI antidepressants), elevates mood. Low serotonin levels can trigger depression. Sleep reduces stress and its associated hormones. Inflammation and blood pressure are consequently reduced.
   - Try to work with your natural circadian rhythm, which relates to cortisol levels. Cortisol levels peak at sunrise and ebb around 10PM. Optimal physical and mental repair occurs when the sleep cycle is 10PM to 6AM.
   - Sleep in a completely darkened room to ensure sufficient melatonin levels. Melatonin, made in the pineal gland, aids sleep, suppresses tumor growth and is one of our body's best and most ubiquitous anti-oxidants. Low levels

6 Ghrelin and leptin are important hormones that regulate appetite. Good sleep patterns and exercising regularly allow you to produce plenty of leptin. High leptin levels signal appetite satisfaction. You feel full. If you avoid exercise or lack sleep, whether through apnea or poor sleep hygiene, grehlin becomes your main appetite controller. Its insistent signal tells you to eat constantly, which leads to weight gain. Those who treat apnea often lose significant weight

from sleep deprivation or exposure to lights late at night are linked to high blood pressure and reduced immunity.

11. **Reduce oxidation and free radical exposure.** Consume antioxidants throughout each day. While normal metabolism and daily living constantly produce free radicals, habits like smoking flood the body with them. As tissues accumulate free radical damage, their deterioration makes them vulnerable to disease. You can reduce free radicals by limiting activities that cause them and ingesting foods rich in nutrients that bind with and neutralize them. See the chart of ORAC values at the end of the Chapter Five.

Gary Null, a popular anti-aging author, states, "Free radicals perhaps do their greatest damage through a process of fusing DNA and protein molecules, referred to as cross-linking. Unlike the other contents of cells, the body cannot produce new strands of DNA. The best it can do is to repair them, but it can't always do that. In addition to damaging DNA, cross-linking results in essential proteins becoming stiff and therefore unable to function correctly. This process is responsible for many of the symptoms most often associated with aging – cataracts, wrinkles, brittle bones, kidney failure, hardening of the arteries, and immune deficiency. Cross-linking is particularly prevalent in diabetics, as glucose fuels the process, and helps explain why diabetes is a disease recognized for its severe premature aging effects." [xiii] Of course he is referring to AGEs and glycation.

12. **Laugh often!** Dr. Lee Berk of Loma Linda University in California studied the effect of laughter on three kinds of white blood cells: lymphocytes, granulocytes, and monocytes. The research involved a group of participants who were shown a humorous video that produced mirthful laughter. Blood levels of various white blood cells were measured before, during, soon after, and even the day following the laughter-producing video exercise. They found white blood cells and their products increased during laughter; this statistically significant increase often extended into the next day, implying the effect may be long term. Significant increase was noted in lymphocyte products such as natural killer cells

and gamma interferon that specifically attack viral and tumor cells. Antibodies, those B-lymphocyte products that provide immunity against certain diseases, also increased. Laughter also lowers blood pressure, reduces stress hormones, and triggers the release of endorphins, the body's natural painkillers.[xii]

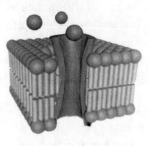

"Pores" in cell membranes open and close to release toxins and admit nutrients. Researchers observe that when a person is angry, these pores are tightly closed. Nutrients cannot enter; toxins cannot exit. These pores open when one is happy, open more when one is meditating or praying, and open most when one laughs with gusto!

13. **If you smoke, stop.**

14. **Manage your oral care daily!** Seek regular professional care to monitor and treat oral health.

15. **Enjoy music you love.** It can dilate arteries as much as aerobic exercise.

# Goals

> *"Worms will not eat living wood where the vital sap is flowing; rust will not hinder the opening of a gate when the hinges are used each day.  Movement gives health and life. Stagnation brings disease and death."*

> **~ Traditional Chinese Medicine proverb ~**

People who are casual about life – who live life without goals – are often unhappy people. Those who strive to grow and change know they must not set themselves up for failure by stating poorly defined goals. When you set a goal, state it in terms you can measure or count. If you tell yourself, "I am going to exercise more this year," you are setting yourself up for failure. "I will walk two miles on Mondays, Wednesdays, and Fridays, before work," is an attainable goal.

# Heavy Metal: Mercury Toxicity and Planned Obsolescence

*"All truth goes through three steps.*
*First, it is ridiculed.*
*Second, it is violently opposed.*
*Finally, it is accepted as self-evident."*

**~ Arthur Schopenhauser, German philosopher ~**

Many will disagree with the information presented here about silver fillings – the amount of mercury they emit on a daily basis, their retention in the body, their toxicity, and the safe removal techniques many dental professionals advise. However everyone should be aware of the issues that matter to those opposing mercury fillings, if only to understand and address their concerns.

Most of us know the American Dental Association (ADA) and the FDA supported mercury fillings for over a century and a half. The powerful ADA still does. As I presented to Jeff Shuren, the man in charge of the "amalgam rule" at the FDA in March 2011, mercury-based fillings are never stress-reducing restorations – the preparations required of them destroy the enamel webbing that distributes stresses. The material allows no connection of the tooth "from side to side, front to back, top to bottom". Amalgam fillings initiate cracks and set teeth up to fail. I mentioned the Delta Dental Insurance company's study showing the "economical" lifetime cost of these fillings is in excess of $2000.00 per tooth in 2003 dollars - more if these teeth need crowns or root canals. The true costs should concern us all. This planned obsolescence grants no savings by any measure. I asked him to help dentists abandon their drills and inadequate, late-stage methods of determining decay.

Though more and more people seek care from dentists who aspire to preserve teeth in their most natural and functional state and who know stress reduction needs to be engineered into tooth repairs – that is, from dentists trained in Minimally Invasive and Biomimetic Dentistry – the questions of toxicity and longevity remain as long as people house these relics in their mouths.

Even though the FDA stated in May, 2011 that they plan to "phase out" mercury fillings (Why not an outright ban? ), many of us must make decisions about what they want to do with these archaic technologies and materials.

In "Boom Times for Dentistry, But Not for Teeth," Alex Berenson of The New York Times railed against our two-tiered system of oral health care wherein the poor continue to receive mercury fillings while upper-income Americans receive non-toxic alternatives.[xv] On the other hand, Danaher, the parent company of Kerr, the largest manufacturer of mercury amalgam filling material, said two-tiered dentistry is a good thing for lower-income Americans and institutional recipients.[xvi]

Wall Street was aware of the firestorm over mercury filling safety concerns as far back as October, 2007. Then, an equity research report prepared by Jon D. Wood and Brandon Couilliard of Bank of America Securities analyzed the political landscape and suggested the industry would be more profitable abandoning mercury fillings. At the time, the report said JP Morgan foresaw the FDA would likely limit mercury filling use when it issued a ruling in 2009, a ruling many sought since the FDA classified all other dental materials 30 years prior. That report was rich with trivia about the dental use of mercury. An example: "The EPA report also suggests more than 1,000 tons of mercury already lie in patients' mouths, accounting for more than half of all the mercury sitting in products." [xvii] Manufacturers expressed concerns that legal risks threatened their assets should they continue to support use of mercury fillings. A first-time vote among Danaher shareholders, showed nearly 17 percent wanted to phase out the production of their mercury filling material.

In late 2009, the FDA ruled mercury fillings do not release enough vapor to be harmful, yet upgraded its risk from a Class I to a Class II, or medium risk medical device.[7] This was a dishonorable ruling, since a judicial order mandated the FDA to classify mercury amalgams in good faith and according to standards set on their own web site. This web site set standards in 2008 and disclosed very plainly the effects of dental mercury. This web site has been removed but it specifically stated dental mercury could cause neurological harm to children and fetuses in the form of nerve problems, brain damage, learning disabilities, and other nerve disorders. The FDA ruling did not protect women, young children, and fetuses, even though the judicial ruling required it.

According to records obtained by the Freedom of Information Act, Consumers For Dental Choice attorney Charles Brown pointed out:

---

[7] Most "upper tier" dentists do not place mercury in their families' or client's mouths. A common saying is, "The only place I can legally put mercury is in your mouth or in a hazardous waste container."

- "While owning stock options in Henry Schein Inc., Commissioner Margaret Hamburg participated in the amalgam rulemaking, presiding at a July 1 policy meeting "to secure feedback from the Office of the Commissioner" and to discuss the rule's "next steps." Having received over a million dollars as a corporate "director" of Schein, one of the biggest retailers of amalgam stock to dentists, Hamburg repeatedly disregarded warnings to stop her participation. These warnings came from an admonition from her financial advisor, and two letters from me. Furthermore, the ethics contract she signed required her to recuse herself.

- Hamburg sidekick Joshua Sharfstein entered at the last minute to rubber-stamp the rule that covers up the mercury and conceals warnings of neurological harm to children and unborn babies that the FDA had already agreed to admit to. Sharfstein has become so knee-deep in this morass that he cancelled a meeting with Congresswoman Diane Watson, who demanded an explanation for such a horrible rule.

- After Hamburg complained to her corporation (Schein) that, "there are constraints on my activities while I hold any interest in Schein," Schein officials offered her a special favor. They agreed to cancel the options before their expiration date – something even Hamburg's financial advisor had said was not possible – so that the Commissioner could start regulating Schein sooner. Hamburg agreed and the deal was signed on July 28 – the day the amalgam rule was announced.

- Henry Schein benefited enormously from the rule. Its stock jumped immediately by $1.50 after the ruling. In an e-mail exchange, the Commissioner "severed" her relationship to Schein (two days after the rule was announced), but assured Schein's general counsel that she hoped her "friendships" at Schein "will outlast the period of my recusal." In response, the general counsel noted that Schein is "indebted" to her for her "service" at FDA.

- The Commissioner's husband, Peter Fitzhugh Brown, was marketed to the American people as an "expert in artificial intelligence." Actually, he is a hedge fund trader, an officer at Wall Street colossus, Renaissance Technologies. Hamburg secretly enlisted Peter Brown into FDA's inner circle to participate in FDA deliberations as to how to deal with the amalgam rule's fall-out, where he could advise agency press aides and policy makers and be advised by FDA lawyers – and get valuable insider information for his day job. (An FDA Commissioner has a huge impact on stock values of major corporations.) Renaissance Technologies traded $6 million in Schein stock during the second quarter alone."

This is past history, but I mention it here to show that policy people at the FDA and other agencies do not always make decisions based on the best interests of the general population.

There is much to do before there is an outright ban on amalgams. Once we do, we will be years behind Canada (1996) and England (1998). Though many groups and politicians were outraged at the 2009 ruling, the American Dental Association was pleased that the decision of whether to use mercury-laden fillings is where it needs to be – between the dentist and the patient.[xviii] I hope these dentists are giving their patients enough information to obtain true "informed consent".

What is all the fuss all about? In fact, what is a mercury filling? It turns out most Americans are not quite sure.

## Consumer Awareness About Mercury Fillings

Zogby International[1] conducted national telephone and region-specific interactive surveys in New England and California regarding consumer attitudes on dental fillings and mercury for a report.[xix] Here are a few of their findings:

- "Most Americans (76 percent) do not know mercury is the primary component of amalgam ["silver"] fillings.
- Americans overwhelmingly (92 percent) want to be informed of their options with respect to mercury and non-mercury dental filling materials prior to treatment.
- The majority (77 percent) of Americans would choose higher cost fillings that do not contain mercury if given the choice.
- Close to half (47 percent) of all Americans think mercury pollution poses a serious problem for the environment.
- More than two-thirds (69 percent nationally) of New Englanders would support a ban on mercury amalgam fillings for children and pregnant women."[xx]

**Note:** In the October 2003 *Journal of the American Dental Association*, the ADA recommended dentists consistently use informed consent. "As every dentist knows, it is a good risk management practice to discuss the risks and benefits of a proposed treatment plan with a patient before starting treatment.

In many cases, the dentist has a corresponding legal obligation to obtain informed consent from a patient before beginning treatment."

1 The International Academy of Oral Medicine and Toxicology hired Zogby International among others, to conduct this study. Their estimated margin of error is +/-2.9 percentage points with margins of error higher in sub-groups. Their sampling and weighting procedures have been validated through its political polling: more than 95 percent of the firm's polls have come within one percent of actual election-day outcomes.

## What Does This Mean to You?

All dental materials represent some risk. Information must be the basis for how a person assesses the risks versus the benefits for themselves. If you have (or accept before the phase out reaches you) mercury-laden repair materials, what are the most relevant questions?

- How much mercury vapor is released from mercury fillings?
- Do we accumulate only safe levels of mercury from our dental fillings?

The privately held dental trade organization, the American Dental Association (ADA), continues to contend that the mercury making up half of each silver filling is stable. They insist only about .03 micrograms/day of inorganic mercury vaporizes from a silver filling. Other privately held dental trade organizations have decried the use of dental mercury for decades. Dental trade groups that prefer biocompatible restorative materials include organizations such as the IAOMT International Academy of Oral Medicine and Toxicology, the International Academy of Biological Dentistry and Medicine (IABDM), the International Association of Mercury Safe Dentists (IAMFD), and Dental Amalgam Mercury Solutions (DAMS). These groups call mercury-laden fillings a timed released poison that emits far more vapor than the ADA contends. A few dissenting voices are presented in *"The Roots of Disease: Connecting Dentistry and Medicine"*: [xxi]

- "The Environmental Protection Agency, the World Health Organization (WHO),[8] and the textbook, *Goodman and Gillman's: The Pharmacological Basis of Therapeutics*, estimates vaporization rates of about 3 to 17 micrograms/day.[9]
- In the EPA's 1997 report to Congress, the highest body burden of inorganic mercury comes from amalgam fillings.[xxii]
- The consensus average estimate for absorbed mercury vapor for a person with an average of eight occlusal (chewing surface) fillings is 10 micrograms, which is probably a low estimate. (A new study by Dr. Haley is noted below and suggests even higher vapor releases.)
- The U.S. Public Health Department has an MRL (minimal risk level) for chronic mercury vapor exposure at 0.28 micrograms/day. The WHO asserts there is no safe level for mercury exposure."

Dr. Boyd Haley,[10] Professor of Chemistry and Biochemistry at the University of Kentucky, is another dissenting voice. He refuted the ADA's position as it was stated in a letter to Congress in 2001.[xxiii] Haley also conducted *"A Study on the Release of Mercury from Dental*

---

8 From: *The World Health Organization's List of the Main Sources of Mercury: Source: Daily Intake of Mercury (mcg):* Vapor released in micrograms/$M^3$

| | |
|---|---|
| Amalgam Filling: 3.8 - 21 | Chewing food: 68 |
| Fish: 3.0 | Brushing teeth: 272 |
| Other Foods: 3.6 | Placing amalgams: 2000 |
| Water: 0.05 | Removing or polishing amalgams: 4000 |
| Air: 0.04 | |

9 A bill reintroduced into the House of Representatives on May 1, 2007 (renumbered: HR2101 IH) contends the WHO numbers for mercury release from amalgam fillings have been revised upwards. People can receive between 3 to 27 micrograms/day per filling. Access at: http://thomas.loc.gov/cgi-bin/query/z?c110:H.R.2101.IH:

10 Dr. Haley was an NIH Postdoctoral Scholar in Physiology at Yale Medical School. His academic appointments are professor in the College of Pharmacy and the Department of Biochemistry of the University of Kentucky Medical Center and Chair of the Department of Chemistry. He is currently focused on the biochemistry of Alzheimer's disease and on the role mercury toxicity may play as a major exacerbating or causal factor for this and several other neurological diseases.

*Amalgams Made from Different Manufactured Materials and Produced by Nine Different Dentists.*" [xxiv] The edited summary states, "Mercury emissions/cm² of surface area [about the size exposed in one, one-surface occlusal filling] of dental amalgams prepared by nine different doctors and from mixtures from three different manufacturers were measured in water at room temperature, 23 degrees Celsius, three months after placement to allow for total aging and the loss of surface bound mercury... Daily emission was 4.5 to 21 micrograms/ cm², much higher than previously estimated values offered by the ADA."

Dr. Haley noted that, "The level of mercury emission was not stimulated by brushing or manipulation of the amalgam." This is important because our body's mercury accumulation increases each time we eat, clench, chew gum, or drink hot beverages. Proximity to dissimilar metals (like gold) also enhances vaporization. This is why amalgam manufacturer's safety sheets used to say[11] amalgam fillings are contra indicated for placement next to gold. Even at the lowest levels exhibited in this study, without the physical and chemical manipulation of the material that constantly occurs in the mouth, the mercury exposure at these rates is considerably higher than acceptable biocompatible levels. The currently accepted "reference dose" for methyl mercury set by the EPA is 0.1 micrograms/kg body weight/day. [xxv] Oral and intestinal bacteria methylate the mercury form released by amalgams.[xxvi xxvii xxviii xxix] Methyl mercury is more toxic than inorganic mercury because it easily binds to cells. That means current acceptable limits for the following people are:

| Weight | Acceptable Limit |
|---|---|
| 120 pounds (54.43 kg) | 5.44 micrograms/day |
| 150 poungs (68.04 kg) | 6.80 micrograms/day |
| 200 pounds (90.72 kg) | 9.07 micrograms/day |
| 250 pounds (113.4 kg) | 11.4 micrograms/day |

People are likely exposed to more mercury from their fillings than they suspect. Remember: heat, chewing, and proximity to other metals

---

11 Unlike less contentious times over mercury implant safety, now all MSDS safety sheets present their amalgam product geared toward the safety of practitioners using their product, not that of the end user. Safety material is presented as though mercury is the sole ingredient of their product. Stringent safety guidelines for product handling are required for dentists.

hastens mercury vaporization. A dramatic video dubbed "Smoking Teeth = Poison Gas" illustrates mercury vapor release from a twenty-five-year-old filling at rest and while being stimulated by pressure and heat. It can be accessed through a link on the International Academy of Oral Medicine and Toxicology web site.[12]

The IAOMT, the IABDM, and the IAMFD biological dental associations named above, disagree with the ADA's position on mercury filling safety. They maintain extensive websites to disseminate their views, including alternative information on mercury toxicity, the political controversy surrounding its use, and other immune system challenges addressed by biological dentists.[13] These sites list member dentists by area. Biomimetic dentists belonging to the Academy of Biomimetic Dentistry (ABD) also eschew amalgam fillings, but for mechanical reasons. Refer to Chapter 13. The ABD lists credentialed biomimetic dentists on their web site as do I.[14] Caveat: not all biomimetic dentists are trained in integrative medicine principals and vice versa. As always, you must prioritize your needs and desires and be sure to ask for what you want.

---

12 http://www.iaomt.org/

13 These organizations explore additional immune system challenges such as the role of extractions and other dental traumas, root canals, implants, particularly titanium implants, and cavitations, explained in more detail in chapter one.

Root canals: as mentioned elsewhere, sterility is as crucial to a successful root canal as it may be impossible to achieve. *The Roots of Disease: Connecting Dentistry with Medicine* by Robert Kulacz, DDS and Thomas E. Levy, MD, JD, and *Root Canal Cover Up Exposed – Many Illnesses Result*, by George Meinig, DDS review these ideas. Go to http://articles. mercola.com/sites/articles/archive/2010/11/16/why-you-should-avoid-root-canals-like-the-plague.aspx to see Dr. Meinig's views.

Implants: Many European and some U.S. dentists eschew titanium implants in favor of zirconium ceramic ones for the same reason they avoid mercury fillings. Titanium implants are not electrically or biologically inert. They constantly release ions into the body, perhaps contributing to autoimmune problems, inflammation, and metal sensitivities. When other metals are present, corrosion rates accelerate. As with all dissimilar metals present within an electrolyte (as saliva is), the system becomes a battery. These currents can cause cellular disruption locally (cancer) and possibly elsewhere.

Noted biological dentist Hal Huggins recommends low level insulin growth factor injections to help bone and nerves heal after wisdom tooth or cavitation surgery. Refer to his book *PZI: Protamine Zinc Insulin/Non Diabetic Uses for Insulin* to review other healing aspects of *low* level insulin injections. He also offers DNA bacterial testing of samples found in cavitation sites and individualized biological compatibiity tests of dental materials.

14 www.AcademyofBiomimeticDent.org./ www.mouthmattersbookcom

## How Toxic Is Mercury?

People know mercury is deadly and are starting to realize even low-level mercury accumulations alter brain function and damage nervous systems and hearts. In response to consumer pressure, cosmetic and medicinal product manufacturers have removed or reduced mercury levels in many of their products. Mercurochrome, calomel lotion, and mercury-filled thermometers were removed from the market long ago. Vaccine manufacturers struggle to reduce thimerosal (49 percent by weight mercury compound) levels. Consumers know to limit certain fish intake due to toxic mercury accumulation in piscine tissues.[15] Are humans immune from similar mercurial accumulation in their tissues?

Only uranium is more toxic than mercury. Lead and arsenic are considerably less toxic.[xxx] As with any heavy metal, one of the keys to mercury's toxicity is its affinity for sulfur. Sulfur bonds dictate the shape of many proteins. Mercury can deform and inactivate proteins. Mercury vapor easily penetrates the central nervous system. Low dose mercury accumulation alters brain function and damages nervous systems and hearts.[xxxi xxxii xxxiii] Mercury is thought to trigger specific diseases in people with a genetic predisposition to them. Implicated diseases are lupus,[xxxiv xxxv] scleroderma,[xxxvi xxxvii] multiple sclerosis, chronic fatigue, fibromyalgia, psoriasis, oral lichen planus, eczema, allergies, and asthma. Neurological consequences include autism and the neurofibrillar tangles of the brain, amyloid plaques, and other markers found in Alzheimer's disease, exacerbation of Parkinson's disease and ALS (Lou Gehrig's disease).

It is established that mercury inhibits kidney function[xxxviii] and damages the heart via numerous routes including impairing its electrical functions. Mercury levels in heart tissues of individuals who died from idiopathic dilated cardiomyopathy (an enlarged heart due to unknown causes) were found to be, on average, 22,000 times higher than in individuals who died of other forms of heart disease.[xxxix] Mercury is associated with high blood pressure, birth defects, learning

---

15 A Centers for Disease Control (CDC) report shows how close some people already come to exceeding "safe" levels of mercury exposure. It says, "Approximately 10 percent (6 million) of U.S. women have mercury levels within one-tenth of potentially hazardous levels, indicating a narrow margin of safety for some women." This seems particularly pertinent when we consider miscarriage and birth defect potential, nursing, and childhood immunizations, many of which still contain thimerosal.

disabilities, heart arrhythmias, weight gain, cold feet and hands, fatigue, and disrupted hormone function. High mercury levels can lead to decreased sex drive and impotence. Women with estrogen-positive breast cancers who take Tamoxifen and other estrogen suppressors should know that mercury mimics estrogen. Men and parents of males might also be concerned since there are so many other estrogen-creating triggers in our environment.[16]

Those undergoing cancer treatment often suffer yeast overgrowth. Most do not know that yeast (Candida) has a strong affinity for mercury. Candida becomes more virulent as it absorbs mercury and invades the cell walls of the intestines. This is why many holistic doctors suggest reducing mercury exposure and mercury chelation as part of cancer treatment.

As always, our young are particularly vulnerable. A University of Calgary School of Medicine study implanted radioactively labeled mercury fillings into pregnant sheep. This mercury showed up in the hearts and brains of the mothers and unborn babies within days. The mercury levels were exceptionally high in the unborn babies' pituitary glands.[xl]

To demonstrate how mercury vapors destroy brain neurons, the Department of Physiology and Biophysics, Faculty of Medicine at the University of Calgary released a video.[17] They report the level of mercury exposure used in the test was well below those levels found in many humans with mercury/silver amalgam dental fillings.

---

16 Another estrogen mimic is the bisphenols (BPAs) found in plastic. BPAs leach into food and water at all temperatures, but heat accelerates leaching. Microwaving food in plastic is a bad idea. The abundant estrogen-mimicking compounds now in our environment are just one reason why girls now begin menstruating earlier and why generally, men have four times the risk of a lower sperm count and twice the risk of lower sperm motility if they have detectible levels in their blood, as ninety percent of Americans do. BPAs also increase te risk of type 2 diabetes and cancers. Governments around the world, including China have already banned BPAs.

Be aware that many of the white filling resins that often replace mercury fillings contain BPAs. Again one must compare risks and benefits. Some companies like Heeraeus make BPA-free resins. Many contain fluoride.

17 http://www.youtube.com/watch?v=VImCpWzXJ_w

## What Are the Global Implications?
## Recycling Waste

The improper disposal of amalgam dental waste and its impact on the environment is another source of concern. Conditions and attitudes have changed since the ADA formulated its position on amalgam fillings about one hundred and fifty years ago. As global efforts continue to bring about a successful decline in mercury use and pollution, the percentage of dental contributions to mercury pollution steadily increases. The EPA estimates dentists purchase 34 tons of mercury per year. In fact, they are the nation's most unregulated users and third largest purchaser of mercury.

What happens to the 1,000 tons of mercury already residing in people's mouths, referenced in the Bank of America Securities analysis? Many European countries regulate mercury more stringently and require amalgam separators in dental offices. Amalgam separators separate the toxic metals removed from patients' mouths from the wastewater that subsequently enters public water supplies. No such requirement exists in the U.S. therefore most dental offices do not have amalgam separators.[18] The mercury discharge into sewers per dentist without amalgam separators is approximately 270 milligrams per day.[xli] Another study released from the Michigan School of Dentistry estimated dental mercury is responsible for approximately fourteen percent of mercury discharged to streams, lakes, and bays as reported by the previously referenced EPA report.[xlii] The FDA has yet to accomplish an environmental assessment of dental use of amalgams.

---

18 After a long and contentious battle, this from Charles Brown, National Counselor for *Consumers for Dental Choice*, "The American Dental Association has reversed its long-standing opposition to dentists installing technology to catch the mercury they don't put in patients' mouths. The ADA has ended its whining that dentists have no duty to spend $700 to address the destructive pollution that they -- the nation's #1 mercury polluter -- cause. On October 2 [2007] in San Francisco, its House of Delegates voted to mandate mercury separators in every dental office. Consumers for Dental Choice has long endorsed separators, because after mercury fillings are banned, dentists must continue to remove this toxin from people's teeth for a genera-tion to come.

19 Many of them have read the compiled studies of Bernie Windham and others. His extensive web site contains links to papers with over 3,000 medical or government agency studies documenting dental amalgam exposure toxicity. It is listed in the ap-pendices of this book.

This heavy metal has serious neurological consequences and is implicated in an enormous number of immune system dysfunctions,[xliii] [xliv xlvi xlvii] heart problems, and hormonal disruptions. For these reasons and because mercury binds to so many cells and organs, each person must decide how to limit mercury exposure. Despite the official position by the FDA and the ADA on dental amalgam stability and safety, many people choose to replace their mercury fillings.[19] Doing so vaporizes massive amounts of mercury, which can be inhaled and absorbed. While perhaps as many as half of all dentists no longer place mercury fillings, and therefore call themselves "mercury-free dentists," most are not yet "mercury-safe dentists." Safe removal protocol should be considered at all times.

There is a rise in the number of dentists taking mercury removal courses around the country. A starting protocol some dentists follow can be found in the appendices of this book. Many practitioners follow more elaborate precautions. Some of these are:

- Making sure the intestinal tract is at peak performance so it can optimally excrete excess mercury
- Providing pre-treatment vitamin C infusions, stopped the day of mercury filling removal to avoid interactions with anesthesia, then restarted
- Providing additional air purification in the office
- Supplementing with activated charcoal or chlorella to help eliminate released mercury. Chlorella is taken separately from vitamin C.
- Taking zeolites, which chelate low levels of heavy metals and other toxins. Chelated materials are then excreted.

The highly charged political debate over mercury toxicity in humans will certainly continue as it has for decades. This is because its related health and financial costs could be astronomically expensive.

**Notes:** The material in this section is not representative of the views held by the majority of dental professionals. To understand dentistry's more widespread views, visit their trade association's web site: http://www.ada.org/.

Regardless of how dentists view mercury filling material, all dental professionals must face it every day. I respect that they choose to put themselves in harm's way every time they go to work, in the spirit of trying to bring health to others.

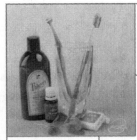

# 16

## RISK IS NOT DESTINY: SIMPLE SOLUTIONS

*"What gets us into trouble is not what we don't know.
It's what we know for sure that just ain't so."*

~ Mark Twain ~

**Explore: Fast and Easy Solutions!**

1. The onslaught of erosive foods.
2. Saliva's role.
3. Understanding fluoride:
   a) How fluoride works.
   b) How the intent of water fluoridation collides with reality. We are overdosed!
   c) Aluminum fluoride complexes, their abundance in today's America; their negative influence over critical life processes.
4. Alternative, safe ways to rebuild teeth and change their chemistry.
5. Strategies that discourage decay and gum disease.
6. Brushing myths, busted. Have you upgraded your style lately?
7. Everybody's favorite word.
8. Coping with chronic bad breath.

## Who Is In Charge?
## DDS Stands For Doctor of Dental Surgery

Once our teeth erupt, they are our body's most durable structure. Most people would be less casual about protecting their teeth if the commonplace practices of "drilling and filling" teeth with sometimes biologically incompatible materials were more correctly referred to as the surgical amputation of a rotten body part. It would be great if

your main contact with highly trained dentists was for therapy
designed to enhance function and improve your smile's attractiveness
rather than to "drill and fill" rotten teeth, usually destroying their
intricate structure in the process. Do consider a second opinion from a
minimally invasive, biomimetic dentist if treatment recommendations
require removing solid tooth structure. It may save you thousands of
dollars and your long-term health.

As discussed in the previous chapter, cost and time are just two
things to consider when one contemplates dental surgery. Because
there are downstream consequences to some of the biologically
incompatible materials dentists use to replace diseased tooth structure
as you will see in a moment, prevention trumps remediation. This
chapter describes what happens when a tooth decays and addresses
some common prevention strategies. Expect more surprising twists.

## GARRETT AND CHRISTOPHER
## Sip All Day? Decay Your Way

Some time ago I designed a pro-health program for preteens. I outlined
the seeds of the program to two boys returning to our practice after a ten-
year absence. When last I had seen them, their ages were four and five.
After their parent's divorce, financial constraints excluded professional
dental care. At fourteen and fifteen, they were not the ages or gender
known to have a sharp focus on personal health and responsibility.

Nonetheless, we explored their mouths with the video camera. I let
the boys' perceptive questions guide our discussion. When I explained
"wound management" theory to them, they were as fascinated with it as
most adults tend to be. Then, while looking at an image of the youngest
child's teeth, they asked how cavities form. I decided to describe the

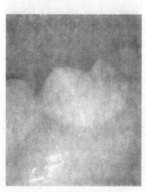

process by using drinking soda as an
example, accurately guessing they consumed
high quantities of soft drinks. I did this not
because of what I saw on the screen, but
because of statistics of which I am aware. A
lively discussion followed.

I pointed to a typical biofilm mass I saw
in the image and said, "Garrett, without
testing, we can't know what varieties of
bacteria are in your mouth but one likely
germ is *strep mutans*. Several bacteria types

produce acids after metabolizing sugars, but *s. mutans* are usually the predominant type. Like you may be, these bacteria are addicted to sugars! As soon as their favorite food is available, they begin processing it. One byproduct is a strong acid. They love to wallow in the acid they make. As you observe, the bacteria are often quite successful.

"I assume you've studied acids in school, so you know they corrode materials. Oral bacteria in biofilm produce acids that continuously dissolve minerals and organic matter from teeth. Worse, these bacteria store sugars internally. This means that if plaques remain, acid production can last hours after you've had your treat. Saliva eventually neutralizes the acidic pH, but it can take hours. This is one reason why it is important to stay hydrated. In the absence of medical problems, adequate, quality water intake ensures adequate saliva. Saliva maintains balance another way. When you eat properly, it contains abundant calcium, phosphate, and magnesium minerals. Where you teeth are plaque-free, saliva is able to replace dissolved minerals. About ninety percent of Americans do not receive that benefit in between their teeth because they leave plaque there almost 100 percent of the time!

## Suggested Water Intake Formula

At least forty percent of Americans are on the verge of dehydration. Ninety-nine percent of the molecules in our body are water molecules. Dozens of health articles focus on water's important role in weight loss. While individual needs vary and expert opinions conflict, one common formula offers a sensible baseline that accounts for individual need: Personal weight divided by two equals the base number of ounces of water a person needs to drink daily. If you exercise, are exposed to high ambient heat, and/or drink diuretic beverages, you require more.

Example: a suggested baseline daily intake of about 60 ounces of water – almost half a gallon – is suggested for a person weighing 120 pounds. A web site whose results correlate with this "rule of thumb" is found at: http://www.calculatorslive.com/Daily-Water-Intake-Calculator.aspx. It is best to hydrate between meals because liquids taken with food dilutes stomach acids and enzymes necessary for digestion.

Note: Some doctors and studies currently degrade the importance of water intake, but they overlook oral health. None of these studies considers oral processes and saliva's role in them. The quality of water is equally important, Review Chapter Fifteen.

"Since you mentioned you drink at least one soda a day, you should know even diet carbonated drinks corrode the teeth. Most sodas are flavored with citric and phosphoric acids. Also the "fizz" of dissolved carbon dioxide creates carbonic acid. A pH of between 2.4 to 3 makes these drinks quite corrosive to teeth.

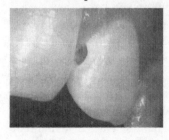
"Here is an image showing the teeth of a person who drank a soda a day. You can see the etched enamel. As minerals leach from a tooth surface, the surface loses its luster and begins to look like frosted glass, as you can see above the obvious hole. As acids continue to etch the tooth, it can turn yellow, then brown.

Microscopically, strong enamel looks solid. Corroded enamel first looks like stacked pipes that have lost the glue holding them together. A corroded area can lose about fifty percent of its mineral structure before the latticework crumbles and requires repair. A lesion usually receives professional repair when the intact surface collapses. Until then, a balance exists between corrosive and protective factors. You have enormous control over the balance. "When I run a dental instrument over unetched healthy teeth, it feels as if I'm dragging it across a smooth mirror. On etched surfaces, it's so porous it feels like a rough sidewalk. I often help clients sense and hear it too.

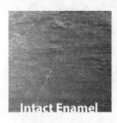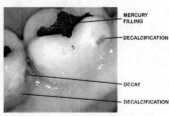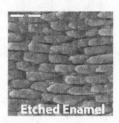

Intact Enamel — MERCURY FILLING — DECALCIFICATION — DECAY — DECALCIFICATION — Etched Enamel

[Pointing to center image/tooth on the left, labeled decay.] "Here's a question: where would you place the margin of the filling to repair this tooth? Dentists prefer to be conservative, but should the filling margin lie within the area of compromised, honeycombed tooth? How long might it last before the edges crumble? The filling would be like a hard ball bearing sitting in a pool of grease."

Garrett cringed, but asked me to continue.

CAROL: "Concerning cavities, it's not about how much sugar you eat, it's how often, how long it's in your mouth, and if plaque is present to convert it to acids. That's why chewing sugared gum, eating sticky candies and dehydrated fruits, sucking candy and breath mints, or sipping carbonated beverages or drinks like Gatoraide® is far worse than one quick snack or an occasional sugary drink.

### Experiments for Grade Schoolers:
### Egg In Vinegar /Oral pH Testing After Sugar Ingestion

When my child was in the first grade, I taught her class about tooth decay. I asked the teacher to cover a hardboiled egg with vinegar early in the day as preparation for a class experiment. After lunch, I conducted another experiment. First, I asked each child to check the pH (a measure of acidity or alkalinity) of his or her saliva with special pH testing strips.[*]

Some children's oral pH was already very acidic. I then divided the class into two groups. One group snacked on nuts while the other group snacked on candy. Those with low pH saliva (due to mouthbreathing, poor diet, or other causes) were necessarily in the candy group.

I used a modified number line to explain acidity to these young children. Seven was "neutral" and equated to "zero" on the number line. Anything above 7 was alkaline; anything below was acidic. The further from pH 7, the stronger the acid or base. I told them the vinegar covering the egg had a pH of five. Later that afternoon, we rechecked the pH of their mouths. Many of those eating candy watched their oral pH plummet to below pH 5.5, the pH at which acids begin to erode teeth. The oral pH of the half of the class who had eaten nuts remained close to a neutral pH 7. I was pleased the children who had eaten candy noticed their mouths were at least as acidic as the vinegar without having to prompt them.

All afternoon we monitored the eggshell and the children's oral acidity. By the dismissal bell, the eggshell had almost disintegrated! The children who originally had been unhappy to be in the "nut" group were crowing to the unhappy "candy" group. Some in the "candy" group were disturbed to leave school with their mouths still in such an acid state. Years later, they reminded me how much they learned that day.

---

[*] The most accurate testing strips are the pHion Diagnostic pH Test Strips. They are more accurate for saliva than for testing urine. Order from: http://www. phionbalance.com/. Chemicals on litmus papers are unhealthy so do not put testing strips in your mouth.

"To illustrate my point, let me tell you a decades old story. A friend of mine kept a jar full of M&Ms® in her dining room. Her habit was to enjoy one or two every time she passed. It seems innocuous, but she passed it at least seven times a day. Eating fourteen little M&Ms® doesn't seem like a huge transgression, but even though she kept hydrated and so maintained adequate saliva, her mouth was probably rarely in a "safe" pH range. She could have viewed her next dental visit as a disaster, but she was able to make the most of a bad situation. She had so many cavities it became reasonable to consider a whole mouth makeover including orthodontics. She finally had the opportunity to help create the mouth she always wanted. Today, her mouth smiles as beautifully as her eyes do. But I wouldn't want to encourage this kind of path to a more attractive, functional smile!

"There are many things you boys can do to create your own oral story. They are fast, effective, and easy to work into your daily routine."

## Take Five: Routines to Protect Your Smile and Health: Decay Reduction

You know decay and repair are dynamic processes and that cavities are a preventable infectious disease. You learned that several kinds of bacteria use simple carbohydrates like sugars and refined flours to leach roughly half of a tooth's minerals away before typical dental intervention. If you know how to balance your oral chemistry, you can keep excessive damage from occurring.

American diets have changed substantially over the last sixty years. One change is the dramatic shift towards acidic and carbohydrate-laden foods that cause oral and systemic acidity. Acidic sodas, fruit juices, and sports drinks have largely replaced water and milk consumption. Even processed foods incorporate acidifiers because they retard bacterial growth.

Becoming dependent on acidic convenience foods has significantly – both directly and indirectly – increased the erosive burden we put on our teeth. Our dietary habits now tip the scales toward decay.

The following table shows the acidity (pH) of various popular beverages. Of course this chart cannot account for the acidifying effects of the acids and sugars on one's body as they deplete buffering reserves.

| Beverage | pH Level |
|---|---|
| A. Carbonated | |
| Lemon-flavored soft drinks | 2.6- 3.2 |
| Cola drinks (excluding root beer) | 2.4- 3.2 |
| Root beers | 4.0- 4.61 |
| Low-calorie cola drinks | 2.8- 3.39 |
| PowerAde | 2.7 |
| Gatorade | 3.1 |
| B. Fruit Juices | |
| Orange | 2.8- 3.6 |
| Apple (contains malic acid) | 3.4- 3.8 |
| Grapefruit | 2.9- 3.4 |
| Pineapple | 3.3- 3.7 |
| Lemon | 2.0- 3.2 |
| Tomato | 4.0- 4.6 |
| Sweetened Grapefruit | 3.1- 3.4 |
| C. Bottled Waters | |
| Natural Mineral Water- still | 7.8 |
| Natural Mineral Water- carbonated | 4.2- 4.8 |
| Spring Water- still | 6.8- 7.8 |
| Spring Water- carbonated | 4.2- 4.8 |
| Table Water-still | 6.8- 7.8 |
| Table Water- carbonated | 4.2- 4.8 |
| D. Milk | 6.5- 6.8 |

Car battery acid has a pH of 1.0. Note only milk and non-carbonated water have non-erosive pH levels (close to a neutral pH of 7). Even many bottled waters have an acidic pH of 4. Tooth demineralization occurs at a pH of 5.5 and below. The pH of drinks is not the only factor causing dental erosion. Another factor is a drink's ability to neutralize acids, called its buffering capacity. Energy drinks, sports drinks like Gatoraide®, and Mountain Dew® have the strongest potential for tooth erosion. Sodas are acidulated with phosphoric acid. Gatoraide uses citric acid. This makes the tooth run a calcium deficit even though pH is different. For this reason, Coke is actually "better" than Gatoraide! Arghhh. This splits hairs that should not need splitting.

The incidence of cavities in seniors is high, accounting for half of all known new cavities. As we age, our lifestyles catch up with us. A lifetime of stress, processed foods, and medications of all kinds show up as depleted saliva with few minerals. Acid-loving bacteria that cause gum disease and decay thrive. Acid buffering and micro-repair slow or catastrophically stop. Type 2 diabetes and Sjögren's syndrome join the over 700 medications that severely curtail the protective flow of saliva. It doesn't have to be that way.

Exposed roots caused by bone and tissue loss around teeth are at highest risk for decay since the body of a tooth including the roots are roughly only 70 percent mineralized. As you have seen, exposed tooth roots are an overlooked cleaning challenge. Since enamel is roughly 98 percent mineralized, the enamel coating over the crowns of teeth makes them far more resistant to acids than their roots. One-third of all adults over the age of 45 have root surface cavities. Half of adults over 65 do. By 2010, nearly half the U.S. population will be in this over-65 bracket. How can these people keep their teeth intact?

If I had my way, everyone would be air polished and scanned with a Diagnodent or Acteon for early diagnosis every six months. If necessary, suspect areas would be treated with Sylc air abrasion, ozone, and a supersaturated solution of minerals or remineralizing nanoparticles. Everyone deemed at risk would have their own personally fitted ozone trays through which a dental professional could circulate ozone.

Think of the benefits to the aged, those with crippling arthritis or other physical disabilities, and even those with mental disabilities that make optimal self-care difficult. And hey, I wouldn't treat my cavity-free children any other way.

But we are not there yet. So what can the rest of you do while you are waiting for politics and education to catch up with what you want for yourselves and your loved ones?

We could all make better food choices. We could eat fewer fermentable carbohydrates and processed, acid-forming foods. We could seriously reduce calorie and acid exposure by rethinking our beverage habits. Most of us should drink more water. I encourage monitoring your salivary or urine pH to determine and modulate your risks. Modify risks until your saliva is routinely about pH 6.8. (Order pHion Test Strips from http://www.phionbalance.com/.)

In the meantime are there ways to protect your teeth? Of course! But first, let us take a detour and give a sacred cornerstone of dental prevention a fresh look.

## Stealth Marketing

Most of us know that Americans who "supersize" fast foods when they order them, increase profits for food processors, agribusinesses, and chain restaurants, while at the same time, they supersize their own waistlines and destroy their health. We unintentionally ingest staggering amounts – far more than we ever intended – of sugars including high fructose corn syrup, trans fats, and other detrimental "flavorings" like MSG, refined salts and AGEs. Are we also ingesting more fluoride than was intended? Can we get too much of a good thing? *Is* fluoride a good thing?

Writing about fluoridation for first edition of *Mouth Matters,* was difficult. I was a strong fluoridation advocate for most of my professional career. I had to accept that I had been blindly advocating a medication that I had not thoroughly examined for myself. Since I chose to advocate for whole body health and I knew there was controversy over the policy, I knew it was past time to study it further.

What I learned shocked me as much as it did Dr. Hardy Limeback, head of preventive dentistry at the University of Toronto, as he delved into the subject for the Environmental Protection Agency and publicly reversed his pro-fluoridation stance years ago.

An increasing number of educated people have serious concerns about fluoride's ubiquitous presence in our lives. Calls for "Fluoridegate" hearings are effectively being heard around the country. As Civil Rights leader, Dr. Durley, wrote to Georgia legislators, "I support the holding of Fluoridegate hearings at the state and national level so we can learn why we haven't been openly told that fluorides build up in the body over time (and) why our government agencies haven't told the black community openly that fluorides disproportionately harm black Americans."

He continued, "The National Research Council (NRC) of the National Academy of Sciences has designated kidney patients, diabetics, seniors, and babies as 'susceptible subpopulations' that are especially vulnerable to harm from ingested fluorides. Black citizens are disproportionately affected by kidney disease and diabetes, and are therefore more impacted by fluorides.

"Fluoride chemicals, added to 96% of Georgia's public drinking water supplies are meant to prevent tooth decay, especially in the poor. Yet, 61% of low-income Georgia third-graders have tooth decay compared to 51% from higher income families.[i] Despite fluoridation, tooth decay is higher in blacks[ii] along with fluoride overexposure symptoms - dental fluorosis or discolored teeth."

Former U.N. Ambassador Young has also expressed concerns about the fairness, safety, and full disclosure regarding fluoridation in letters to Georgia's minority and majority legislative leaders. "We have a cavity epidemic today in our inner cities that have been fluoridated for decades."

Young further stated, "I am most deeply concerned for poor families who have babies: if they cannot afford unfluoridated water for their babies' milk formula, do their babies not count? Of course they do. This is an issue of fairness, civil rights, and compassion. We must find better ways to prevent cavities... My father was a dentist. I formerly was a strong believer in the benefits of water fluoridation for preventing cavities. But many things that we began to do 50 or more years ago we now no longer do, because we have learned further information that changes our practices and policies. So it is with fluoridation."

An American Association for Justice Newsletter for trial lawyers describes potential fluoride legal actions based on personal injury, consumer fraud, and civil rights harm.[iii]

In a letter to their state's Health Commissioner, a bipartisan group of Tennessee legislators expressed their concern about fluoridation's undesirable impact on babies and other groups.[iv]

A bipartisan group of New York City Council Members has also introduced legislation to stop fluoridation in NYC.[v]

But my experiences in working with Austin City Council on the issue show we have an uphill battle. They listen carefully. They ask good questions. It is clear they don't have a science background. They seem ill equipped to be making this decision as they struggle with the studies and the principals. The further we go in this process, the clearer it is: these people should not have to be making what is essentially a blanket medical decision for everyone in the Central Texas Region. It is absurd this power is left up to them. All they can do is rely on the principle of "deferred expertise".

The problem with deferred expertise is that there are political agendas to consider. If nothing else, consider the legal issues facing them, as noted above... consumer fraud, personal injury and the like.

While political and legal wheels grind, you may want to know more, so you can make an informed decision for yourself and those you love. The next few pages will synopsize some of what we now know.

## Drink Contaminant-Free Water

Henry Dark Photography/Joe Peterson

| | | | | | | | | | | | | | | | | | |
|---|---|---|---|---|---|---|---|---|---|---|---|---|---|---|---|---|---|
| H | | | | | | | | | | | | | | | | | He |
| Li | Be | | | | | | | | | | | B | C | N | O | F | Ne |
| Na | Mg | | | | | | | | | | | Al | Si | P | S | Cl | Ar |
| K | Ca | Sc | Ti | V | Cr | Mn | Fe | Co | Ni | Cu | Zn | Ga | Ge | As | Se | Br | Kr |
| Rb | Sr | Y | Zr | Nb | Mo | Tc | Ru | Rh | Pd | Ag | Cd | In | Sn | Sb | Te | I | Xe |
| Cs | Ba | * | Lu | Hf | Ta | W | Re | Os | Ir | Pt | Au | Hg | Tl | Pb | Bi | Po | At | Rn |
| Fr | Ra | ** | Lr | Rf | Db | Sg | Bh | Hs | Mt | Uun | Uuu | Uub | | Uuq | | | |

Fluoride's position in the Periodic Table of Elements determines the properties that contribute to its successes and failures in human health and disease. According to Dr. Mark Winter, chemistry professor at the University of Sheffield, "Fluorine is the most electronegative and reactive of all elements. It is a pale yellow, corrosive gas, which reacts with practically all organic and inorganic substances. Finely divided metals, glass, ceramics, carbon, and even water burn in fluorine with a bright flame." [vi] Fluoride will react with almost anything and is considered highly toxic. Another college chemistry professor, Dr. Anne Marie Helmenstine says, "The recommended maximum allowable concentration for a daily eight-hour time-weighted exposure is 0.1 ppm." [vii] Chemists understand these to be well-known facts.

Fluoride's reactivity with all human tissues[1] and its ability to deeply penetrate them due to its tiny size[2] lies at the heart of the controversy that has raged for decades around water fluoridation. Today's fluoride promoters, including the Centers for Disease Control and many current

---

1 Even if fluoride were biologically compatible with human health in every other way, the fact that fluoride sets off massive oxidation reactions in the human body is counter-productive for the purpose of reducing inflammation.

2 Fluoride can cross the powerfully protective blood-brain barrier to enter the highly sensitive pineal gland. In 1997, Jennifer Luke confirmed in her PhD. thesis, that fluoride accumulates in the human pineal gland. In animals (Mongolian gerbils), fluoride lowers melatonin production and shortens the time to puberty.

Fluoride is a part of many prescription medications; its presence contributes to these medicines' successes and failures. For instance the powerful fluoroquinolone class of antibiotics, such as Cipro and Levaquin are associated with tendon toxicity and an increased risk of tendon ruptures. A Class Action lawsuit against their manufacturers is ongoing.

dental professionals, concede fluoride's benefits to teeth are derived from topical exposure, not ingestion.[3] Fluoridation was originally promoted to work the way most people still think it does: the original fluoride promoters suggested that children drinking artificially fluoridated water would incorporate it into their developing teeth to enhance their ability to withstand acids. Under this model, the window of opportunity for this tooth-building benefit is from birth until age eight, at most.

Now that theory has been debunked, fluoride promoters have switched their promotion tactics. They contend that even the lower fluoridation concentration they now recommend[4] could enhance remineralization as it passes over teeth before swallowing. They also suggest ingested fluoride enters saliva, which can increase exposure time to about 20 minutes.[ix] The following study addresses this theory. It shows topical benefits are limited.

In this study, sodium fluoride penetrated the depth of biofilm to reach tooth surfaces only when plaque was exposed to fluoride continuously for thirty minutes. The researchers who conducted it suggested fluoride applied with viscous toothpaste would further slow penetration. They contended that since cavities occur "at inaccessible stagnation sites where plaque removal is difficult" their results show limited topical use for fluoride's anti-decay intent.[viii] The authors noted 30-minute contact was impractical.

As a hygienist of three decades, I concur – cavities occur in the grooves of teeth, in between them, and at the gum line – all places most people overlook during home hygiene. The fluoride ion will not make it to the tooth structure as it passes over the tooth while drinking, much less stick around for 30 minutes. This is but another reason we should

3 An article in the Journal of the American Dental Association, "The Science and Practice of Caries Prevention" (Featherstone, 2000;131(7): 887-899) summarized this fact, well-known in dental circles since the 1990's. Children growing up in "optimally" fluoridated areas have about 100ppm (parts per million) incorporated in their teeth, though a thin layer of enamel at the surface might have 1,000 to 2,000ppm. In these ranges there was no difference in the way teeth dissolved in acids, compared to teeth formed in non-fluoridated areas. "Only when fluoride is concentrated into a new crystal surface topically during remineralization (repair) is it sufficient to beneficially alter enamel solubility." Featherstone outlines how fluoride disrupts the metabolism of bacteria as it passes over teeth and how it helps teeth remineralize under acidic conditions.
4 As of January, 2011, the government officially lower the recommended limit for fluoride in public water supplies to .7 ppm, conceding we now know Americans receive it from multiple sources. I note they always point to fluoride's presence in dental products, never to the pesticide or food-borne sources.

move away from current models of care. Remember: only ozone gas delivers *predictable* remineralization. *It is not enough to provide minerals.*

A *Scientific American* article, "Second Thoughts On Fluoride" reintroduced a new generation to the fluoride controversy.[x] The article, which reviewed the vitriol expressed on both sides of the debate, pointed out that this was America's first environmental health controversy. The original debate was so politicized it polarized every group involved. Serious opponents became "rabid crackpots" and advocates were "communists" with a plan to poison America. Community water fluoridation advocates generally prevailed. Over time, the controversy evolved into something of a sacred belief system for many.

Many professionals realize we should adopt a more targeted and voluntary approach to fluoride use. Many people argue the Safe Water Drinking Act mandates this. These same people believe selective topical application should be emphasized over involuntary ingestion, where harm can and does occur. As with mercury, fluoride is found in multiple unexpected sources, dosages are higher than many professionals and policy makers anticipated, and toxicity to the most susceptible is underrated.

## Are You Underdosed? Don't Worry… Be Happy!

The stated original goal of artificial fluoridation was that it deliver one milligram (mg) of fluoride every day to each child living in the U.S. Promoters said this amount would incorporate throughout children's developing teeth, thereby strengthening them and making them more decay-resistant. Decades ago the following was assumed:

- Each child drinks one liter of water/day.
- Children would have no other source of fluoride exposure.

These assumptions were then translated into a universal medication "dosage". Our politician's desired *dose* for each child is one mg total daily exposure. Unfortunately, they set this dose as a concentration, that is: one part per million (1 ppm). The two should never be confused. One might argue that if politicians and policy-makers can make this basic a science error, they have no business formulating and enforcing a medical policy. In fact, in January 2010, the new guideline that suggests lowering city water fluoridation levels to a maximum of .7ppm was a response to the realization that we are all exposed to multiple fluoride sources.

When doctors prescribe medications, they evaluate weight, individual need, additional exposure sources and medical history. They then set medication doses accordingly. This protection is not granted with fluoride since it comes to us through artificial public water fluoridation and many other sources. Monitoring dosages is impossible. Even more unusual for a medication: at this universal concentration, no margin for error exists to protect the most vulnerable populations against adverse effects.

At the allowed contaminant level set by the EPA (four ppm) some of the population is at risk, therefore many say it violates the criteria mandated by the Safe Water Drinking Act. It was known as early as the 1940s that two mg of fluoride a day caused objectionable levels of dental fluorosis to occur. Nonetheless city water supplies began supplementing drinking water, thus foods and beverages processed with fluoridated city water, with roughly one ppm of fluoride to attain the desired 1mg/day goal.

American children aged 12 to 15 with some level of fluorosis climbed to 41 percent in 2004 from 23 percent in 1987, according to the most recent data available in the National Health and Nutrition Examination Survey. Only 8.7 percent of adults in their 40s studied had fluorosis. Fluorosis should be considered a biomarker for its concentration in various body systems, though the CDC says the only objectionable side effect of too much fluoride is dental fluorosis. As stated in the kidney chapter, when we are healthy, we excrete about half of the fluoride we ingest. Someone with damaged kidneys can only excrete about twenty percent. Where does the rest of it go?

## The Dose Makes the Poison

In the U.S., fluoride exposure is uncontrolled and unavoidable, no matter where you live. Many Americans drink more than one liter of water or water-based beverage each day, which easily doubles or triples their daily dose.[5] Further, anyone can easily exceed the "recommended" dosage since we drink additional beverages and

---

5 Some populations have substantially higher water intake. These include athletes, outdoor workers – especially in the South – pregnant and lactating mothers, those with diabetes and other medical conditions, and military personnel. U.S. Army hydration requirements for warm weather training are .47-.96L/hour, with a daily maximum of 12 quarts.

eat foods contaminated with fluoride. This is because they are either processed with fluoridated water or treated with post-harvest fumigants like synthetic cryolite (sodium aluminum fluoride, a particularly damaging compound), or sulfuryl fluoride, which first gained approval in 2004. Current Environmental Protection Agency (EPA) tolerance levels for synthetic cryolite on produce, is seven ppm. Kiwi fruit is the exception. Its residue tolerance level is 15 ppm.

The EPA regulations tolerate historically high levels of fluoride residue on crops. The chart below highlights its tolerances. For more information, see: http://www.fluoridealert.org/pesticides/sf.documents.html.

| FOOD PRODUCT | EPA'S TOLERANCE LEVEL FOR FLUORIDE RESIDUE FROM SULFU-RYL FLUORIDE IN PPM/July 15, 2005 |
|---|---|
| Barley | 45 ppm |
| Legumes (all beans) | 70 ppm |
| Cheese | 5 ppm |
| Coconut | 40 ppm |
| Coffee | 15 ppm |
| Herbs | 15 ppm |
| Nuts (exception peanuts) | 10 ppm |
| Nuts, peanuts | 15 ppm |
| Oat, flour or rolled | 75 ppm |
| Oat, grain | 25 ppm |
| Popcorn | 10 ppm |
| Rice, grain | 12 ppm |
| Wheat, flour | 125 ppm |
| Wheat, germ | 130 ppm |
| Wheat grain | 40ppm |
| Powdered eggs | 900ppm |

**Factoid:** The amount of fluoride in one glass of water at 1 ppm is the same as that found in the suggested pea-sized amount of fluoridated toothpaste. The warning label on the back of all fluoridated toothpastes say to call the poison control center if you swallow it. Many people have no choice about swallowing that amount with their drinking water.

*Fluoride in Drinking Water: A Scientific Review of EPA's Standards*, is a critical report issued in 2006. In 2003, the EPA ordered the National Research Council (NRC) to conduct a review of the EPA's established maximum fluoride contamination levels in drinking water. The NRC panel was particularly instructed *not* to review artificial fluoridation.

As the researchers reviewed the data, they assigned tea a pesticide residue concentration of 897.72 ppm for dried or powdered tea[xi] considering it more appropriate than the five ppm level the EPA used for brewed tea in a 2004 analysis. Interestingly, a half cup of tea was the assumed daily dose in their exposure tables – tables that still reflect substantial overdosing – even though tea drinkers rarely drink only half of a cup of tea per day.

The National Research Council further advised that in their exposure tables, "the exposure from foods treated with sulfuryl fluoride is not applicable."[xii] In other words, allowances for the pesticide sulfuryl fluoride were not considered in their data tables since limits were being rewritten at the time of the report. After reviewing the abbreviated data table above, one can see how this omission would skew the data in that report by a wide margin. Additionally, all food-processing facilities, such as canneries, bottlers, dairies, mills, bakeries, and packagers are allowed to fumigate to a 70-ppm residue fluoride tolerance – and in the U.S. and Australia, while food is still on the premisis.[6] Anyone curious as to why pesticides contain fluoride?

The 2006 release of the NRC report finally galvanized the American Dental Association to warn the public about overexposure of infants to fluoride – months after the report's release. Were *you* alerted the American Dental Association issued a statement that no child under 12 months of age should have his or her formula mixed with fluoridated tap water? The message was so poorly publicized, even most dental professionals are still unaware of its warning. Do you know how to obtain safe water? Are dental professionals able to guide you?

Fluoridating water supplies and adding it to so many products is consistent with the American mind set: if some is good, more is better. But this policy has had unintended and unforeseen consequences. As early as the 1990s, some dental professionals voiced concerns about the mineral's unhealthy concentration levels in processed foods such as juices, which are most heavily ingested by young children and who by nature have lower tolerances to toxins.

---

[6] See: http://www.fluoridealert.org/sf/index.html to see the broad range of facilities and circumstances under which the EPA allows a 70 ppm fluoride tolerance.

In February of 1997, the Academy of General Dentistry advised dentists to warn parents that their children should not drink excessive amounts of juice due to its high fluoride content. This followed studies published in professional journals showing ready-to-drink juices may contain up to 6.8 ppm fluoride,[xiii][xiv] and infant foods may have as much as 8.38 ppm.[xv]

The ADA also published a series of studies about overexposure due to the widespread use of fluoridated water, fluoride dentifrice, dietary fluoride supplements, and other forms of fluoride.

## What Are Fluoride Overdose Risks?

With all the report's shortcomings, *Fluoride in Drinking Water* called for the Environmental Protection Agency to lower their standard maximum fluoride contamination in drinking water to reduce fluorosis[7] in children. Until that point, fluorosis was considered simply a cosmetic, not a health effect. The NRC report acknowledged the standard did not protect infants and young children against dental fluorosis. It also emphasized that research gaps exist, which cover a wide range of possible negative health effects for susceptible populations.

Concerns arising from the National Resource Council of the National Academies 2006 report include the following:

**Neurotoxocity and Neurobehavioral Effects.** In his review of the report, Dr. R.J. Carton[8] said, "Fluoride has adverse effects on the brain, especially in combination with aluminum. Seriously detrimental effects are known to occur in animals at a fluoride level of 0.3 mg/L in conjunction with aluminum."[xvi] Do you cook with aluminum pots and pans? If you do, the aluminum will react with the fluoride in your cooking water and on your produce to form aluminum fluoride (AlFx) compounds, which you will then ingest. Do you eat produce or drink wines made from grapes fumigated with cryolite, also known as sodium aluminum fluoride? What fluoride compound does your city use to fluoridate water? Call your water department. You might find that – as

---

7 Fluorosis is responsible for the discoloration, pitting, and weakening of the crystalline structure of enamel and dentin (the body of the tooth underlying the enamel) of teeth. If the dentin is weak, the tooth is weak. Severe fluorosis involves enamel loss.

8 RJ Carton, PhD, is an environmental scientist who has worked for over 30 years in the U.S. federal government writing regulations, managing risk assessments on high priority toxic chemicals, and providing environmental oversight of medical research conducted by the government.

many cities do – they add aluminum fluoride compounds to your public water supply. Fluoride increases aluminum uptake in humans.

The review cited four studies from China indicating children living in communities with high fluoride had lower IQs. It suggested this could happen as aluminum fluoride (AlFx) complexes form. Aluminum and fluoride have a powerful affinity for each other.[9] These complexes mimic the structure of phosphates that influence enzyme activities in the brain. The review also suggests a possible association with autism. There are now more than 24 studies showing links between excessive fluoride and lower IQ.

**Reported increase of rare sarcomas in young males with increased fluoride ingestion.** Dr. Carton's NRC review included an assessment of pre-publication data from a major study undertaken at Harvard to look into this association. It found a positive link between exposure to fluoride in drinking water and the incidence of osteosarcoma (bone cancer) in young males. This study took five years to be published, but amidst strong controversy, it is finally available.[xvii]

**Hormonal effects.** Low thyroid function, called hypothyroidism, is at near epidemic levels in the U.S. Is fluoride overexposure partly to blame? In Europe, overactive thyroid function was treated with low doses of fluoride to reduce function until the 1970s. The thyroid must be saturated with iodine to function. All of the halogen group of elements in the Periodic Table above iodine displace iodine in the thyroid. Ordered from smallest element size to largest, these are: fluorine, chlorine, and bromine. We drink chlorinated and fluorinated water and breathe its vapors. We consume bromine in many processed foods, and

---

9 As an internal group of EPA scientists expressed in their journal: "AlFx complexes interact with all known G-protein-activated effector enzymes. G-proteins take part in an enormous variety of biological signaling systems, helping control almost all important life processes [For example, beta endorphins, discussed earlier, interact with these G proteins.]… It appears probable we will not find any physiological process, which is not potentially influenced by AlFx… Pharmacologists estimate that up to 60 percent of all medicines used today exert their effects through a G-protein signaling pathway. The synergistic action of fluoride and aluminum in the environment, water, and food can thus evoke multiple pathological symptoms. AlFx might induce alterations in homeostasis, metabolism, growth, and differentiation in living organisms. An awareness of the health risks of this new ecotoxicological phenomenon, an increasing load of aluminum ions and fluoride, would undoubtedly contribute significantly to reducing the risk of a decrease in intelligence of children and adults, and many other disorders in the 21st century." (*Inside the Fishbowl.* NTEU Chapter 280. U.S.EPA, National Headquarters. January/February 2003; 19(1)

we are liberally exposed to bromine- and fluorine-based pesticides and bromine-based flame-retardants. If your core temperature is consistently below 98.6, it is likely you have low thyroid function. It could be your thyroid is not saturated with iodine because it has been displaced with the other halide elements. Iodine deficiencies are also associated with elevated risk of prostate and breast cancer and fibrocystic breast disease.

Dr. Carton's review suggested the NRC Report had many research gaps. In particular, he was concerned about those involving the thyroid gland, whose hormones regulate growth and metabolism. He states, "Decreased thyroid function is an adverse health effect, particularly to individuals with inadequate dietary iodine [estimated to be at least 12 percent of the U.S. population]. These individuals could be affected with a daily fluoride dose of 0.7 mg/day. This is less than the amount already in the diet." [**Note:** This statement was made prior to approval of extensive use of sulfuryl fluoride as a food pesticide.]

**Bone Fracture/Skeletal Fluorosis.** Remember, teeth reflect internal conditions. Teeth and bones are a target for fluoride. Fluoride increases the skeletal requirement for calcium and can result in a general state of calcium deficiency and secondary Hyperparathyroidism. Again, from Dr. Carton's review:

- Moderate dental fluorosis is an adverse health effect occurring at fluoride levels of 0.7 to 1.2mg/L, the levels of water fluoridation.
- The Lowest Observed Adverse Effect Level (LOAEL) for bone fractures is at least as low as 1.5 mg/L and may be lower than this figure.
- Stage II and Stage III skeletal fluorosis may be occurring at levels less than 2 mg/L.
- Stage I skeletal fluorosis, defined as arthritis, clinically manifested as pain and stiffness in joints, is an adverse health effect which may occur with a daily fluoride intake of 1.4 mg/day. This amount is less than the amount the average person already obtains in their diet in non-fluoridated areas. The Maximum Contaminant Level should be zero.[xviii]

**Dental fluorosis.** Fluorosis in teeth occurs when children ingest excessive fluoride during tooth formation. I warn my clients their teeth are more brittle than those without fluorosis. I suggest they avoid crunching hard foods and ice. As with skeletal bones, mineral density does not necessarily translate into strength or fracture resistance.

**Effects on the digestive system, liver, immune system, and kidneys.** Possible ill effects of fluoride on these systems and organs have been inadequately studied. I introduced kidney damage via fluoride ingestion in Chapter Ten of this book. Despite the fact that many studies suggest associations between fluoride exposure and adverse kidney effects, the NRC committee generally concluded research on these topics was still insufficient. (Currently, dialysis centers filter fluoride out of water used for dialysis because failing kidneys cannot filter fluoride well, thus accelerating kidney damage. The National Kidney Foundation, once listed as fluoridation advocates, no longer support fluoridation. They "take no position" on it.)

Ingested fluoride has a particular affinity for skeletal bones as they remodel. About half of ingested fluoride of a person without kidney damage is stored in the body. Some accumulates in teeth, the pineal gland of the brain, and other organs, but more than 90 percent is stored in skeletal bones. This should be of particular interest to older women because post-menopausal women no longer have the bone-sparing benefits of estrogen. As a result, many take bisphosphonate bone-sparing medications, which lead to increased bone density and brittleness, just as fluoride ingestion does. This only compounds the risks for skeletal fractures these woman face.

Dr. Hardy Limeback, head of preventive dentistry at the University of Toronto, and a *Fluoride in Drinking Water* research panel member, is one of many former advocates of water fluoridation who have reversed their position on fluoride safety and efficacy. He said, "A lifetime of fluoride ingestion in areas where water is 'optimally' fluoridated (1 ppm) can change the quality of dentin and bone and may increase fracture rates for both." [xix]

Bone samples taken from Toronto residents (where water is fluoridated at 1ppm) showed altered architecture, which decreased bones' resistance to compression. Skeletal bones had higher density but a lower mineral content, which increased their brittleness. Dr. Limeback asserts the study shows fluoride lowers compressive strength and resilience, or toughness, of bone. He continues to speak out against water fluoridation. [10]

10 Grass Roots and Global Video in association with Fluoride Action Network hosts a sample interview called Leading Dental Researcher Speaks out Against Water Fluoridation at: http://video.google.com/videoplay?docid=-3153312008186362773.

Kathleen Thiessen, another NRC fluoride toxicology review panel member and a senior scientist at SENES Oak Ridge, Center for Risk Analysis, also believes water fluoridation is a reckless policy on many counts.[11]

The NRC report states, "The EPA's Maximum Contaminant Level Goal for fluoride (MCLG) was set only to protect against the adverse health effects of crippling skeletal fluorosis (Stage III)." It admitted, "Stage II skeletal fluorosis, the symptoms of which include sporadic pain, joint stiffness, and abnormal thickening (osteosclerosis) of the pelvis and spine, also constitutes an adverse health effect." Many consider joint pain and stiffness early warning signs of a body super-saturated by fluoride.

The report also notes that fluoridation remains far from universally practiced. Most Western European countries have ceased, or never practiced, water fluoridation for various reasons. A final quote from the report states, "The extent of the benefits of water fluoridation to oral health also has received some scrutiny. An overall reduction in caries has been observed in fluoridated and non-fluoridated communities in the United States; more recent studies suggest water fluoridation has become less important and effective in preventing caries when compared with the findings of earlier studies. Some of this research has attributed the smaller differences in caries prevalence between fluoridated and non-fluoridated communities to the widespread use of fluoride toothpaste and other preventive dental care, and to better nutrition."

For those interested in mechanisms of fluoride action, a research paper released in 2010 by Gazzano et al describes how fluoride creates excessive free radicals, inhibits enzymes,[12] interacts with G-proteins, (a primary cell signaling device), affects bone remodeling, and many other negative effects.[xx]

**Note:** For those who understand our bodies run on electricity, fluoride encourages a suboptimal voltage and is acidifying.

---

11 An interview with Dr. Thiessen can also be accessed at http://www.fluoridealert.org/articles/thiessen-interview/.

12 Enzymes run about 100,000 chemical reactions per second in our bodies. Fluorine, the most reactive element, deactivates enzymes. Fluoride salts are commonly used in biochemistry to inhibit enzyme activities. Enzyme chemists were the first opponents of fluoridation decades ago. Fluoride either bonds to Mg, Zn, or Cu on the active center of enzymes or it forms a competing hydrogen bond, changing the enzyme's shape. In biology, function follows form. If a molecule's shape is wrong, it will not function as it should. Through fluoride's ability to interfere with hydrogen bonds, it changes the shapes of other molecules as well, also rendering them useless.

## Where Do Cities Obtain Fluoride?

Ninety-two percent of the communities who medicate city water with fluoride, do so with industrial grade hydrofluorosilicic acid or sodium silicofluorides. These silicofluorides are by-products of phosphate fertilizer manufacturing. Phosphate ores naturally contain about two to four percent fluoride as well as other Class I toxins like lead, uranium, cadmium, and arsenic. To extract the phosphate from ore, it is treated with sulfuric acid. The process creates a steam that carries the toxins to pollution scrubbers. The unrefined toxic wastes removed from these pollution scrubbers are then sold to cities across the United States to fluoridate public water. Despite evidence showing silicofluorides enhance the uptake of lead into the brain,[xxi] fluoridation proponents argue toxin levels are virtually undetectable after adequate dilution.

In a summary from the previously mentioned *Scientific American* article, John Doull, professor emeritus of pharmacology and toxicology at the University of Kansas Medical Center, and chair of the NRC committee said, "We've gone with the status quo regarding fluoride for many years – too long, really – and now we need to take a fresh look. Many of these questions are unsettled and we have much less information than we should, considering how long this (fluoridation) has been going on. I think that's why fluoridation is still being challenged so many years after it began. In the face of ignorance, controversy is rampant."

Paul Connett, a chemistry professor at St. Lawrence University and the executive director of the Fluoride Action Network[13] said, "I absolutely believe it's a scientific turning point because now everything's on the table. Fluoride is the most consumed drug in the U.S., and it's time we talked about it."

To summarize, fluorine is more reactive than chlorine. It liberally creates free radicals, a major cause of inflammation. Fluoride's deep penetration plus its oxidation and inflammatory effects may contribute to joint pain and stiffness among other inflammatory effects.

*"An error does not become a mistake until we refuse to correct it."*
**~ Orlando Battista, Chemist ~**

---

13 http://www.fluoridealert.org/

## Shifting the Balance From Destruction to Reconstruction

Chapter Thirteen describes how tooth structure is not static – that tooth enamel and dentin can repair themselves given the right circumstances.

Saliva is naturally loaded with calcium and phosphate minerals. Those minerals are not there to aggravate you or provide a career path for hygienists, though personal experience causes most to think otherwise! The plaque barrier can inappropriately mineralize, but the ideal target for these minerals is bare tooth structure. When a tooth is cleared of plaque biofilm, demineralized areas incorporate these natural and safe minerals that constantly bathe the mouth, thus repairing the micro-damage acids cause. Of course, beyond a certain point, dental professionals need to help the process along.

When teeth are kept plaque-free, are rarely exposed to simple carbohydrates or acids, and are allowed to bathe in the healing natural minerals provided by adequate saliva, breakdown and repair are in balance. But when age, prescription drugs and/or diseases such as Sjogren's syndrome, Parkinson's, or diabetes compromise saliva, the natural repair process is interrupted and breakdown exceeds repair. Minimally invasive techniques described in Chapter Thirteen offer powerful help to everyone. But what can you do to support the therapy or do for yourself if that kind of help is unavailable? To help shift the balance toward repair, promising new technologies offer improved protection and rebuilding without fluoride. Three of these choices are:

**Decay Reduction: NovaMin®.** NovaMin® is a fluoride alternative with multiple oral benefits. This calcium phosphate technology also may remineralize teeth desensitize exposed roots.

Surgeons used Novamin's mineral delivery system for years to enhance bone regeneration. The material from which NovaMin® is made was first used in the 1960s to repair the broken bones of our military during the Viet Nam War in a product called NovaBone®. Dental surgeons subsequently used it as PerioGlas® to enhance healing after extractions and periodontal surgery. Studies show that toothpastes with NovaMin® provide more than twice the tooth protection compared to brushing with toothpaste alone.[xxii xxiii] Beyond rebuilding and desensitizing teeth, NovaMin® has antimicrobial properties against some microbes associated with gum disease and cavities.

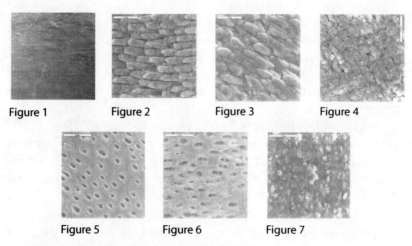

Figure 1          Figure 2          Figure 3          Figure 4

Figure 5          Figure 6          Figure 7

**Figure 1.** Intact enamel with no demineralization
**Figure 2.** Demineralized enamel after acid attack
**Figure 3.** Enamel treated with prescription strength (1100ppm) fluoride
**Figure 4.** Enamel treated with NovaMin®
**Figure 5.** Exposed root surface. Clenching, aggressive brushing, or chemical or physical trauma cause tooth flexing. This leads to gum recession and subsequent root exposure. Nerves run through each tubule and can be exposed, which can cause acute sensitivity. Occluding the tubules with various minerals insulates the nerves from the oral environment. Common therapies include using over-the-counter (OTC) sensitivity reducing toothpastes, professionally applied desensitizing fluoride, OTC and prescription fluoride, Recaldent®, and NovaMin® used professionally or at home. See a professional to be certain sensitivity is not triggered by decay or another serious oral condition.
**Figure 6.** Root surface treated with Recaldent®
**Figure 7.** Root surface treated with NovaMin®. The tubules are significantly occluded.

Dr. Collins Restore toothpaste is one of the few toothpastes available over-the-counter in the U.S. containing calcium sodium phosphosilicate (as NovaMin®). Check online for shifting availability of toothpastes containing this ingredient. This paste also contains titanium dioxide and the foaming agent sodium lauryl sulphate, an ingredient known to cause mouth sores in some people. Why do Americans need opaque, foaming toothpastes?

I use a 50/50 mix of a NovaMin® powder (Sylc)/sodium bicarbonate when I air polish. The NovaMin® reduces sensitivity and begins to diffuse minerals into the teeth. The baking soda cleans. The Caphosol generic I apply afterwards further encourages calcium ion diffusion into sensitive dentinal tubules and demineralized lesions.

**Decay Reduction: Recaldent®.** A prescription toothpaste (Prospec MI Paste) with Recaldent® delivers highly soluble calcium and phosphate minerals to plaque and tooth surfaces, making them available for future remineralization. These minerals release only when the mouth is slightly acidic. Recaldent® may strengthen demineralized lesions, reduce sensitivity, and buffer plaque acids, but long-term clinical studies must prove these roles. Recaldent® is derived from milk casein it so should not be used if you have a milk protein allergy. Those who are lactose intolerant can use it. Its use directly after ozone therapy is limited because it works best at around a neutral pH. Ozone alkalizes.

**Decay Reduction: BioRepair or Carifree® CTx3 Gel.** Size matters. Enamel is comprised of specifically oriented hydroxyapatite (HAP) crystals in the 20–40 nanometer range. The size, shape, and orientation of these native crystals grant both mechanical strength and biological protection to teeth.

Most products commonly used to counter enamel and dentin erosion, such as fluoride, work by slowing down acid dissolution of tooth enamel while increasing surface hardness. As mentioned in Chapter 12, most remineralization agents are unable to reconstruct the lost crystalline structure of enamel. Remineralizing agents found in most over-the-counter dental products such as amorphous calcium phosphate (ACP) and conventional hydroxyapatites (cHAP) are so large (hundreds of nanometers), and are incorrectly shaped so they cannot orient themselves into enamel to give it the strength and decay resistance of native enamel. Additionally, they adhere too poorly to be incorporated, thus they are unsuitable for enamel repair.

Synthesized 20 nanometer HAP crystals can self-assemble into enamel-like crystalline structures with an unusual ability to bond to natural tissues. These crystals confer superior strength and erosion resistance to a tooth. In fact, newly remineralized areas may be more acid-resistant than enamel! These apatite nanoparticles also help with root surface sensitivity. (For images, see: http://www.carifree.com/dentists/science/documents/ Repairofenamelbyusinghydroxyaoatitenanoasbuildingblocks.pdf)

BioRepair contains the ubiquitous titanium dioxide and parabens present in many popular commercial toothpastes. CariFree includes Sodium Lauryl Sulfate. We can't have it all – yet. BioRepair and the children's CTx3 version of CariFree omit fluoride. These are huge steps in the right direction. CariFree is my current top choice for those who want remineralization properties in their toothpaste.

When using rebuilding products at home, first remove biofilms to assure these products reach bare tooth surfaces. I brush with straight baking soda (not baking soda toothpaste) at night to alkalize my mouth, and then use CariFree CTx3 children's toothpaste in the morning.

## Decay Reduction: Xylitol

Xylitol is a sweet-tasting carbohydrate that exists naturally in fruits, vegetables, and mushrooms. An average adult might routinely ingest several hundred milligrams per day as part of a diet rich in fruits and vegetables. Our bodies also produce about five to ten milligrams of xylitol daily as we metabolize our natural blood sugar. Xylitol has no known toxicity, though some people suffer diarrhea if they overdo it. Its use barely affects blood sugar or insulin levels. Numerous studies suggest xylitol's frequent presence in the mouth helps reduce cavities[xxiv] [xxv xxvi xxvii xxviii] however a normal diet is insufficient to produce this protective effect.

As noted in Chapter Fourteen, *strep mutans* and other bacteria in the mouth create erosive acids from simple carbohydrates. Biofilms keep these acids close to the teeth for hours. However, if you regularly use appropriate doses of xylitol, cavity-causing bacteria begin preferring xylitol as a food source over other carbohydrates. Because the bacteria cannot ferment the xylitol, they cannot produce acids.[14] Think of xylitol as junk food for bacteria.

Additionally, the bacteria starve because xylitol does not provide the food they need that they otherwise get from mannitol, sorbitol, honey, sucrose, corn syrup and other sweeteners. Since they thrive only in acidic environments, the bacteria dwindle and demineralization slows. Xylitol also affects these bacteria's adhering properties so they simply flush away into saliva. Xylitol also binds to the molecules that transport sugar into bacterial cells. This unbreakable bond keeps sugar transport molecules from feeding additional sugars to the bacteria, another reason for their demise.

The most common delivery system for xylitol is either chewing gum or lozenges. Gum's advantage over lozenges is that gum stimulates saliva flow more than lozenges. This keeps teeth immersed in the naturally occurring salivary minerals that enhance rebuilding. Nonetheless, lozenges are effective and preferred in some circumstances.

---

14 The key to xylitol's success is its five-carbon alcohol structure. Sorbitol and mannitol are six-carbon structures that oral bacteria can metabolize.

Studies show positive effects after a five minute exposure to one gram of xylitol four times a day over the course of six weeks. This is the minimum. To get the recommended one gram necessary to produce the antibacterial effect, xylitol should be the only sugar listed on a product label. Many brands list xylitol as the third sugar, meaning that gum fails to provide the required concentrations. Xylitol gums or lozenges also help relieve "dry mouth."

Chewing gum or dissolving lozenges four times per day – after every meal plus an extra time – is easy. This schedule is particularly good because the act of chewing stimulates the pancreas to produce digestive enzymes, helpful after a meal, but undesirable at other times.

Many dentists, periodontists, pediatricians, and orthodontists recommend xylitol.[xxix] The California Dental Association suggests patients view xylitol "as part of an overall strategy for decay reduction". This is because, "With xylitol use, the quality of the bacteria in the mouth changes and fewer and fewer decay-causing bacteria survive on tooth surfaces. Less plaque forms and the level of acids attacking the tooth surface is lowered." [xxx]

Researchers wanted to see if reducing cavity-causing bacteria in mothers would diminish decay rates in their offspring by reducing transmission of these bacteria to their children. Study results showed significant delay in establishing cavity-causing bacteria and far fewer cavities in children whose caregivers used xylitol products regularly for the first two years of the child's life compared to those whose caregivers received fluoride or chlorhexidine varnishes applied three times over the child's first five years. The children did not chew gum or receive varnish protection. The significant advantage in bacterial inoculation and decay rates in children whose caregivers used xylitol prevention measures extended well beyond the child's first two years. At five years of age, these children had 70 percent fewer cavities compared to those whose caregivers had received fluoride varnishes.[xxxi]

Xylitol is so effective in preventing decay that some dental insurance plans provide members with discounts on xylitol products. They include:

- Aetna
- Assurant Employee Benefits
- CIGNA
- Delta Dental
- Dentaquest
- Dental Select
- Guardian

Diabetics appreciate it because it has only 2.4 calories/gram compared to table sugar's four calories/gram. Xylitol's glycemic index value (GI) is seven as opposed to sucrose's value of 68 (sucrose is half fructose and half glucose), so substituting xylitol for table sugar could help stabilize blood sugar levels, though I wouldn't recommend it. As with other sugars, it unbalances the ecology of gut bacteria.

Last note: I prefer xylitol derived from birch trees as compared to xylitol derived from corn grown in the U.S.

Xylitol is also used to reduce middle ear[xxxii] and sinus infections.[15] These applications work the same way xylitol works in the mouth – to reduce tissue adherence of harmful bacteria so they cannot colonize. If a person avoids antihistamines and decongestants, the body's natural defenses flush pollutants and bacteria from sinuses, nasal cavities, and eustachian tubes. Many doctors now recommend daily xylitol sprays or washes to clients with chronic sinusitis and ear infections.

**Notes:** In very high doses, it can have a laxative effect, but these are doses well beyond the dental use described here. In one study, a few participants suffered diarrhea occasionally, but most showed no ill effects even at doses of 400 grams/day for two years.[xxxiii] Introducing xylitol slowly usually mitigates this problem. I do not recommend xylitol use as an artificial sweetener in large doses like this because in its effectiveness, it wipes out the rich bacterial life your digestive tract and immune system depend on.

There is some evidence bacteria are evolving to overcome xylitol's effectiveness as well. Stay tuned, but right now it is effective.

Xylitol only gum and mints like Spry gum and mints, Theragum and Theramints, and Zellies are easy to find.

Keep away from pets. High doses can cause hypoglycemia/death.

---

15 A common recommendation is to wipe a wet washcloth through an infant's mouth daily to clear oral tissues. Using Spiffies™ oral wipes (online at www.dentist. net/spiffies-dental-wipes.asp) on babies older than four months helps prevent common ear infections. The major cause of ear and sinus infections is Strep pneumococci, which is closely related to the Strep mutans bacteria. The xylitol wipes work in a similar fashion. To effect change, xylitol enters through the eustachian tubes. Xlear, obtainable at http://www.xlear.com/xylitol-products-ppc1.aspx?gclid=CNzS9PvUob ACFQrf4Aod5F7-XQ, is used by many as a sinus inhaler at the beginning of a sinus infection. Personal experience and feedback from others who have used Xlear has revealed infections often clear up after several days without the use of antibiotics. Eye, nose and throat doctors often recommend xylitol to clear up clients' infections.

## Myth Busting: Brushing to Reduce Cavities and Gum Disease

Most people cling tenaciously to outdated tooth brushing lore. Here are a few dated ideas:

- **Brush teeth immediately after eating, particularly after sugary snacks.** A better strategy is to make sure you brush and floss *prior* to eating. After eating, acids are so intense they soften teeth. It is then easy to brush away weakened enamel crystals. Better: Chew xylitol gum or rinse well after eating to float out food particles. Many clients chew xylitol gum after every meal and after snacks. Gum mechanically removes food particles and stimulates saliva flow. Saliva bathes teeth in reparative minerals and neutralizes the acids eating promotes. All the strategies discussed in this chapter help with the impossible-to-clean grooves in the chewing surface. *Toothbrush bristles cannot penetrate these deep and narrow crevices to remove plaque.* Here, one must depend on decay-resistant enamel and oral chemistry modification to avoid or repair cavities on these surfaces.

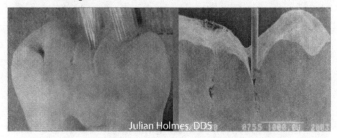

Julian Holmes, DDS

Think of brushing and flossing as a way to "clear the palate." The full flavor of food can be appreciated without the abrupt and strong flavor change of toothpastes afterwards.

- **Toothpaste is essential for removing biofilm.** Brushing with toothpaste gives one a sense of cleanliness, but this is often a result of the strong mint flavorings added to cover odor. Unfortunately, those strong flavorings numb your feedback mechanism. Have you ever noticed your teeth feel fuzzy soon after brushing? Did you think plaque had reformed that quickly? What actually happened was that the numbing effect of the flavorings wore off and you felt the plaque you did not sense and remove the first time!

I suggest you do your most thorough daily brushing without toothpaste. This offers several benefits. First, you are not tethered to a sink, so you can brush anywhere, at any time. Double-tasking while you brush allows you to spend more time doing it and less time resenting it. Many clients do their best biofilm removal in their cars, in front of the television, or while reading books. My children did it as I read to them. Skipping toothpaste frees up your schedule!

Brushing without toothpaste while doing something else adds minutes to the day and can ensure a careful, gentle job. Many people brush haphazardly before they dash from their homes in the morning. This often leads to damage because when people brush quickly, they tend to use excessive pressure and saw horizontally across the teeth. This can contribute to root exposure caused by recession.[16] Because I, too, run late in the mornings, I have worked out a routine. I brush rapidly and lightly with baking soda[17] or a remineralizing toothpaste like Carifree CTx3 at home – mainly to make my mouth feel clean. It is during this brushing that I scrub dead cells and biofilm from all oral skin, particularly from my tongue. (More on that soon.) Then, as I cruise to work, I pull out my "car" brush (ozonated, treated with a UV light, or thrown in the dishwasher after last use) and do a thorough, gentle brushing. It is the brush and our mechanical skills that remove biofilm, not the toothpaste.[xxxiv] I use toothpastes to serve a function, for example: CariFree to remineralize and desensitize in the morning, Thieves or other brands to naturally reduce germs, normalize pH, et cetera.

---

[16] Recession refers to gum line migration away from the chewing surfaces of teeth, usually due to mechanical forces such as clenching. Recession exposes more cavity-prone and sensitive roots. Though not the disease-driven process described at length in this book, the end result is still loss of support for one's teeth. Recession and gum disease are often confused. They both result in loss of tooth support, but are essentially different. One is bacteria/inflammation driven; the other is driven by mechanical stresses.

[17] Baking soda has no additives oral tissues can absorb, is far less abrasive than most commercial toothpastes and is alkalinizing. This is especially important at night. Commercial toothpastes are almost always acidic, a negative. Baking soda also dessicates oral bacteria, deodorizes, and helps remove stains. I like the price and how fresh my mouth feels after I use it.

- **What is old is new again.** One old theory states that brushing our gums stimulates them and makes them healthier. It improves blood circulation and toughens them. For a long time, the dental profession scoffed at this theory and didn't necessarily encourage brushing gums. But new reasons to gently brush the gums – and tongue – are emerging. First, brushing removes the dead cells that emit volatile sulfur compounds (VSCs). Details regarding VSCs follow the flossing section ahead.

  Second, it appears that just as other body tissues (like muscles) strengthen in response to mechanical stress, so do oral tissues. Momentary micro-tears in oral cells may heal in seconds, but before they do, growth factors that repair damage exits the cells. These strengthen oral tissues by triggering new collagen growth and new cells and blood vessels. This appears to occur in all oral tissues during gentle stimulation, including the tongue surface and its muscles.[xxxv]

## Effective Brushing

You would think you had mastered brushing decades ago, but brushing is more complicated than it seems. If this were not the case, teeth's anatomical undercuts and pockets – the primary focus of this book – would not be the continuing challenge they are for most people.

The good news is, once you have studied the pictures from Chapter One and understand your objective, the rest is simple. The hard part is overcoming an entrenched and mindless lifetime physical habit! Nonetheless, I like to describe the principals, then let my intelligent clients tweak them to fit their lifestyle. I refer to my favored brushing technique as "the tip-over technique." Using the idea helps guide brush bristles around the undercut and into the pockets surrounding teeth instead of inadvertently reverting to the nearly universal angle of 90 degrees to the surface of the teeth, which allows the pocket to teem with toxic biofilm.

First, you must choose a brush. For many reasons choose either soft or extra soft. Many people fear a soft brush will not effectively remove a sticky biofilm, but style trumps stiffness and your gums need a light touch. They are fragile, especially if they are infected. Gums can be torn, eroded, and scrubbed away. Brushing delicately will help you avoid disease. Also, the curves of teeth require adaptable, flexible bristles.

Buy brushes from a reputable company. Major American manufacturers "polish" or "end-round" bristle tips to prevent gum damage. Manual brushes can be effective, if time-consuming. Many clients prefer electric brushes for efficiency. When using these, I suggest traditional flat-across-the-top, rectangular-shaped heads whose use is easily adapted to the following description for manual brushes. Given the curves to be negotiated, many patients have difficulty maneuvering round-headed brushes gently into the pocket, though it is possible.

Many appreciate the efficiency and stain removal power electric brushes offer. In addition to mechanical disruption, power brushes like Sonicare, Oral B Braun, and Ultreo incorporate enhanced biofilm disruption via "fluid dynamics." [18] Ultrasonic waves create bubbles that forcefully expand and contract to disrupt sticky biofilms.

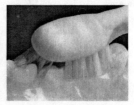

Rotary toothbrushes tend to tear gum tissues. Flat round brushes should oscillate and have fine, pliable bristles that splay easily under gums. MouthWatchers makes an inexpensive, yet effective one. Ultra-fine bristles impregnated with silver nano-particles kill germ populations on the brush head. They can be used without toothpaste, so children's teeth gleam without the usual complaints and whining. Use light pressure.

**Note:** Children are not adept at maneuvering these brushes. They are great for the caregiver to use as a follow-up to a child's brushing. I assisted my children until they were nine years old, when fine motor skills start to emerge.

Use the following effective, simple technique with a manual or rectangular-shaped electric brush:

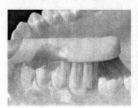 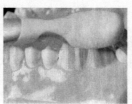

Choose a quadrant of your mouth and scrub across the biting surfaces of your teeth in your normal way. Then, slightly tilt the head of the brush to either the cheek or tongue side of the teeth. (Do not flip your

---

18 Studies show they disrupt the fimbria on individual bacteria, hypothesized as one of the means bacteria communicate and form complex biofilms. I suspect they also disrupt the nano-electrical network, which is another way biofilms communicate as they mature.

wrist to aim at the target surface. No 90-degree angles!) Keep the bulk of the brush on the chewing surface to provide guidance. Otherwise it is easy to slip back into the old habit of brushing at a 90-degree angle to the teeth. Feel the bristles nudge up under the gums; jiggle the brush for a while to break up the biofilm's sticky bonds. Don't scrub the bristle tips as much as vibrate them. Again, a heavy-handed, back and forth sawing action can contribute to recession and root exposure and be less effective.

When you are finished, tilt the head of the brush the opposite way and repeat. That is it. The technique does not vary no matter what area you brush! After scrubbing the back biting surfaces, you can also tilt the bristles down behind the last tooth in the arch and vibrate. In this area, the bristles can be persuaded to go deeper than floss if necessary. While I also floss behind the last tooth of each arch, sometimes the architecture of the gums makes flossing inadequate or impossible here.

Two notes:

- Brushing inside curves with a straight brush is challenging, so most people concentrate on the outside of their teeth. Try to spend at least as much time brushing the inside surfaces of your teeth. The "tipover" technique simplifies the process because it never requires you to fit a straight brush onto a curved surface. Form a pattern. Stick with it. Do not let your tongue discourage you or get in the way. Use the same technique on the inside of the top front and bottom front teeth. That is, split bristles of the brush head between the outside and inside of the teeth, tilt, and jiggle. It really works well.

- When you brush the outside of your top back teeth, you must relax your jaw by closing slightly. Remember the main cheek muscle that allows you to chew with those enormous compressive forces? If your mouth is wide open, this strong muscle will tightly hug your back teeth and your brush will not fit. When you close down about halfway, you create enough room for a few bristles to tip over and scrub the outside surface. [View instruction video on www. mouthmattersbook.com.]

A widely known and loved Austin music legend returned to our office recently. His story inspires many. During his initial visit, he displayed moderate to advanced gum disease. We reviewed the oral pocket tissue concept with the camera and he seemed completely engaged. I expected to see significant healing within three months of initial treatment because he enthusiastically embraced the idea of oral/ whole body health and his role in it. I did note, however, that his wife accompanied him on the visit. I knew he devoted himself to caring for her since her severe slide into Alzheimer's disease. They never left each other's side.

Despite comprehensive initial therapy, his first follow-up visit showed no particular healing or improvement in self-care. I was somewhat surprised because I anticipated he would fully collaborate in his care. But I also know sometimes it takes repetition, time, and the right circumstances. I knew he was focused on his wife's care.

Between his second and third visit, it had been necessary for him to find a comfortable and caring home for his wife where she could receive the care he could no longer adequately provide. Because of his sorrow and stress, I expected poor home care and continuing unhealthy gums. But his teeth were impeccably clean and gum health was restored. He had filed all my recommendations; he just was unable to immediately act on them. The moment he could start readjusting his priorities, he began carrying a toothbrush and flosser in his back pocket. He used them effectively – once a day and without toothpaste! Like Molly, he was obsessive and he loved it. He could feel the difference. His success story is but one of hundreds, but I smile every time I tell it.

The point is his oral health did not return until he actively participated with targeted, if simple, daily self-care. A professional's role is merely to facilitate clients' roles in controlling their own health.

## Oh No! Here comes that @*&## Word Again! Flossing Is Not a Four-Letter Word

An archaeological dig in Madrid uncovered two human molar teeth judged to be about 63,400 years old. According to paleontology professor Juan Luis Asuarga, finding "grooves formed by the passage of a pointed object, (which) confirms the use of a small stick for cleaning the mouth," [xxxvi] suggests "between the teeth clean" is not a new idea!

Like many, I wish I had grown up knowing about flossing. When I was a child, in the sixties, I remember seeing a roll of good old J&J

waxed dental floss sitting around in my parent's bathroom drawer. I assumed it was just one of those things grown-ups had around we were not supposed to know about. I was not quite sure why it was there. I never saw them use it and I believe the roll I saw as I headed off to college was the same one I had noticed as a child. I used it awkwardly once or twice, feeling a little grown up as I sneaked in to use some after eating corn on the cob to remove the offending fibers.

I was introduced to flossing in dental school. I hate to admit it, but it took a while for the message to sink in. I've often wondered how anyone my age got the message or began the habit in those long ago days. We simply didn't grow up with flossing, so I know how difficult it is to jump-start the habit.

Most clients are quite self-deprecating when it comes to flossing. They blame themselves for being lazy or forgetful. I believe there are more realistic reasons for not flossing regularly. It is often not a habit that has a scheduled time, but more than anything I think most people have an aversion to putting their fingers into their mouths. For others, I think it is a lack of confidence in flossing ability. Flossing is technique-sensitive and takes some coaching and practice to reduce the awkwardness. Even the best dental practices do not often take the one-on-one time necessary to observe and coach clients regarding technique. As a result, most people are self-taught and it shows. Some are so inexperienced they have a hard time finding the spaces between their teeth!

We all want a perfect smile and product advertisers make the most of it. Their extensive advertising has given hygienists and their preventive messages some credibility. People are finally thinking about their teeth. They seek beautiful smiles but seem to do any number of things besides flossing: rinse, WaterPik®, toothpick, inter-dental brush, Hydrofloss®… Studies don't always back my observation that the most superior results come from flossing. After looking at the pictures in Chapter One, perhaps you can see why I like flossing. A slim tool is required to slip under the gums both to stimulate them and to remove the biofilm. Some devices do clean between teeth, but most cannot reach into the crevice. Still, if flossing simply will not work for you, there are many acceptable substitutes. I highly recommend using ozonated oils like $O_3$ Skincare in conjunction with Gum Soft-Picks as an adjunct.

Many clients prefer to use their fingers to manipulate floss. Most men seem to prefer floss holders because of large or awkward hands.

Women love them too. There are many kinds of flossers on the market to suit all needs and budgets. Most clients (including the musician just mentioned) credit their flossing habit to the long-handled Johnson and Johnson Reach holder. Though he is a master guitarist with extremely capable fingers, he prefers not to put them in his mouth. He found this flosser large enough for his hands to grasp.

The small "U-shaped" disposable floss cartridge is positioned at a 90-degree angle to the handle. This makes all the difference. As with sliding any floss between teeth, teasing it through tight contacts at a slant works better than trying to pop it through from directly overhead.

For those who do not use flossers, floss with texture, such as Oral B's Ultra, adds efficiency. Nonetheless, Gortex-covered flosses provide strength when tight teeth make shredding a frustrating issue. If one must use slick floss, I suggest more repetitions up and down teeth. Some dental flosses are impregnated with tea tree or other oils, VSC neutralizing agents and whitening additives or polishing agents.[19] Automated flossing devices cannot be dismissed.[xxxvii] They may not be as ideal as manual flossing, but they do disrupt much of the bacterial burden. See the appendices for more flossing suggestions.

People with arthritis, mental incapacities, inadequate dexterity, or not enough fingers to floss or use other adjuncts can benefit extraordinarily by evaluating the suggestions outlined in this book and elsewhere for changing their terrain – making their bodies and mouths inhospitable to harmful bacteria.

## Chlorhexidine: A Magnet for Bacteria?

Many doctors think chlorhexidine helps solve a number of oral health problems. Studies show rinsing with prescription chlorhexidine for two weeks significantly reduces cavity-causing bacteria and keeps them from recolonizing for up to six months.[xxxviii] Since most damaging oral microorganisms are gram negative, and chlorhexidine is gram positive, the two are magnets for each other. Chlorhexidine compromises bacterial membranes, so bacteria with cell membranes die. Its use in controlling bacteria responsible for gum disease is even more favored by dental professionals. Two well-known negative consequences of chlorhexidine use are staining and altered taste perception for the

---

19 For instance, StaiNo has an entire line of aluminum oxide impregnated inter-dental as well as a "stain eraser." For more information call 845-887-5746 or go to www. staino.com.

duration of its use. Careful hygiene, particularly with an electric toothbrush, can control staining problems.

Chlorhexidine may not be the best solution however. It also kills beneficial bacteria, such as those on the back of the tongue that convert nitrates to the blood-vessel-dilating nitric oxide (NO), discussed earlier. Further there are many highly destructive bacteria (such as the spirochete *Treponema denticola,* one of 53 oral spirochetes) that have an adaptive life phase that has no cell wall for either chlorhexidine or antibiotics to destroy. When these products are used, active forms of spirochetes enter stealth mode. They begin to "go underground" by morphing into these cell wall deficient forms that are up to five times smaller than their active form. They become invisible to the immune system.

Several strong reasons preclude daily use. It seems that, as with xylitol and antibiotics, some microorganisms are developing a resistance to chlorhexidine. Researchers worry that opportunistic pathogens will establish themselves as the microflora of the mouth shifts.

Two significant caveat is that chlorhexidine interferes with fibroblast activity, an important component of healing gum disease. CloSYS® does not. It is alcohol and sodium laurel sulfate-free, and compared to chlorhexidine rinses, has similar bacterial kill/recolonization rates. Another consideration: blood inactivates chlorhexidine.

To reiterate, because ozone overcomes all the above objections, I use many ozone modalities.

As with any therapy, terrain trumps all. Keep your immune system strong.

## VSCs and Bad Breath: Certain Mouthwashes and Tongue Scraping are an Answer

Tongue scraping is one habit not well embraced in our culture. Because of its rough surface, the tongue harbors huge numbers of bacteria and dead cells. As oral cells decompose, they emit volatile sulfur compounds (VSCs).

VSCs, the source of many people's chronic bad breath, stink due to the sulfur content. VSCs help bacterial toxins enter oral tissues and slow healing by suppressing our body's ability to make DNA, collagen, and other proteins. VSCs also increase inflammation. Soon after this discovery, an instrument that measured VSCs was developed. Dentists across the country use the resulting Halimeter® machine for client treatment and for halitosis studies. Treatment for chronic breath problems thus detected usually includes a series of professional tongue scrapings and various special mouthwashes designed to reduce VSCs. Clients also receive instruction on how to keep the tongue clean and uncoated.

There are various methods for cleaning the tongue at home. Many people simply brush the top surface as vigorously and thoroughly as possible with a toothbrush. Those who choose to use tongue scrapers usually report better results compared to brushing. Pertinent studies back them up. Using a tongue scraper generally reduces tongue residues that produce hydrogen sulfide gases by 75 percent. Toothbrushes reduce them by about 45 percent.[xxxix] Some people effectively use the front edge of a spoon turned upside down. The most difficult to reach part of the tongue – the most posterior part by the throat – is the part that needs the most attention. It helps to lean forward over the sink and extend the tongue as far out as possible for cleaning.

Another source for VSCs is the oral pocket tissue where pockets are more than 4mm deep. For many people, realizing that treating gum disease can reduce the social pressures of bad breath helps them prioritize oral health.

VSC-reducing mouthwashes recommended by dental professionals usually contain chlorine dioxide,[20] sodium chlorite, or zinc. Zinc is the most recognized and effective VSC neutralizing agent. I discourage most mouthwashes and toothpastes because they are acidic. Acids and alcohol are counter-productive because they increase dead cell volume. Many dentists prefer zinc-based TheraBreath or SmartMouth to reduce VSCs. Consult your dental provider or look online for other choices.

My symptom-based choice once again for a serious halitosis problem is ozonated oil. Stout tasting, brush your tongue fast and furiously, then rinse. You will feel fresh.

It is important to clean your mouth and tongue before using mouthwash. Gargling helps rinses gain access to the throat and back of the tongue. These strategies can make an enormous difference in people's lives. Once a person overcomes an acute halitosis problem, they usually have no need to use these mouthwashes – or ozonated oils on a daily basis. They use as needed.

---

20 An example is CloSYS. CloSYS rinses and toothpastes are sodium lauryl sulfate-free and alcohol-free. For more information call 800-643-3337 or visit www.rowpar. com.

## Dietary Contributions

Other suggestions relate to diet. Garlic and onions are famous for causing bad breath because they create sulfur compounds similar to VSCs. When anaerobic bacteria extract sulfur compounds from amino acids, it smells like rotting food.

In the mouth, anaerobic bacteria produce sulfur from various ingested foods. Acidic foods and beverages such as sodas, coffee, citrus, and other fruit juices cause bacterial populations to explode. Sugars add additional fuel to these bacteria. This is why it makes little sense to feed oral bacteria sugary mints to control bad breath.

For some, dense protein foods are especially problematic. For others, over-eating meats causes bad breath. Others should avoid dairy products, particularly those who are lactose intolerant. Of course, anything that causes dry mouth causes cellular death. This includes smoking, many medications, alcohol-containing mouthwashes, and alcoholic beverages. Some solutions:

- **Stay hydrated.** Bacteria thrive in dry conditions. If dry mouth not related to diabetes or medications is a continuing problem, chewing gum helps stimulate saliva production. TheraBreath has an oxygenating chewing gum and breath mint that contains zinc and fights anaerobic bacteria. Xylitol is one sweetening ingredient. Xylimelts, Salese and Dentiva lozenges also help and are discussed in the next section.
- **Eat parsley, fennel, or anise after meals.** The chlorophyll and essential oils in them fight anaerobic bacteria. Many products now contain essential oils. A good one offered only through dental offices is: Tooth and Gums Tonic®, made by the Dental Herb Company®. Young Living makes a wonderful non-prescription rinse called Thieves. There are many others.
- **Some people brush with toothpastes containing essential oils like rosemary, peppermint, or myrrh.** I bypass the Thieves mouthwash and simply drop Thieves oil (clove, lemon, cinnamon bark, eucalyptus, and rosemary essential oils) on the back of my tongue and swish.
- **Eat raw food to clean out your digestive system and mouth.** David Wolfe offers recipe books and an online presence to

help you start your raw food journey – with delicious recipes you cannot tell are raw. Start drinking green smoothies. Hundreds of recipes are available online.

- **Reduce oral acidity.** Acids in foods and beverages such as coffee decrease oxygenation of bacteria, which leads to VSCs. Anaerobic bacteria thrive in acidic environments.
- **Yogurt and unpasteurized fermented probiotics** may help because they allow lactic acid-loving bacteria to compete with VSC-producing bacteria.

**Halitosis note:** Bad breath in the morning is common because we produce less saliva at night. This allows bacteria to thrive and VSCs to concentrate. Mouth breathers suffer more than those who sleep with their mouths closed.

The mouth is not the only source of bad breath. Nose, sinus, and tonsil inflammation can also contribute. In these cases, many find relief by using xylitol in a different form. As previously mentioned, I suggest Xlear with xylitol, which is found in many health food stores. When one sprays or inhales Xlear into the nostrils, it reduces bacterial numbers because they can no longer feed or adhere. Washing the sinuses daily with a neti pot and sterile water also helps.

Bad breath also derives from diet and gastric disturbances. Foods such as garlic, onions, spicy foods and alcohol respire from the lungs for hours after ingestion, often informing social acquaintances of earlier food choices. In rare instances, serious illnesses can cause oral malodor.

## You Don't Miss it Until It's Gone
## Saliva's Contributions

Saliva is our most important weapon against dental diseases. When young, we take this oral lubricant for granted. But as we age, saliva's mineral content and consistency can change. If you take one of the more than 700 medications whose mouth-drying effects compound age-related saliva loss, you miss saliva's myriad properties. Here are a few reasons saliva is crucial to oral health:

- Saliva heightens taste and aids swallowing.
- Saliva buffers and dilutes acids to maintain a neutral pH

environment. When humans chew, think about or smell food, stimulated saliva flow should double or quadruple. Released bicarbonate ions buffer the mouth's acidic environment.

- Saliva helps rebuild teeth after carbohydrate ingestion triggers acid attacks. Calcium, phosphate, and other minerals supersaturate saliva.
- Saliva lubricates oral tissues. Remember the last time you were nervous and you felt like you were chewing on cotton? It is not comfortable, is it? This is why public speakers always have water available when they lecture. It is a poor substitute, but it helps.
- Saliva is loaded with bacteria-fighting immunoglobulins and proteins.
- Saliva helps clear carbohydrates.
- Salivary enzymes initiate digestion.
- Saliva helps maintain tissue integrity. Cancer patients often say the loss of saliva is the worst side effect of therapy. Since tissues become sticky, rough and may even bleed and tear, it often causes depression and keeps them awake at night. It also increases their risk of tooth decay, which in turn raises their chances of bone death in treatment areas should extractions become necessary. (Of course Caphasol and ozone therapy vastly improve these situations.)
- Proteins and lipids (fats) in saliva form a protective organic membrane on the tooth's surface.
- Saliva contains many cancer "tags" and other disease markers.

More than 90 percent of the 32 million adults in the U.S. suffer dry mouth because they take certain medications. Other causes of dry mouth include dehydration, smoking, mouth breathing, autoimmune diseases, oral surgeries that compromise saliva ducts, radiation therapy, diabetes, oral yeast infections, and hormonal fluctuations (menopause). In acute cases, dry mouth patients complain that oral tissues burn and that swallowing and speaking are difficult.

Most clients are unaware their mouths are excessively dry because they unconsciously adapt coping skills to deal with cotton mouth. Healthy saliva production equates to about a liter per day. Stop and note: do you have a pool of saliva under your tongue right now? You should. To definitively check for adequate saliva flow, find a graduated (measured and marked in milliliters) test tube. An hour after eating, drinking, chewing gum, brushing or flossing, flow all the saliva you produce during a timed five minute period into the tube. Divide the total volume taken by five. Normal, unstimulated flow should be between 0.3 and 0.4 ml/minute. If less than 0.1 ml/minute, stimulate your saliva flow by chewing on unflavored paraffin wax for five minutes and repeat. This will help you learn if you have compromised saliva gland function. One to two ml/minute of stimulated flow is optimal. Less than 0.7 ml/minute is abnormally low and puts you at risk for discomfort and decay. Examine your saliva. It should be clear and thin, not cloudy, thick, and ropey.

Your dental professional can suggest many saliva substitutes. Clients report that, though useful, they are poor substitutes for the real thing. This is when saliva-stimulating efforts become important. Chewing gum can increase saliva flow by ten times for some conditions. It will not help those whose saliva loss is the result of a prescription medication. The effects last for about 20 minutes. Saliva is loaded with natural healing components, so this helps many people. If gum is objectionable, sugar-free mouth mints also stimulate saliva flow, though less vigorously.

Salese ™ [21] soft lozenges can offer substantial relief. These dime-sized tablets take at least an hour to dissolve, and release essential oils, xylitol and other proprietary ingredients that fight dry mouth and plaque. The base material of the lozenge keeps your mouth moisturized. If you have minimal saliva, sip water. The lozenge helps retain the moisture. **Note:** Salese currently contains sucralose (Splenda®) in addition to xylitol. A more natural substitute, I recommend Xylimelts, available at Amazon and elsewhere. A biodegradable adhesive helps hold them in place for safe night time use.

Another good product is Rain™ Dry Mouth Spray, a Spry product. This spray is infused with moisturizing xylitol, aloe vera, and a form of calcium (glycerophosphate) that reportedly improves tooth remineralization. Use it as often as desired. All these products alkalize.

Saliva production stops for a short time after eating sugars, when you are most at risk because bacteria are already beginning to convert sugar to acids. Thus, the common habit of chewing xylitol gum after a meal is a good one. Saliva's most effective properties like buffering, ion-remineralizing, and carbohydrate-clearing capabilities work best then. Gum also helps with the mechanical removal of plaque and food from the teeth's chewing surfaces. Chewing gum for 20 to 30 minutes after sugar exposure will help bathe teeth in natural mineral ions while at risk.

21 Available through www.nuvorainc.com or by calling: 877-530-9811.

If you suffer a dry mouth, refer to Appendix V-D.

Dental researchers have reversed their position on gum chewing. It is no longer considered harmful to the jaw joint as once believed. Further, chewing gum is now being used as a vehicle for many beneficial additives and medications. Some of these are chlorhexadine, bicarbonate, calcium phosphate, zinc, vitamin C, methadone, miconazole (anti-fungal), xylitol and – for smoking cessation therapy – nicotine.

If your gums are healthy, the five minutes it takes to properly brush and floss every day are sufficient for you to maintain oral health. If your gums are diseased, your dental team can help you heal. More ideas are presented in the self-help section. The steps outlined in this chapter are simple steps, especially considering all the potential social and health benefits they reap!

## Looking In From the Outside

In closing, I will share a different cultural perspective. Americans often take their culture for granted. The suggestion to floss is always good for an eyeball roll. Dental health information is perceived as being incredibly boring – that is until it becomes the most important thing in one's life.

On the other hand, I have noticed that people from Asian cultures tend to express an eagerness to know what Americans have to offer. Regarding oral health, they usually follow suggestions scrupulously. I particularly enjoyed the response of a Chinese graduate student at the University of Texas. Though only in her mid-twenties, she had gum disease including moderate bone loss and inflammation. We used two long visits to initially treat her disease. Her gums responded beautifully. Her self-care quickly became meticulous. Months later, she shared an inspirational story.

She was so excited by her treatment results, she contacted her mother who lives in a remote Chinese village and shared what she had learned. She followed up by sending her mother this amazing string Americans use to clean between their teeth and instructions on how to use it.

Her mother was initially skeptical, but because she loved her daughter and respected her intelligence, she began to floss. As days turned into weeks, she noticed changes that delighted her. Areas in her mouth that had previously caused her pain were now comfortable! Although I do not know the details of her original condition and wonder how the results could be so beneficial without professional dental intervention, I appreciate the fact that flossing caused positive changes.

The mother shared the technique with all her sisters who told all their friends. As a result, the graduate student sends much more floss to China than she ever intended. What a lovely ripple effect!

*"Your Health…"*

*In a small village at the foot of the Himalayas lived a wise old man. People from miles around sought his counsel. A group of children decided one day they would mock this respected figure. They planned to expose his knowledge to ridicule. The plan was to bring a bird, hidden behind the back of one of the boys. The boy would ask if the bird was alive or dead. If the old man said alive, the boy would crush it to death. If he said dead, the boy would release the bird. And so one day the group approached the old man. One boy came forward to the village father and said, "Father, what do I have in my hand?" "A bird," he answered. "Is it alive or dead?" The old man looked up slowly and said gently, "It is in your hands."*

*"…Is in your hands."*

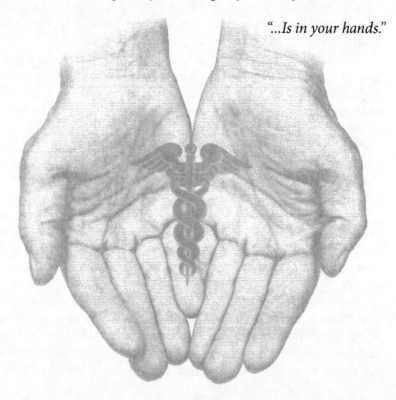

# 17

## RESTRUCTURING TO MEET THE FUTURE!

**Explore:**
1. Is your dentist's office headed for the future?
2. Does it affect how comfortably you will age?
3. What is at stake individually and nationally if we continue to discount knowledge, prevention, and the role dental hygienists can play? Can we afford the burden of cost and misery if we continue with the status quo?

## Two Current Models

My experience tells me dental practices are basically organized in one of two ways. If the dentist heading the practice values prevention, it becomes the cornerstone from which all other activities derive. These are the few dentists for whom integrative medicine is second nature. They are not the "tooth carpenters" who approach their patients' health or mouths on a piecemeal basis. An initial visit will begin with a serious look at overall health and nutrition. Deviations from wellness are discussed. Oral health is assessed within the context of general health.

In this model, oral assessments are thorough and involve at a minimum: repeatable, accurate diagnosis of tooth health, the relationship of the upper and lower teeth to each other, joint function, habits that interfere with correct tooth function including clenching habits, oral posture, cancer screening, evaluation of the teeth's support structure, pH and oral hydration conditions. As dentistry begins to treat oral diseases as physicians treat disease, they will increasingly blend molecular diagnostic lab work into their clinical practices. They will request genetic susceptibility testing and bacterial profiling as needed. Discovering and treating the source of disease will become

more important than treating the symptoms. Working together, the
practitioner and the patient will co-diagnose and establish goals and
a treatment plan together. These offices more frequently collaborate
with other health care providers for their clients' ultimate health
outcomes. Needs are addressed on a "whole mouth/whole body"
model. Physicians and dentists collaborate to guide the direction of
prevention, supported by the hygienist.

More typically, offices are organized on a piecemeal "menu-driven"
basis. These practices are steered by insurance and remediation.
During the initial contact a full mouth series of x-rays is taken; decayed
teeth are identified and scheduled for repair. A cleaning is scheduled
during which a gum disease examination is often performed. The teeth
are either "cleaned" at that time or rescheduled for a series of therapy
appointments. Prevention discussions are haphazardly relegated
to cleaning appointments as the interests of the hygienist and client
dictate.

As you can see, just as dentistry is considered discretionary
medicine, preventive dentistry is often considered discretionary
dentistry. Neither approach serves the public well. How did this
happen? Should you care? Does dentistry's internal politics affect you?

I'm afraid it does. "Realizing how and why dental hygiene began
is an important step in making decisions about dental care delivery in
today's society," [i] says Christine Nathe associate professor and graduate
program director at University of New Mexico's hygiene department.
She observes the recommendations suggested by the Surgeon General
in the report *Oral Health in America* closely mirror the original theories
advanced for the new profession of dental hygiene, created in 1913.

These address the same principals outlined in this book. Clearly
progress is painstakingly slow. Christine Nathe continues, "I suggest
the principal reason is that hygienists have never been allowed to take
the role originally envisioned for them – a role eloquently outlined in
the first textbook for dental hygienists *Mouth Hygiene* (edition 1-4,
**1916-1934**):

'The dental hygienist was created from the realization that mouth
hygiene was a necessity and that the average dental practitioner could
not give sufficient time to it and that the toothbrush alone would never
produce it... The present need of the dental profession in solving the
public health problem of mouth hygiene is an immense corps of women
workers, educated and trained as dental hygienists, and therefore

competent to enter public schools, dental offices, infirmaries, public clinics, sanitariums, factories, and other private corporations, to care for the mouths of the millions who need this educational service... The actual results secured by dental hygienists in private and public services, particularly in public schools, affords incontrovertible proof of the value of dental hygienists...' "

Yet currently, strict supervision regulations keep dental hygienists largely confined to private practice under the supervision of a dentist. Please remember about half of all Americans do not access dental care regularly. The central tenet of the dental hygiene profession – prevention through education – became fragmented as these regulations were implemented. And this was almost as soon as the dental hygiene profession was created!

## What is at Stake?

What are the costs of ignorance? One of the driving forces behind this book is my dismay that preventive voices are muted while the incidence of degenerative diseases and their personal, societal and financial costs skyrocket.

I am dismayed I never heard or saw Laura Bush mention oral health while tirelessly working to educate women about their heart disease risks. I am dismayed that the current political debates surrounding health care ignore oral health. I am dismayed that any number of excellent health books about diabetes, anti-aging, maintaining mental acuity as we age, nutrition, immune system boosting, heart disease and so on, ignore oral health. I am dismayed at how few cardiac units advise patients they discharge to clean up their oral health. I am especially dismayed there is no cohesive national program of oral health developed for or required in our public school systems.

In the face of overwhelming research showing simple preventive solutions can vastly improve general health, most hygienists are alarmed by organized dentistry's continual efforts to downgrade entry-level professional education standards for hygienists. Hygienists understand that doing so attracts less qualified and motivated candidates into the profession. Private practice settings offer a comfortable living, often with less than a full-time commitment. It affords a wonderful lifestyle, yet cannot offer opportunities for professional advancement.

Without a well-defined and serious commitment to integrate prevention into private practices, the most deeply committed and talented are often lost early to other careers. Those hygienists that stay do not always have a burning desire to continually evaluate and apply new research, nor are they often encouraged to.

The general public has an abysmal lack of knowledge about their mouths. Obviously, few understand its overall importance to their health. Certainly most do not grasp the political ramifications of its delivery. This does not apply to just children or the poor. The ignorance cuts across all socioeconomic lines. In the light of new integrative medicine concepts discussed in this book and the more permanent, less invasive dentistry we now have available and the serious consequences of the ignorance of them, I believe dental hygienists must be allowed to play a more active role in prevention, treatment, and education. To meet future needs economically, hygienists need to be better educated, not less educated. And they need the freedom to practice in more settings and be able to offer more early intervention services.

I am disheartened that the efforts to reduce educational standards will have a profound impact on the public's health and pocketbooks as professional dental organizations continue to be successful. I hope this book not only will raise individual awareness and health, but also will raise public awareness of the significant stakes involved, both personally and nationally.

As many physicians say, "The time to treat a heart attack is not in the emergency room of a hospital, but long before it happens." Hygienists are well positioned to help change statistics on this disease and others discussed in this book through massive prevention and early intervention efforts. Again, if "most patients visit their doctors when they are ill and dentists when they perceive themselves as well," hygienists can screen for many serious diseases of which patients are unaware.

I would like to see hygienists expand their usefulness and legally take their places in broad-based school prevention and treatment programs as originally envisioned.

I would like to see hygienists play a larger role in nursing home and hospital settings where they can play a significant role in assisting residents avoid the respiratory diseases common and dangerous in both settings.

I hope hygienists some day gain the right to accomplish early fissure decay diagnosis (Chapter 13) outside of traditional dental settings, now that advanced tools can deliver reproducible and predictable results that far exceed the current twenty-five percent diagnostic accuracy common today. If we really think broadly, now that anesthetic and dental drills need not be involved, I see no reason hygienists with advanced training can even gain the right to intervene early.

Yet our profession continues to fight "preceptorship" (on-the-job training of hygienists by dentists) throughout the country. It may be a losing battle. Who loses most? Do you think this could affect you or your loved ones?

### How do you know dentistry is in favor of on-the-job training?

Organized dentistry has been trying to give on-the-job training programs for dental hygienists a foothold for more than 10 years now, but recent actions taken by ADA's House of Delegates show that the dental association is intensifying its efforts to make on-the-job programs a reality. In recent years, ADA's House of Delegates – its policy-making and governing body – voted to support the Alabama Dental Hygiene Program (ADHP), an on-the-job program that trains individuals to perform traditional dental hygiene duties. The delegates also voted to provide assistance to state dental societies that are trying to change laws to make such programs legal, and to urge state dental boards to accept on-the-job programs as adequate preparation for direct patient care.

And this is just the federal activity. On the state level, last year Kansas passed a law to allow dental assistants to clean teeth above the gum line, a cosmetic procedure that does nothing to prevent periodontal disease and stop the threat of bacteria spread throughout the body.

### Why would dentists support something that could harm patients?

We can't speak for dentistry, but some dentists, clearly unhappy about the ADA actions, suggest it is a financial and political issue.

**What's wrong with on-the-job training as long as dentists know what they're doing?**

That's just the problem. Dentists don't have the time to train a hygienist in the office, and typically they don't know very much about the preventive skills in which dental hygienists specialize. Dentists specialize in restorative duties like filling cavities.

Usually dentists spend very little practice time on periodontics – the diagnosis and treatment of the gum and bones that support teeth. In fact, in many dental schools, it is dental hygienists who teach preventive procedures to dental students and preventive topics are a small portion of dental students' course of study.

Another problem is that patients won't even know the trainees providing care are not fully qualified.

**Is there a shortage of dental hygienists? I've heard that's the reason dentists are in favor of reducing the time it takes to become a dental hygienist.**

Dental groups who are in favor of shifting dental hygiene duties to other workers usually say they are doing it because they believe there is a national shortage of dental hygienists. However, such claims are not borne out by the statistics. In fact, the number of dental hygiene program graduates has exceeded dental school graduates for the past decade.

There are certain areas of the country, especially rural areas, where there aren't enough dental hygienists, but then, these are the same areas that have too few dentists. Restrictive supervision laws for dental hygienists are the number one barrier to access to oral health care. Since dental hygienists must practice with dentists, they are forced to go where the jobs are instead of where patients need them." [ii]

## How Do We Move Forward?

A few states allow additional advanced certification for hygienists who are to deliver mid-level health care in under-served areas. This is dentistry's version of a nurse practitioner. It is a start, though there are practical concerns. The places advanced practitioners can practice are often so severely restricted, they might find it hard to run a profitable business. How are they to be reimbursed? Will it be cost effective to earn a graduate degree?

Because many training programs have been diluted, this advanced level certification makes good sense, though even this is being fought. So far, there are no proposals to allow completely independent practice by hygienists. I strongly see this as a future need. Not only will this draw highly motivated and professionally oriented people into the field, eager to excel on their terms, it will offer the general population more choice. I believe competition breeds excellence; excellence generates pride and excitement. Too many of our best practitioners leave the profession due to boredom – a lack of challenge, appreciation, and advancement opportunities. It is a waste of educational dollars and a sad loss of experience.

Until the last decade, I did not have a strong opinion about independent practice. I know hygienists are subject to their employer's priorities, which often keeps them from delivering what they consider key services. I once considered client convenience a priority. I did not want clients to have to see two different oral caregivers. I now think the public should have options.

## Self Determination and Expanded Roles

I personally believe allowing hygienists to govern themselves, accredit their own schools, and have the opportunity for independent practice would bring more mutual respect between dentists and hygienists, improve the level of preventive care most patients receive, and allow more avenues for preventive messages to reach the public.

Along with the ADHA, I strongly believe *more* education, not less should be required for entry-level positions. I hope this book clearly makes this point.

Our population is aging and they are doing so with more diseases, many of them tied to oral health. Well-educated and motivated hygienists can not only potentially alert patients to signs and symptoms they observe that suggest heart disease, stroke risk, adverse pregnancy outcomes, diabetes or sugar metabolism problems, they are trained to understand the complex treatment ramifications that must be considered. Hygienists often have a role in smoking cessation programs when practices allow it. Well-educated hygienists are capable of the enhanced level of communication necessary in whole body health collaborative care models.

Many hygienists envision a larger role in health care as research continues to augment and reinforce integrated preventive health models and early intervention. Not only do they see the profession taking and monitoring vital signs, but eventually providing bacteriological testing, ordering genetic testing, monitoring blood glucose levels, and screening for innumerable "high impact" diseases by examining biomarkers present in saliva. So far, promising research by Dr. Li et al, at the University of California, LA Dental Research Institute is looking at these disease biomarkers in saliva: cardiovascular disease, cancer (lung, prostate, ovarian, and colon), Alzheimer's, osteoporosis, cerebrovascular diseases, nephritis, septicemia, chronic respiratory diseases, chronic liver disease, and pneumonitis.[iii] Again, the mouth is a "mirror of the body" and oral fluid is the perfect surveillance tool for health and disease. Hygienists are well positioned to take on a larger role in health care, perhaps even being key liaisons between some specialties. This can only occur with augmented education.

It should concern us all that diluting educational standards for entry-level dental hygiene is swimming against the tide of progress. More education is the predominant trend in the health care industry. Occupational therapists and physical therapists are moving towards master's degrees and speech pathology is moving towards doctorate degrees for entry-level positions.

Meanwhile baccalaureate degree programs for dental hygiene are closing throughout the country while lesser schools are flooded with applicants. Coupled with the disenchantment causing many well-trained hygienists to leave the field – their education dollars and resourcefulness wasted – to seek more fertile and challenging career opportunities, improving America's oral health looks bleak if hygienists aren't able to politically reverse present trends.

Do you think this could affect you?

## The Need is So Great There is Room for All

Here I would like to digress with personal thoughts and observations. People across all socioeconomic lines avoid dental care due to fear, cost, and lack of trust in the dental profession. I think dental hygienists could provide an introductory level of care that would help reduce all these difficulties. They could provide the critical education necessary to both improve people's dental and overall health and give them more confidence in dentistry as a profession. I especially think it could funnel needed restorative care for under-served populations to dentists earlier in the disease phase therefore decreasing the need for complicated, expensive, and traumatic repairs. I think dentists would actually experience increased business and people would suffer less.

I understand dentist's biggest fear might be hygienists will become the "gatekeepers" of dental care. I appreciate their concerns and they may not be unfounded. I have two rebuttals. First, gate keeping is a common occurrence throughout business systems. For instance general dentists are frequent gatekeepers for dental specialists. To compete for business, specialists have to be the best they can be to live up to the trust placed in them by their referring doctors.

Second, competition between hygienists in independent practice could also keep hygienists at the top of their game. Presently it is easy to get away with a lackadaisical attitude. I have abundant faith in our consumer-driven, free market economy that allows choice. I believe competition would encourage a higher level of engagement by dental hygienists. I also believe patients have the capacity to decide for themselves if they like the doctors to whom they are referred and for that matter, the hygienists they choose. Competition is the way of business in our market-driven economy. It is the main counterbalance to protective policies!

Something to consider: About 6000 dentists retire a year while 4000 enter the field. Requiring hygienists to work only under dentists in private practices seems to unreasonably restrict care. I envision hygienists being allowed to work for various medical providers in the future. I imagine gum disease screening and counseling could be helpful in many medical settings.

I suspect hygienists in independent practice can offer an economic advantage for preventive and introductory care due to low business overhead. I would not want to imply the same pressures of running a commercial enterprise could not also impact professional standards of hygienists. But I do have faith in people's abilities to choose what they want for themselves in a free market system.

Last, giving hygienists the right to practice privately would not preclude hygienists from practicing freely within a dental private practice, as in the current system. There is room – and need – for both. I assume many patients, dentists, and hygienists would prefer the status quo. But with such vastly underserved populations, I see room for allowing both modes of practice. With independence from dentists, there would be more leeway to independently develop and run prevention programs outside of a restoration-based commercial enterprise that would not leave hygienists crosswise with various current state dental practice acts.

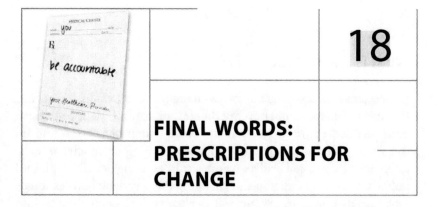

**18**

# FINAL WORDS: PRESCRIPTIONS FOR CHANGE

*"I have come to the conclusion that politics is too serious
a matter to be left to the politicians."*

**~ Charles DeGaulle ~**

Dear Reader, as you finish reading I hope you will not see these last pages as a conclusion. It should be a beginning. They are intended as a three-part prescription for informed action.

- First, to help you deal with the condition of your mouth as an element of your overall health.
- Second, to encourage concerned professionals to keep reprioritizing prevention within dentistry, and oral health within preventive medicine.
- Finally, a plea for all of us as citizens to insist that oral health be made part of America's quest for an equitable, science-driven health care system that balances prevention with early intervention.

When I started the reflection and research leading to this project I was cautioned that a book about what goes on in people's mouths was, to put it mildly, "unusual." But I knew I had something to say that went beyond a personal wellness book or hand-wringing over the shocking number of poor people in this prosperous nation who have ruined mouths and the number of not-so-poor people who are not far behind.

What I hope to do with this book is to challenge the manner in which we think about the health of our mouths – personally, professionally and politically.

## What is Easy, What is Hard

In one sense the easy part involves changing your personal behavior; the stories I shared about how my clients took control tell us people can grasp the concept of prevention and change their behavior – if given the opportunity and some caring guidance. It is much, much harder to influence professional leaders who resist integrating dental health into public preventive medicine and changing the way dental professionals integrate disease prevention, oral health, and biocompatibility into their practices.

In my view, leadership of the health professions may represent entrenched interests, but should not be confused with the eyes-wide-open selfish interests found in many regulated industries. They are professional leaders who believe they are well educated, well informed and well intentioned.

Ultimately, they follow where scientific findings lead them. If they are too slow, public opinion, lawmakers, or liability law prods them. It won't be easy, but mercury, fluoride, and the dentistry of a long-ago era will likely go the route of what we now know to have been dangerous, damaging, ineffective, or over-prescribed.

## Is There a Prevention Imperative?

Turning the corner on matters of technique will be easy for professional leaders in comparison with the issues they face on re-organizing their professions to meet the disease prevention challenge. The role of dentistry in disease prevention seems as ill defined in medical practices as the role of prevention is in the practice of dentistry.

Yet in the Surgeon General's ground breaking 2000 report on oral health in America, it is estimated children lose over 50 million hours from school and adults 160 million hours from work annually from dental illness and professional visits.[i] Pain from toothaches is a significant public health problem affecting approximately 22 million adults during any six-month period in the United States.[ii]

Research and clinical experience tells us long-term consequences of poor oral health often leads to:

- Remedial treatment of dental diseases preventive care could have forestalled or minimized.
- Accelerated treatment costs for exacerbated chronic inflammatory diseases.
- Broken down mouths resulting in compromised nutritional, social, and work status.  Poor nutrition leads to an overall decline in health, especially among the elderly.

These all accelerate health care costs. They can be prevented. As medical research conclusively demonstrates ways in which a healthy mouth can be a vital part of disease prevention, public awareness, health professionals, and public policy are not keeping up.

In the continuing national debate on proposals for life-changing reforms on the scope, focus, and cost of health care in America, preventive medicine is getting some well-deserved attention, but oral health is barely a blip on the screen.

## True Health-Care-Dollar Savings?

When Maryland eliminated Medicaid reimbursement to dentists for treatment of adult dental emergencies in 1993, the rate of emergency room visits for dental problems rose by 12 percent and medical care costs rose.[iii] Is it likely this represented a net savings? Hardly likely.

The costs to the Medicare system increase as many disadvantaged patients continue to live with untreated oral health problems and its associated pain. Since dental diseases are not self-limiting, it is difficult to grasp the emotional and physical toll of these diseases on their sufferers.

We know incalculable funds, both public and personal are squandered when we ignore prevention. It is cost prohibitive to treat advanced oral infections and deadly inflammatory diseases. As these diseases advance, employee absenteeism erodes productivity and performance. It is interesting to note that loss of productivity provided the primary impetus for creating prevention oriented dental hygienists at the turn of the 1900s! What happened? What can be done?

## Sacred Cows and Silent Epidemics

It is going to take something more than knowledge to deal with the simple enough notion that the health of our mouths is tied to the health of our bodies and we should act accordingly. There are some sacred cows on the road around which professional and political leaders must maneuver.

Some say our American Constitution, democracy, and market economy combine to create the freedom and wealth that make us the envy of the world. Our system helped finance my early education, underwrote most of the research I have been talking about, and gives me the freedom to speak up and even write a book on matters I care about.

But in a market-driven economy, those who provide products and services do so within a framework where costs must be controlled to produce profits. In a real-world health care setting, cost control concerns can creep beyond savings on utilities, administration, etc. and extend into cutting service and compromising quality – sometimes with ramifications that frustrate providers and leave patients at risk or worse.

I believe dealing honestly with the interaction between the cost and quality of health care is at the core of the debate over America's health care system as well as so many health-related decisions we make in our own lives. The sacred cow often blocking the path to reform is the "bottom line."

## Personal, Professional, and Political Challenges Beyond Sheer Ignorance

I hate to say it, but all who bother to check will tell you most people are health ignorant. The situation is appalling in a wealthy and relatively literate country barraged with information outlets. But we cannot educate ourselves out of the silent epidemic undermining our oral health; there are professional reforms needed to move dentistry and oral health out of the shadow; there are complex policy challenges that pertain to all this.

Let us start with our personal lives where for most of us, fear and procrastination all too often dominate our approach to oral care. It is common to postpone seeing a dentist until something is wrong – far too often because we budget our households on a (flawed) business model. It is flawed because it does not include investment in prevention – taking the kind of measures my clients learned. But most people do not have a prevention regimen and many hygienists are not able to invest the time I was able to dedicate to keep clients and their families "out of trouble."

I believe every health care provider I know, professionally or personally, would agree we must be governed by strict rules and high standards. That is what we expect, our clients expect, and society has come to demand. But there is a commercial dimension to almost all professional offices in America. No matter how much compassion and wisdom lies beneath our investment in education and research or how high we have raised the bar on professional standards and ethical conduct we cannot escape "the bottom line."

## The "Bottom Line" and the Status Quo

Like it or not, policy makers, professionals and patients themselves must sometimes make decisions based on what can be afforded, not just what is needed. The status quo is tethered to that "bottom line." With this book I hope I am illuminating what can be at stake: that so-called "economic reality" can have lethal consequences or cause us to pay a price far in excess of the costs we save.

The new bywords in dentistry over the last decade have been "evidence based practice." Simply put, it means taking a fresh look at ideas and practices as science brings new realities. Unfortunately it does not guarantee change. In the professional and public policy world I believe the greatest enemy is complacency – inaction when we know better. Much complacency is cost–inspired, these quiet compromises we make when the balance sheet is brought out and the bottom line drives decision-making.

Three good examples of such complacency are the slow adoption of micro-dentistry/MID by the American Dental Association, thus the dental schools, the amalgam controversy discussed in Chapters 13 and 15, and the problems we face in solving the problem of fluoride over-ingestion because of its unexpected concentrations in processed foods and beverages, fluorine residues from pesticides/fungicides used on our crops, its presence in our water, prescription medications, toothpastes, mouthwashes, and other sources. In those situations I believe our recurring quandary over quality care versus economic reality is about ready to burst forth dramatically. In spite of an increasing body of scientific research that accompanies a growing chorus of concern there seems to be little action being taken in regulatory and professional quarters.

### The Mercury Challenge

An editorial response to a recent New York Times article by Charles Brown, National Counsel for Consumers for Choice:

In "Boom Times for Dentistry," [iv] reporter Alex Berenson explains the economic forces that lead to abysmal oral health care for America's working poor. By focusing on public relations, political aggrandizement, and amassing wealth for dentists, he thinks the American Dental Association bears primary responsibility. By controlling the process of who gets appointed to dental boards, the ADA and its state affiliates use this power effectively to prevent competition from dental hygienists, those willing and able to serve the poor.

Barenson suggests the nation's two-tiered system of oral health care is manifested in the continued use of mercury amalgam – which the ADA deceptively calls 'silver fillings' – on lower-income Americans, while upper-income Americans receive non-toxic alternatives. This duality was characterized by an NAACP witness testifying before Congress as 'mercury for the poor and choice for the rich.'

It is his further opinion that one message drawn from this first page story that blames the ADA and the dental boards for using their powers to block competition and hence deny low-income children basic oral health care, is it should "end the ADA's ridiculous position that mercury fillings are the only way to serve the poor – the facts are that (the) ADA blocks the very programs that will serve the poor." I might point out one again, that if the ADA cared about the poor, it would encourage legal changes allowing hygienists with advanced training greater independence to provide expanded preventive services and insist dental schools abandon the teaching of techniques proven not to work, in favor of procedures that do.

In spite of the history of its contentious rise to acceptance in the US, mercury-based amalgams at one time served as an inexpensive material with good compressive strength that was easily placed in a wet environment. Now that we have safer materials, techniques, and bonding agents for advanced lesions, the higher initial costs and skill levels they require should not impede them from becoming the new minimum standard. At the very least informed consent should be required.

I believe the FDA was slow to act, only hinting at a phase-out in March of 2011, because it understood significant interests in our economy could face huge financial threats should official policy change overnight. One only has to remember the enormous tobacco lawsuit settlements to imagine what liability settlements and court costs could be incurred. Depending on how the amalgam challenge is finally met, shock waves may yet travel through the insurance industry, the regulatory bodies, the amalgam manufacturing companies, and the dental profession as tort claims mount, safety parameters are set, alternative dental materials approved and replacements are demanded at an ever-growing pace. We also need to consider how we will handle all the extra environmental waste as more and more people demand replacement of their mercury fillings.

The health care/insurance crisis facing American consumers and health care providers is rooted in our complacency. We are complacent about public and personal health education. We as individuals often do not take an active role in promoting our own health or that of our families. Government subsidizes agribusinesses that produce mostly junk food. We do not find opportunities to exercise, cook healthy meals, and deeply relax. We accept insurance policy dictates as treatment guides. For instance, if an insurance policy only covers the cost of the less expensive amalgam filling in a posterior tooth, we accept amalgams as our treatment choice, unwilling or unable to pay for cost differences. Or are we uninformed about the different treatment options available?

An active part of the health care debate revolves around just that point. Should there be a high level of health care available to all, or should health care be socially and financially stratified based on preventive knowledge and ability to pay? This is a difficult question.

Too often patients and medical professionals have passively accepted compromises dictated by a commercially dominated approach to health care, a pattern of self destructive abdication that is letting third party private insurance companies dictate care levels. (If dental care were part of Medicare, which it unfortunately is not, you could add "bureaucrat" as another "third party.")

Doctors already realize they face real world challenges and dilemmas as they try to remain financially viable and competitive in commercial practices. To avoid the dilemmas insurance dependency can create, many medical students are choosing cosmetic dermatology and other elective procedure-oriented practices that by definition, are not covered by insurance. In dentistry, many practices also emphasize elective cosmetic work, partly for the same reason. Cosmetic dentistry helps them meet that bottom line.

These practices are having a harder time making ends meet as demand for cosmetic dentistry dwindles in challenging economic climates. This may provide the perfect opportunity for these practices to switch to accurate, early diagnosis and intervention. The speed, ease, and comfort of MID dentistry could create the high volume some of these practices need to survive.

By now I hope most informed Americans have learned what health providers know but do not enjoy saying – total reliance on existing health insurance arrangements to secure comprehensive medical care will involve sacrifices in the scope and quality of your treatment and protection. A few insurers have looked at that infamous bottom line and something good has come of it – they are covering some disease protection measures because they help restrain costs. They see that providing dental benefits are essential benefits for maintaining total health.

A friend has looked at what other industrialized nations offer their residents and says, "health care in America can be the best or the worst in the world, depending on where you are, what you can afford and what ails you."

As most countries have been adopting the notion that everyone has a right to receive health care, the core ingredients of our model reflect our economic system. Elements are: individuals make informed choices about who will treat them, a free-market economy prevails among competing providers, protection is provided by a self-sustaining insurance system, there is a preference for enlightened self-regulation and minimal regulation or any intervention by government.

## Insuring Change

Recently, it appeared America's political leaders in both parties were ready to make good health an explicit right to be enjoyed by everyone and supported in some measure by the federal government. Reform of how health insurance protection could be provided to all Americans was at the center of a great debate in Washington and across the country.

The passion our elected officials brought to the debate signals a decline in the public complacency that nurtured unfairness and inefficiency in how we deal with our health care. Polls showed that how they pay for medical care is a top priority among people.

Hopefully one day, investment in preventive medicine will be given the strategic importance it is due. Unfortunately there are impediments – complex issues that make dentistry the neglected stepchild of organized medicine and allow prevention to be secondary to a dental practice and practically non-existent in the public realm.

I know we can "get it right" if we work at government. Those baby steps we have taken over the years toward a national framework of protection have given us some good, though flawed, institutions: The National Institutes of Health, the Centers for Disease Control, and the Food and Drug Administration. The Medicare system may have some flaws in what it fails to cover, but operates with an overhead level that is roughly half of what private insurers require.

In all of this – the personal, the professional, the political – we will get what we work for and will suffer from what we failed to stop when we knew better.

## Rx – The ABCs of Taking Action
### A. As Patients – Take Charge!!

But don't think for a minute you don't need professional help – you do. Self-help can only go so far and treatment of many dental problems can only be found in a dental setting. That is true as well for adopting a systematic prevention program for your mouth and gums.

If you opened this book it means you are probably interested in taking care of yourself and if you read it all, you understand the role your mouth plays in your overall health. Educating yourself and making informed choices is more critical than it ever has been. I have offered a number of examples of how clients I have served have taken charge of their oral health. I have tried to tell you why all the self-care, diet and behavioral issues matter.

And I hope you don't wonder why I spend so much time talking about things like diabetes and heart disease and hormones. All body systems are tightly interconnected in a complex biological dance. What I am trying to do is to help you understand the urgency and importance of becoming that dance's choreographer.

---

Date: *Now!*

$R_x$ for personal care:

1.  *Brush gently with a soft brush into the oral pocket tissue daily.*
2.  *Find a workable strategy for regularly cleaning in between your teeth.*
3.  *Use strategies to maintain adequate saliva.*
4.  *Limit simple carbohydrate intake.*
5.  *In all ways try to enhance your immune system.*

*Your Healthcare Provider*

---

## B. As Professionals – Speak up; Heal Yourselves!

In the preceding chapter, I touched far too briefly on some changes that must be made in dentistry, disease prevention and the organization of our health care system. Although some will disagree, I believe dentistry continues to be a stepchild of the medical establishment, to the detriment of all the health professions and the health of the public. The oral health of a patient is a vital part of his or her wellness. When they fail to be guided by that assertion I believe they are short-changing their patients and their profession.

There are problems associated with the curious wall that divides dentistry and other medical professions. First and foremost I believe is the manner in which we pay for health care in our public and private Medicare systems. The professions involved in this system are organized and have well financed administrators and lobbyists. They are served by professional schools and have the ear of those who make laws and set the rules. They don't need me to tell them what to do.

Within most dental offices I know, dentists determine the role of prevention for their clients. Much of the preventive care is left to the dental hygienist – to be accomplished only incidentally as time, interest, and rapport between client and clinician allows during "cleanings" – the procedure reimbursable by insurance. I have had exceptional opportunities in my career, but most hygienists I know do not feel empowered by their profession or their employers to actively plan a patient's approach to prevention. The problems of prevention within a dental office are much more than office politics involving the hierarchy of dental health professionals. It goes to the core of what dentistry is about and where it stands within preventive medicine.

As a health consumer, you can speak to these professional issues and should do so.

You don't have to stop there. In our country, you can still speak truth to power and sometimes see things happen.

---

Date: *Now!*

$R_x$ What you could and should demand of your health care system:

1. Ask to schedule a meeting in your dentist's office to discuss a plan to treat your problems comprehensively, one assuring your dental and general health. If you have particular general health concerns, insist on discussing them as they relate to your oral health. These concerns may be ones introduced here or in other areas of your life.
2. Ask your MD if he has a report from your dentist on what has shown up in various screenings and x-rays of your mouth.
3. Expect and ask for a continuing dialogue between your medical and dental providers. Be an active participant yourself in these concerns.

*Your Healthcare Provider*

## C. As Citizens – Speak Up, Write . . . Vote!

*Some men see things as they are and ask why?*
*I dream things that never were and ask, why not?*

~ **John Kennedy** ~

In our blessed American democracy, we all get to participate in political life if we want. And we don't have to if we choose not to. We take the latter choice at our peril when sweeping changes are being made in how we are governed and what government does for us – or to us, as some prefer to say. This may be one of those times; some say there is a sea change underway in the way we organize and deliver health care in America.

Do not think you can't be heard; you can, but you will have to work at it.

So many years in Austin, the state capitol of Texas, has given me an opportunity to know more than a few legislators, lobbyists, and even some people who followed Presidents Johnson and Bush to Washington. Most will tell you some ideas find their way into the mix of public policy that are outside the focus of the powerful lobbyists. Sometimes they are just so compellingly important they trump interest group politics.

Even if what you want requires the attention of someone way, way up the ladder, keep in mind what House Speaker Tip O'Neil once observed – "ultimately, all politics is local."

What should we ask for? Whom should we ask? How do we ask? We need to change our mind-set about health on many levels. We need to focus less on "Big Pharma's" disease mongering direct-to-consumer advertising for their pharmaceutical products. We need to think of how and why we subsidize the agribusinesses that provide us with the junk foods that destroy our health. Industrialized foods may seem economical, but they are responsible for much of the sixteen percent of our gross domestic product we spend on managing disease. When companies spend more on health care than they do on producing their product, it affects our global competitive edge. We must begin to exercise caution within our own families, our communities, and in our country.

In the same way, when consumers demand cosmetic dentistry, it becomes available. If we seek long-lasting smiles at an economical cost, dentistry will respond. It is how our system works. We need to think holistically about how to find the balance and prevention that is so lacking in most of our lives. This book has offered a smorgasbord of reforms I am interested in seeing take place. You may not agree with some or any of it. Or you may just decide to exercise your right to remain passive. But don't make the mistake of thinking you can't make a difference. You can!

---

Date: *Now!*

$R_x$ As a citizen, if you want to get involved in public policy, there are many of great resources.

- *There are any number of useful "how to do it" books for citizen lobbyists. A popular one is: The Citizen's Guide to Lobbying Congress by Donald E. deKieffer*
- *Websites that push a particular agenda make citizen action easy. A little cruising the Internet will reveal these. An example: if you are interested in stopping water fluoridation, go to: http://www.fluoridealert.org/ to sign petitions and find other ideas. Citizen lobbying books will help you plan steps to take as you define positions you want to act on.*

*Your Healthcare Provider*

# GLOSSARY

**A1c (or A1C):** A test that measures a person's average blood glucose level over the past 2 to 3 months. Hemoglobin is the part of a red blood cell that carries oxygen to the cells and sometimes joins with the glucose in the bloodstream to form AGEs. Also called hemoglobin A1C or glycosylated hemoglobin, the test shows the amount of glucose that sticks to the red blood cell, which is proportional to the amount of circulating glucose. Self-testing is available.

**Acidosis:** A condition in which the blood pH is reduced below 7.35. It can occur when the kidney loses its ability to excrete acid, so urea and creatinine build up in the blood. It also occurs when one gets inadequate oxygen, whether due to strenuous exercise, starvation, a shift from using sugar for energy to using stored fatty acids as occurs in diabetes, or hypoventilation as occurs with respiratory distresses.

**AGEs:** Acronym for advanced glycation (glycosylation) end products. Simple carbohydrates convert to glucose for use in the human body. Like sugars, glucose is very sticky. If it circulates too long in the blood supply, it begins to clump with blood proteins and fats. White blood cells can gobble up some of these ruined proteins, but most AGEs accumulate and damage the body in many ways, like damaging blood vessels and complicating diabetes. AGEs are very pro-inflammatory.

**Albuminuria:** A condition in which the urine contains more than normal amounts of a protein called albumin. Albuminuria may be a sign of nephropathy (kidney disease). Gum disease also drives albumin spillover into urine.

**Allele:** DNA sequences that code for a gene on chromosomes. Humans have paired chromosomes with two copies of each gene – one allele will be donated by the mother, one allele by the father.

**Amalgam:** Also known as "silver filling" material. For 180 years, the restorative material of choice making up about 75 to 80 percent of all tooth fillings. The mixture contains about 50 percent elemental mercury by weight and also 35 percent silver, tin copper and zinc. Elemental mercury is highly volatile at room temperature and produces an easily absorbed vapor.

**Anaerobe:** An organism that can live in the absence of oxygen.

**Antibiotics:** Compounds that inhibit or destroy life.

**Antibodies:** Proteins made by the body to protect itself from "foreign" substances like bacteria or viruses. People exhibit type 1 diabetes when their bodies make antibodies that destroy its own insulin-making beta cells.

**Antioxidants:** Antioxidants help protect cells against free radical damage. Free radicals are produced continually as one breaks down food, exercises, is exposed to radiation, or inhales respiratory irritants like tobacco smoke. Just like oxygen oxidizes steel into rust, free radicals damage cells by stealing electrons from the first thing they encounter like cell walls, DNA, etc. Losing these electrons is called oxidation. Free radical damage causes tissues to degrade and diseases to begin. Because oxygen is toxic to biological tissues, it is crucial to have antioxidants run interference for your tissues.

**Aorta:** The first segment of blood vessel that connects to the heart. It carries the oxygenated blood that is exiting the heart that circulates around the body to nourish it with oxygen and other nutrients.

**Artery:** Arteries carry oxygenated blood away from the heart.

**Atherosclerosis:** Clogging, narrowing and hardening of the body's large arteries and medium-sized blood vessels with mineralized plaques. It is an inflammatory response designed to heal blood vessels. It is a slowly progressive disease wherein damage can accumulate for decades, but eventually atherosclerosis can lead to strokes, heart attacks, eye and kidney problems.

**BDNF:** Brain Derived Neuroropic Factor. BDNF supports existing nerves, stimulates the growth of new ones, enhances neurotransmission and supports normal brain structure. It is critical for long-term memory storage. Stress, inflammation and poor diet decreases levels and may be linked to depression. Other conditions associated with low levels of BDNF are schizophrenia, obsessive-compulsive disorder, dementia, and Alzheimer's. Exercise and a diet rich in omega-3s and low in simple carbohydrates increase levels. Depressed people have low levels of BDNF.

**BON (Bisphosphonate Osteonecrosis of the Jaw):** Death of the jawbone, driven by the class of prescription drugs called bisphosphonates like Fosamax, Actonel, and Boniva. Also known as BONJ.

**Chelation Therapy:** The use of agents like EDTA, DMPS, and DMSA that detoxify the body by combining with poisonous heavy metals in the bloodstream by means of a chelate. Chelates bind to the metal and are then excreted. Special therapists oversee the chelation process. Zeolites for instance, are a low-level binder to heavy metals that can be safely used at home.

**Chorioamnion:** The complex that comprises both the chorion and the amnion. The amniotic sac consists of two membranes: 1) the outer membrane, the chorion, contains the amnion and is part of the placenta and 2) the inner membrane, the amnion, contains the amniotic fluid and the fetus.

Chorioamnionitis is an inflammation of the chorion and amnion. It is usually caused by a bacterial infection and is a common cause for brain injuries in newborns.

**Chirodontics** combines both chiropractic techniques and dentistry in order to help with head, neck, facial, and cranial problems. There are several different systems working in the body. Because they compensate for each other, often difficult dental patients are easy chiropractic cases and difficult chiropractic patients are simple dental orthopedic cases. When these teams work together, they are termed Chirodontics. Typically, these teams incorporate nutrition and lifestyle counseling to achieve true health.

**Chromium:** Chromium is necessary in trace amounts. Hexavalent chromium (+6) is biologically toxic. Trivalent chromium (+3) is critical to the metabolism and storage of carbohydrates, protein and fat and enhances insulin's actions. Good sources are brewers' yeast, broccoli, and whole grains. Very little is absorbed, though vitamin C and niacin enhance uptake. Infections, high sugar intake, and stress deplete chromium. A chromium deficiency raises insulin requirements. Antacids and corticosteroids my inhibit absorption. Beta-blockers, corticosteroids, insulin, and anti-inflammatory drugs like NSAIDS may increase chromium absorption. NSAIDS can enhance the effects of medications. Fluoride inactivates enzymes that contain chromium.

**Collagen:** The tough fibrous structural protein that gives cells their external structure. It is found in cartilage, ligaments, tendons, fascia, bone and teeth. It is responsible for skin strength and is a major component of artificial skin. Vitamin C is crucial in collagen production. It is why vitamin C deficiency causes scurvy. Gums deteriorate and bleed easily without strong connective tissue, skin discolors, and wounds do not heal.

In the autoimmune/collagen tissue diseases of rheumatoid arthritis or lupus erythematosus, the surrounding tissues become inflamed as healthy collagen fibers are systematically destroyed by the immune system.

Many bacteria and viruses either destroy collagen or interfere with its production.

**Collagenase:** A set of enzymes involved in degradation of collagen. *See MMPs.*

**Crohn's disease:** Likely an autoimmune disease; the lining of any part of the digestive tract remains inflamed in sufferers. Expression of the disease depends on the part of the GI tract affected. Often, absorption of nutrients is reduced.

**Cushing's Syndrome:** A disease in which the pituitary gland stimulates the adrenal gland to release excessive cortisol. Secondary hyperadrenocorticism has a different cause, but the same outcome.

**Diabetic ketoacidosis (DKA):** An emergency condition in which extremely high blood glucose levels, along with a severe lack of insulin, result in the breakdown of body fat for energy and an accumulation of ketones in the blood and urine. Signs of DKA are nausea and vomiting, stomach pain, fruity breath odor, and rapid breathing. Untreated DKA can lead to coma and death. It is one of the conditions that can happen especially to type 1 diabetics.

**Diabetes mellitus:** A condition characterized by hyperglycemia resulting from the body's inability to use blood glucose for energy. In type 1 diabetes, the pancreas no longer makes insulin and therefore blood glucose cannot enter the cells to be used for energy. In type 2 diabetes, either the pancreas does not make enough insulin or the body is unable to use insulin correctly.

**Dopamine:** A neurotransmitter released by the brain's hypothalamus. It stimulates the sympathetic nervous system, which leads to increases heart rate and blood pressure. It is a motivational chemical based on *anticipation* of a reward, not necessarily receiving the reward itself. As such, it is associated with the pleasure centers of the brain and addictions. Behaviors such as anticipating eating certain foods, taking certain drugs such as cocaine and amphetamines, having sex, and so forth increase dopamine levels. A study showed that in mice with genetic consistently high levels of dopamine, there was a great desire for sweets compared to mice with lower levels of dopamine, but they did not necessarily show a greater enjoyment of them. (Peciña S, Cagniard B, Berridge K, Aldridge J, Zhuang X. **Hyperdopaminergic mutant mice have higher "wanting" but not "liking" for sweet rewards.** *J Neurosci* 2003; 23 (28): 9395–402.

**Endothelium:** The internal lining of all blood vessels. Plaques and atheromas form here to narrow blood's channels. Bacteria can easily invade this lining.

**Endotoxins:** A structural component of bacteria that has the potential to be toxic to the host when the bacteria die. LPS or lipopolysaccharides are the classic example. Most gram-negative bacteria release them. A cascade of chemical reactions happens, eventually leading to the release of infection mediators and nitric oxide that leads to endotoxic shock.

**Fibroblasts:** Formative cells that moderate wound healing. They secrete the proteins that form collagen and elastic fibers and the substance between the cells of connective tissue. Gingival fibroblasts are critical for the reconnection of damaged gum tissue to tooth structure.

**Fibronectin:** Fibronectin is excreted by fibroblasts and plays a role in cell adhesion and wound healing.

**Gastrectomy:** Partial or complete surgical removal of the stomach.

**Gastrointestinal tract (GI tract):** The organ system that accepts and digests food, absorbs the nutrients and expels the waste. It encompasses the mouth, the anus, and all the organs in between.

**Glomerular filtration rate:** Measure of the kidney's ability to filter and remove waste products.

**Glomerulus:** The capillary bed that is part of the blood filtration unit of the kidney.

**Glucocorticoids:** Steroidal hormones produced in the adrenal gland's cortex are involved in the metabolism mainly of carbohydrates, but also of fats and proteins. Receptors for glucocorticoids are found in almost all living cells, so its effects are far-ranging. Cortisol (hydrocortisone) is the predominant natural hormone. Many synthetic corticoids are created in the lab and frequently prescribed for their anti-inflammatory and immunosuppressive properties to treat autoimmune diseases, arthritis and dermatitis. Excessive levels of glucocorticoids in humans produce Cushing's disease. Manifestations of Cushing's disease include hypertension, diabetes, obesity in the presence of muscle wasting, and thin skin. Insufficiencies of cortisol produce Addison's disease in which lethargy, diarrhea, and cardiovascular diseases can be present.

**Glucagon:** A hormone produced by the alpha islet cells of the pancreas. Like insulin, it plays a major role in maintaining normal glucose concentrations in the blood. Insulin influences the liver to store some sugar as glycogen, which is quickly released for energy use when blood sugar levels fall. Glucagon may play a major role in insulin resistance.

**HDL "cholesterol" (High density lipoprotein):** A carrier for cholesterols. HDLs are actually the smallest of the cholesterol transporting molecules. Their density is a result of having more protein than fat (45-50 percent protein). They transport cholesterols from foam cells in atherosclerotic plaque back to the liver for recycling or degradation by bile into bile acids after which they are excreted. HDLs also transport cholesterol to the ovaries, testes, and adrenal glands to make various steroid hormones. Its reputation as a "good or protective cholesterol" comes from its ability to remove cholesterols from atherosclerotic arteries after they have healed. As with LDLs, HDLs vary in size with the largest being correlated to the highest level of protection. Electrophoresis and NMR spectroscopy tests refine whether one simply has a high number of total HDLs or has a large concentration of large protective HDL particles. Those with high HDL are less likely to have dementia.

However, new evidence shows "all HDL is not functionally equivalent. The authors of recent studies have shown that infection, inflammation, diabetes, and coronary artery disease are associated with dysfunctional

HDL. HDL can lose its protective activities through a variety of mechanisms, including, but not limited to, altered protein composition, and oxidative protein modification mediated by the enzyme myeloperoxidase, and lipid modification." (Smith JD. "Myeloperoxidase, inflammation, and dysfunctional high-density lipoprotein." *J of Lipidology* 2010; 4(5): 382-388.)

**Heterozygous:** Having two different alleles of the same gene, each allele representing one parent's contribution to the cells complete genome. Loss of heterozygosity (LOH) is often due to the loss of a tumor suppressor gene at a particular location. However genes can also be deleted, converted, mitotically recombined or just lost.

**Hyperparathyroidism:** Four little glands, the parathyroid glands, piggyback on the thyroid gland and produce a hormone called PTH or parathyroid hormone. This hormone is involved in keeping the blood calcium, phosphorus, and vitamin D levels optimal. Calcium is important to many body functions, including muscle contraction, skeletal strength. Hyperparathyroidism is excessive production of parathyroid hormone (PTH) by the parathyroid glands. When calcium levels are too low, the body responds by increasing production of parathyroid hormone. This increase in parathyroid hormone causes more calcium to be taken from the bone and more calcium to be reabsorbed by the intestines and kidney. When the calcium level returns to normal, parathyroid hormone production slows down. Some symptoms are: Back pain, blurred vision, depression, Fatigue, increased thirst and urine output, muscle weakness, and nausea.

**Inflammatory mediator/messengers:** Various molecules that are released by the immune system in response to harmful stimuli. These stimuli can be from damaged cells, irritants, and autoimmune reactions or in the case of an acute infection: external pathogens. They are meant to aid the body in the healing process, but sometimes there is simultaneous destruction and healing in the tissues that occurs over a long period of time. This is called chronic inflammation and the response is quite different from acute inflammation.

Some inflammatory messengers are: C-reactive proteins, monocytes, macrophages, lymphocytes, plasma cells, fibroblasts, TNF-alpha and other cytokines, growth factors, reactive oxygen species, hydrolytic enzymes.

Inflammation also induces high systemic levels of acute-phase proteins. In acute inflammation, these proteins prove beneficial, however in chronic inflammation they can contribute to amyloidosis. These proteins include C-reactive protein, serum amyloid A, Serum amyloid P, vasopressin and glucocorticoids.

High levels of several inflammation-related markers, such as IL-6, IL-8, and TNF-alpha are associated with obesity. During clinical studies, inflammatory-related molecule levels were reduced and increased levels of anti-inflammatory molecules were seen within four weeks after patients began a very low calorie diet. The association of systemic inflammation with insulin resistance and atherosclerosis is the subject of intense research.

**Kidneys:** The two bean-shaped organs that filter wastes from the blood and form urine. The kidneys are located near the middle of the back. They send urine to the bladder.

**Kidney failure:** A chronic condition in which the body retains fluid and harmful wastes build up because the kidneys no longer work properly. A person with kidney failure needs dialysis or a kidney transplant. Also called end-stage renal (REE-nul) disease or ESRD.

**LDL "cholesterol" (low-density lipoprotein):** LDLs are markers for cholesterol and the body's need for them. It is a fat/protein molecule found in the blood that *transports* cholesterols made in the liver to places in the body where it is needed for cell repair. How you eat determines the size of LDL proteins. The very small LDLs, generally from excessive sugar consumption, tend to get stuck in the tiny crevices of blood vessel walls where they oxidize and promote inflammation and scarring. Often, the reason cholesterol is "called" to the sight is because of damage caused by glycation (AGEs), high blood insulin levels found in pre-diabetics, or damage done by the excessive cortisol released when stressed. Nonetheless, this is how LDLs earned their reputation as "bad" cholesterols. Statin drugs lower LDLs, i.e., they "shoot" the band-aids.

**Macrophage:** Versatile components of our immune system that can scavenge LDLs, pathogens, tumor cells, and worn out cells and other debris. They are a critical component of the immune system. They help develop antibodies. They also secrete many important regulatory chemical signals such as interleukin-1s, TNF, enzymes, etc.

**Metastasis:** The spread of cancer from its primary location to other places in the body. The cancer cells break away from the primary tumor and are moved to a distant sight via the lymphatic and circulatory systems.

**Microalbuminuria:** A condition wherein the urine contains small amounts of albumin. Microalbuminuria is an early sign of kidney damage, or nephropathy, a common and serious complication of diabetes. The American Diabetes Associaion recommends people diagnosed with type 2 diabetes be tested for microalbuminuria at the time they are diagnosed and every year thereafter; people with type 1 diabetes should be tested 5 years after diagnosis and every year thereafter. Microalbuminuria is managed by improving blood glucose control, reducing blood pressure, treating gum disease, and modifying the diet.

**Microaneurysm:** A small swelling that forms on the side of tiny blood vessels. These small swellings may break and allow blood to leak into nearby tissue. People with diabetes may get microaneurysms in the retina of the eye.

**MMP (Matrix metalloproteinases):** A set of enzymes whose function is to degrade matrix proteins during tissue remodeling. Collagenases are one group of enzymes that comprise the MMP enzymes. MMPs #s 1, 8, 13, 14 and 18 are mainly described to be in the oral pocket tissue and involved in tissue destruction there. MMP-1 is important in rheumatoid and osteo-arthritis. Doxycyclines at sub-antimicrobial doses inhibit MMP activity, and have been used in various experimental systems for this purpose. It is used clinically for the treatment of periodontal disease and osteoporosis and used to be the only MMP inhibitor widely available clinically. It is sold under the trade name Periostat by the company CollaGenex. Now Oracea and Periostat MR are available. All work well to inhibit MMPs, and lower hs-CRPs and $A_1C$ levels.

**Monocyte:** A white blood cell that has a single nucleus and can ingest (take in) foreign material. (In other words, a monocyte is a mononuclear phagocyte that circulates in the blood.) Monocytes later emigrate from blood into the tissues of the body and there they differentiate, or evolve into cells called macrophages, which play an important role in killing of some bacteria, protozoa, and tumor cells. They also release substances that stimulate other cells of the immune system, and are involved in antigen presentation.

**Neutrophil:** A type of white blood cell, specifically a form of granulocyte, filled with neutrally-staining granules, tiny sacs of enzymes that help the cell kill and digest microorganisms it has engulfed by phagocytosis.
The neutrophil has a lifespan of about 3 days.

**Nephropathy:** Disease of the kidneys. Hyperglycemia and hypertension can damage the kidneys' glomeruli. When the kidneys are damaged, proteins leak out of the kidneys into the urine. Damaged kidneys can no longer remove waste and extra fluids from the bloodstream.

**Nitric oxide (NO):** A signaling molecule in gas form. It is not to be confused with nitrous oxide. NO has a broad range of functions in the body. It is a potent vasodilator that relaxes smooth muscles. Its role in blood vessel dilation helps lower blood pressure and assists penile erection. It regulates the activities of many organs and relaxes the vagus nerve. It assists platelet aggregation and in high concentrations, has direct antimicrobial activity. Mouth breathers rarely make enough.

**Oleic acid:** An acid found in animal and vegetable fats. Though oleic acid makes up 55 to 80 percent of olive oil, only a small percentage is a free acid. Grape seed oil contains about 15 to 20 percent oleic acid.

**OPG:** Osteoprotegerin. Decoy receptors for RANKL. When RANK is released from the osteoblasts, its intended target is the osteoclasts. It is supposed to tell them to release acid into the bone to begin the resorption process. Because of these OPG decoys, it often doesn't reach, them so bone resorption is decreased.

**Oral cleft:** Oral clefts are birth defects in which embryonic mouth (palate) and/or lip tissues don't fuse properly during pregnancy. It appears as a narrow gap in the roof of the mouth or in the skin of the upper lip to the base of the nose. Oral clefts are treatable.

**Osteoblast:** Cells that build bone.

**Osteoclast:** Cells that resorb bone.

**Phagocytosis:** The process by which a cell engulfs particles such as bacteria, aged red blood cells, foreign matter, and other microorganisms. The principal phagocytes (cells that engage in phagocytosis) include the neutrophils and monocytes (types of white blood cells). In Greek, "phago" means "to eat." Phagocytic index is the average number of bacteria or other foreign particles ingested per white blood cell.

**Preeclampsia:** A set of symptoms that occurs in almost 10 percent of pregnancies, it includes high blood pressure, excess nitrogen in the urine, and sometimes swelling of hand, face or feet. The condition is a major cause of death or morbidity in a mother or fetus. Survivors may face liver and kidney damage. Sometimes a placenta that doesn't implant deeply contributes to preeclampsia. In this case the lack of oxygen in the placenta leads to elevated levels of inflammatory mediators. This burden, added to the cascade of increased levels of inflammatory mediators in pregnant mothers with gum disease may be what tips a mother into preeclampsia symptoms.

**Probiotics:** Dietary supplements of live bacteria or yeasts taken to keep beneficial gut bacteria thriving. The theory is that high carbohydrate ingestion and antibiotics reduce "good" bacteria, allowing harmful competitors to thrive. Probiotics, also found in non-pasteurized fermented foods like some yogurt and kefir are often used to treat gut-related yeast infections. There are likely other effects of probiotics at play such as immune system interactions, reduction of some kinds of inflammation, possible reduction in cholesterol levels and blood pressure, and improved mineral absorption. Probiotics are active in the small intestine. Prebiotics work in the large intestine. Probiotics should be matched to the site where the benefit is desired. That is to say, if you want to influence oral bacterial balance, choose a probiotic that contains human-derived natural colonizers of the mouth. If you want to change your gut flora, take probiotics that contain beneficial bacteria known to colonize the gut. Gut bacteria do not noramlly colonize in the mouth. Specialized oral probiotics such as Evora help maintain oral balance.

**Proinflammatory cytokines:** Cytokines are the numerous signaling compounds used in cellular communication. Interleukins, chemokines, and lymphokines are subgroups of cytokines and originally named based on their functions. This no longer holds true. One of their most important roles is the immune response. Proinflammatory cytokines activate the inflammatory response.

**Prostaglandins:** A group of hormone-like substances that regulate inflammation. They can be pro- or anti-inflammatory, based on the types of fats one ingests. The Pro-inflammatory prostaglandins derive from arachidonic acid. Pro-inflammatory prostaglandins ($PGE_2$) stimulate uterine contraction and can clinically induce labor. Prostaglandins are also involved in clotting. In inflammation, COX-2, produced in the blood vessels, stomach and kidneys, is what increases prostaglandin levels. It follows that Cox-2 inhibitors reduce prostaglandin levels. Aspirin works by inhibiting prostaglandin synthesis.

**PT/LBW/Pre-term, Low Birth Weight.** Babies born before a gestation period of 37 weeks with low birth weight – less than 2500 grams or 5 pounds, 8 ounces are PT/LBW. Most babies gestate for about 40 weeks. Very Low Birth Weight describes delivery occurring before 32 weeks and weighing less than 1500 grams. The incidence of these has increased 30 percent over the last two decades with 2006 levels in the US being about 1 in 8, or 12 percent. There are many risk factors such as age of the mother (more than 35 or less than 18), high blood pressure, smoking, alcohol use, diabetes, poor nutrition, lack of prenatal care, multifetal pregnancy, infections of the GU tract, kidney, or mouth, and preeclampsia. (Martin JA, Hamilton BE, Sutton PD, Ventura SJ, Menacker F, Kirmeyer S. "Births: Final Data for 2004." National Vital Statistics Reports, vol. 55, no 1. Hyattsville, Maryland: National Center for Health Statistics, 2006.)

**Rheumatoid arthritis (RA):** A chronic inflammatory disease primarily affecting the lining of joints. Swelling, pain, and enzyme release that digests bone and cartilage characterize this disease. Joint stiffness may occur during end stages. Sufferers benefit from early, aggressive treatment. Because of gum disease's likely role, consistent oral care and systemic ozone therapy could be very helpful, especially in the early phases. In a process called citrullination, the common oral pathogen *P. gingivalis* rapidly converts the amino acid arginine into citrulline. This P gingivalis-mediated citrullination of bacterial and other host proteins in joints may be a key way the body generates antigens that drive the autoimmune response in RA. The immune system cranks up and begins to attack joints, leading to pain, swelling, modified joint architecture, and resulting disability.

**Spina bifida:** A developmental birth defect wherein the neural tube that encloses the spinal cord nerves closes incompletely during the first month of pregnancy. The vertebrae protecting this tube may or may not be fused. Nerve impairment begins at the open defect and below due to lack of development or damage. Folic acid helps decrease the incidence of spina bifida, though there are other risk factors such as diabetes, obesity, genetics, or anticonvulsant medication. Elevated body temperatures from hot tubs, electric blankets, or fevers may also be to blame. Much is still unknown about this defect.

**Stenosis:** abnormal narrowing of a blood vessel.

**TNF-alpha:** (Tumor necrosis factor alpha) TNF-alpha is an inflammatory mediator that stimulates the liver to produce C-reactive proteins (CRP) and other inflammatory mediators. As with other inflammatory events, its short-term presence aids healing. TNF is responsible for the cardinal signs of inflammation: heat, swelling, redness and pain. More troublesome is its chronic presence. It increases insulin resistance, damages blood vessel walls, and raises blood triglyceride levels, thus contributing to atherosclerosis.

**Urea:** A waste product found in the blood that results from the normal breakdown of protein in the liver. Urea is normally removed from the blood by the kidneys and then excreted in the urine.

**Uremia:** The illness associated with the buildup of urea in the blood because the kidneys are working ineffectively. Symptoms include nausea, vomiting, loss of appetite, weakness, and mental confusion.

**Zinc:** Zinc is an essential mineral required for the function of numerous enzymes. When fluoride reacts with zinc in enzymes, it deactivates the enzyme. Zinc also prevents metals like iron and copper from oxidizing cell membranes. It especially maintains the integrity of the blood brain barrier. Since this barrier has a high polyunsaturated fatty acid content, zinc's antioxidant role here is critical. Zinc aids immune function, wound healing, protein and DNA synthesis, and cellular division. Zinc is not stored in the body, so daily intake is important. It is found abundantly in red meat and poultry, though beans, nuts, whole grains, and dairy products contain small amounts. Note that most grains and legumes contain phytates that inhibit zinc absorption.

# SOURCES

[i] "Interview with Gene Simmons." *Fresh Air*. NPR. Philadelphia: WHYY, February 4, 2002.

## INTRODUCTION

[i] Chilton, Floyd H. *Inflammation Nation: The First Clinically Proven Eating Plan to End Our Nation's Secret Epidemic*. New York: Fireside, 2005.
[ii] "Personal Care Market Reports from Packaged Facts." *Consumer Goods Market Research and Analysis from Packaged Facts*. 20 June 2009 (http://www.packagedfacts. com/personal-care-market-c113/).
[iii] Kenneth Kornman. "Healthy Gums and a Healthy Heart: The Perio-Cardio Connection." Gum Disease Information from the American Academy of Periodontology. http://www.perio.org/consumer/perio_cardio.htm (Accessed July 26, 2009).

## CHAPTER ONE
## INTEGRATION: ALL THINGS CONNECTED

[i] Chilton, Floyd H. *Inflammation Nation: The First Clinically Proven Eating Plan to End Our Nation's Secret Epidemic*.
[ii] Albandar, JM,Brunelle JA, and Kingman A. "Destructive Periodontal disease in adults 30 years of age and older in the United States." *Journal of Periodontology* 1999; 70(7):13-29.
[iii] Glassman P, Folse G. "Financing oral health services for people with special needs: Projecting national expenditures." *Journal of the California Dental Association*. 2005; 33(9): 731-40.
[iv] Diringer J, Bonalos K. "Putting Teeth Into Health Care Reform." *Dental Health Foundation/California Primary Care Association. Oral Health Access Council*. June 2007.
[v] Otto, Mary. "For Want of a Dentist. Pr. George'e Boy Dies after Bacteria From Tooth Spread to Brain." *Washington Post*, February 28, 2001, B01.
[vi] Scannapieco, FA, Wang, B, Shiau, H. "Oral Bacteria and Respiratory Infection: Effects on Respiratory Pathogen Adhesion and Epithelial Cell Proinflammatory Cytokine Production." *Anals Periodontol*. 2001; Dec6(1): 78-86.
[vii] Azarpazhooh, A. Leake, JL. "Systematic Review of the Association Between Respiratory Diseases and Oral Health." *J Periodontol*. 2006; 77(9): 1465-1482.
[viii] Scannapieco, FA, Wang, B, Shiau, H. "Oral Bacteria and Respiratory Infection: Effects on Respiratory Pathogen Adhesion and Epithelial Cell Proinflammatory Cytokine Production." *Anals Periodontol*. 2001; Dec6(1): 78-86.
[ix] Okuda K, Kimizuka R, Abe S, et al. "Involvement of Periodontopathic Anaerobes in Aspiration Pneumonia." *J Periodontol*. 2005; 76(11-s):2154-2160.
[x] Adachi M, Ishihara K, Abe S, et al. "Professional oral health care by dental hygienists reduced respiratory infections in elderly persons requiring nursing care." *International Journal of Dental Hygiene*. 2007; 5(2): 69-74.

## CHAPTER TWO
## GUARDING THE GATES

[i] Albert DA, Sadowsky D, Papapanou P, et al. "An Examination of periodontal treatment and per member per month (OMOM) medical costs in an insured population." *BMC Health Serv Res.* 2006; 6: 103. www.pubmedcentral.nih.gov/articlerender.fcgi?artid=1574303 (Accessed July 28,2009.)

[ii] "17.1 Social and Economic Impact of Oral Disease Annual Report -NIDCR/CDC Dental, Oral and Craniofacial Data Resource Center (DRC)." Home Page - NIDCR/CDC Dental, Oral and Craniofacial Data Resource Center (DRC). http://drc.hhs.gov/report/17_1.htm (Accessed June 20, 2009).

[iii] Arumugam M, Raes J, Pelletier E, et al. Enterotypes of the human gut microbiome. *Nature.* 2011 May 12;473(7346):174-80.

[iv] Neufeld KM, Kang N, Bienenstock J. "Reduced anxiety-like behavior and central neurochemical change in germ-free mice." *Neurogastroenterology & Motility* 2011;23(3), 255–e119. DOI: 10.1111/j.1365-2982.2010.01620.x. Accessed May 15, 2011.

[v] University of California Museum of Paleontology. "Antony van Leeuwenhoek." http://www.ucmp.berkeley.edu/history/leeuwenhoek.html(accessed December 12, 2009)

[vi] Kramer JM, Gaffen SL. "Interleukin-17: A New Paradigm in Inflammation, Autoimmunity, and Therapy." *J Periodontol* 2007; 78(6):1083-93.

[vii] Marotte H, Farge P, Gaudin P. "The Association Between Periodontal Disease and Joint Destruction in Rheumatoid Arthritis Patients Extends the Link Between the HLA-DR Shared Epitope and Bone Destruction Severity." *Ann Rheum Dis.* 2006; 65(7): 905-9.

[viii] Abou-Raya S, Abou-Raya A, Naim A. "Rheumatoid arthritis, periodontal disease and coronary artery disease." *Clin Rheumatol.* 2008; 27(4): 551.

[ix] Chung CP, Avalos I, Raggi P, et al. "Atherosclerosis and inflammation: Insights from Rheumatoid Arthritis." *Clin Rheumatol.* 2007; 26(8):1228-33.

[x] Sanchez, Albert, JL Reeser, HS Lau, PY Yahiku, et al. "Role of Sugars in Human Neutrophilic Phagocytosis." *Am J Clin Nutr* 1973; 26: 1180-1184.

[xi] Lee DH, Folsom AR, Harnack L, et al. "Does supplemental Vitamin C Increase Cardiovascular Disease Risk in Women with diabetes?" *J of Clin Nutr* 2004; Nov80(5): 1194-1200.

[xii] Ryan, George, and Julius Torelli. Beyond Cholesterol: *7 Life- Saving Heart Disease Tests That Your Doctor May Not Give You (Lynn Sonberg Books).* New York, New York: St. Martin's Griffin, 2005.

[xiii] Liao F, Li Z, Wang Y, Shi B, et al. "Porphyromonas gingivalis may play an important role in the pathogenesis of periodontitis-associated rheumatoid arthritis." *Med Hypotheses* 2009; Jun72(6):732-5.

[xiv] Kleinewietfeld, M, Manzel A, Titze J, et al. "Sodium chloride drives autoimmune disease by the induction of pathogenic TH17 cells." *Nature* 2013; Apr(496), 518–522.

## CHAPTER THREE
## WHAT'S THE HEART GOT TO DO, GOT TO DO WITH IT?

[i] Czerniuk MR, Górska R, Filipiak KJ, et al. "Inflammatory Response to Acute Coronary Syndrome in Patients With Coexistent Periodontal Disease." *J Periodontol* 2004; 75(7):1020-1026.

[ii] Loos BG. "Systemic Markers of Inflammation in Periodontitis." *J Periodontal* 2005; 76(11-s) 2106-2115.

[iii] "Inflammation, Heart Disease and Stroke: The Role of C-Reactive Protein." American Heart Association; Learn and Live. www.americanheart.org/presenter.jhtml?identifier=4648 (Accessed July 3, 2009).

[iv] Ibid.

[v] "MedlinePlus Medical Encyclopedia." National Library of Medicine - National Institutes of Health. "C-Reactive Protein" http://www.nlm.nih.gov/medlineplus/ency/article/003356. htm (accessed June 20, 2009).

[vi] Lopez-Garcia E. "Consumption of Trans Fatty Acids Is related to Plasma Biomarkers of Inflammation and Endothelial Dysfunction." *The Journal of Nutrition.* 2005; 135(3) 562-566.

[vii] Zhou N, Pan H, Chen H. "Periodontal diseases and elevated serum high-sensitivity-reactive protein." Paper presented to the International Association of Dental Research. Miami, FL April 4, 2009. http://iadr.confex.com/iadr/2009miami/webprogram/ Paper117258.html (Accessed January 1, 2009).

[viii] Ridker PM, Pare G, Parker A, et al. "Loci related to metabolic syndrome pathways including LEPR, HNF1A, IL6R, and GCKR associate with plasma C-reactive protein: The Women's Genome Health Study." *Am J Hum Genet.* 2008; 82(5):1185-1192.

[ix] Kolata, Gina. "Substance Thought to Cause Heart Disease Doesn't, Study Finds - NYTimes.com." The New York Times - Breaking News, World News & Multimedia. http:// www.nytimes.com/2009/07/01/health/01heart.html (accessed July 2, 2009).

[x] Seymour GJ, Ford PJ, Gemmell E. "Infection or Inflammation: The Link Between Periodontal Disease and Systemic Disease." *Future Cardiology.* 2009; 5(1):5-9. http://www. medscape.com/viewarticle/587591 (Accessed June 20, 2009)

[xi] Geerts S, Legrand V, Charpentier J, et al. "Further Evidence of the Association Between Periodontal Conditions and Coronary Artery Disease" *J Periodontol* 2004; 75(9):1274-1280.

[xii] Pucar A, Milasin J, Lekovic V, et al. "Correlation Between Atherosclerosis and Periodontal Putative Pathogenic Bacterial Infections in Coronary and Internal Mammary Arteries." *J Periodontal.* 2007; 78(4): 677-682.

[xiii] Angiogenesis Foundation – *"Understanding Angiogenesis."* Angiogenesis Foundation. http://www.angio.org/ua.php (accessed June 3, 2007).

[xiv] Brodala N, Merricks EP, Bellinger DA, et al. *"Porphyromonas gingivalis* Bacteremia Induces Coronary and Aortic Athersclerosis in Normocholesterolemic and Hypercholesterolemic Pigs." *Arteriosclerosis, Thrombosis, and Vascular Biology.* 2005; 24:1446.

[xv] Kanh XL, Laflamme C, Rouabhla M, *"Porphromonas gingivalis* decreases osteoblast proliferation through IL-6-RANKL/OPG and MMP-9.TMPs pathways" *Indian Journal of Dental Research.* 2009; 20(2):141–149.

[xvi] "Inflammation, Heart Disease and stroke: The Role of C-Reactive Protein." American Heart Association; Learn and Live. www.americanheart.org/presenter. jhtml?identifier=4648 (Accessed July 3, 2009).

[xvii] Ford PJ, Gemmell E, Hamlet SM, et al. "Cross-reactivity of GroEL antibodies with human heat shock protein 60 and quantification of pathogens in atherosclerosis." *Oral Microbiol Immunol.* 2005; Oct; 20(5): 296-302.

[xviii] McGuire MK, Nunn ME. "Prognosis versus actual outcome. IV. The effectiveness of clinical parameters and IL-1 genotype in accurately predicting prognosis and tooth survival." *J Periodontol 1999.* 70:49–56.

[xix] Meisel, P, Schwahn, C, Gesch, D, et al. "Dose-Effect Relation of Smoking and the Interleukin-1 Gene Polymorphism in Periodontal Disease." *J Periodontal* 2004; 75(2): 236-242.

[xx] Bartold PM, Marshall RI, Haynes DR. "Periodontitis and Rheumatoid Arthritis: A Review." *J Periodontal.* 2005; 76(11-s,) 2066-2074.

[xxi] Quappe L, Jara L. Lopez N, "Association of Interleukin-1 Polymorphisms With Aggressive Periodontitis." *J Periodontol* 2004;75(11):1509-1515.

[xxii] Salvi GE, Yalda B. Collins JG, et al. "Inflammatory mediator response as a potential risk marker for periodontal disease in insulin-dependent diabetes mellitus patients." *J Investigative Dermatology* 2004; 123:87-92. http://www.nature.com/jid/journal/v123/n1/full/5602396a.html. (accessed July 8, 2007)

[xxiii] Geerts SO, Nys M, DeMol P, et al. "Systemic release of endotoxins induced by gentle mastication: association with periodontitis severity." *J Periodontal.* 2002; 73(1): 73-78.

[xxiv] Guntheroth WG, "How important are dental procedures as a cause of infective endocarditis?" *Am J Cardiol.* 1984; 54(7): 797-801.

[xv] Pallasch TJ, Slots J. "Antibiotic prophylaxis and the medically compromised patient." *J Periodontol* 2000 1996;10:107-138.

[xxvi] Bender IB, Naidorf IJ, Garvey GJ. "Bacterial endocarditis: a consideration for physician and dentist." *J Am Dent Assoc* 1984;109(3):415-420.

## CHAPTER FOUR
## STROKE/CAROTID ARTERY DISEASE

[i] Friedlander AH, Altman L. "Carotid artery atheromas in postmenopausal women: Their prevalence on panoramic radiographs and their relationship to atherogenic risk factors." *Journal of the American Dental Association* 2001;132(8):1130-1136.

[ii] Desvarieux M, Demmer RT, Rundek T, et al. "Periodontal microbiota and carotid intima-media thickness: the Oral Infections and Vascular Disease Epidemiology Study (INVEST)." *Circulation.* 2005; 111: 576–582. http://circ.ahajournals.org/cgi/content/full/circulationaha;111/5/576. (accessed July12, 2007)

[iii] Engebretson SP, Lamster IB, Elkind MSV, et al. "Radiographic Measures of Chronic Periodontitis and Carotid Artery Plaque." *Stroke* 2005; 36(3): 561 - 566.

[iv] Schillinger T, Kluger W, Exner M, et al. "Dental and Periodontal Status and Risk for Progression of Carotid Atherosclerosis: The Inflammation and Carotid Artery Risk for Atherosclerosis Study Dental Substudy." *Stroke*, September 1, 2006; 37(9): 2271 - 2276.

[v] Brodala N, Merricks EP, Bellinger DA, et al. "Porphyromonas gingivalis Bacteremia Induces Coronary and Aortic Atherosclerosis in Normocholesterolemic and Hypercholesterolemic Pigs." *Arteriosclerosis, Thrombosis, and Vascular Biology.* 2005; 25(7): 1446-1451.

## CHAPTER FIVE
## DIABETES AS AN ACCELERATED AGING MODEL

[i] dePommereau V, Dargent-Pare C Robert JJ. et al. "Periodontal Status in Insulin-dependent Diabetic Adolescents." *J Clin Periodontal.* 1992; Oct19(9 Pt 1): 628-632.

[ii] Gusberti FA, Syed SA, Bacon G, et al. "Puberty Gingivitis in Insulin-dependent Diabetic Children. I. CrossSectional Observations." *J Periodontal.* 1983; 54(12): 714–20.

[iii] Gislen G, Nilsson DO, Matsson L. "Gingival Inflammation in Diabetic Children related to Degree of Metabolic Control." *Acta Odontol Scand.* 1980; 38(4): 241-6.

[iv] Gojka R, Unwin DM, Bennet PH, et al. "The Burden of Mortality Attributable to Diabetes. Estimates for the year 2000." *Diabetes Care* 2005; 28: 2130-2135.

[v] Ryan ME, Carnu O, Kamer A. "The Influence of Diabetes on the Periodontal Tissues." *J Am Dent Assoc.* 2003; 134(Suppl 1) 34S-40S. (accessed June 21, 2009)

[vi] Chilton, Floyd. *Inflammation Nation: The First Clinically Proven Eating Plan to End Our Nation's Secret Epidemic.* New York: Fireside, 2005.

[vii] Shoelson S, Jongsoon L, Goldfine S. "Inflammation and insulin resistance." *J Clin Invest* 2006; Jul 3;116(7): 1793-1801 .http://www.jci.org/articles/view/29069/version/1 (accessed July 26, 2009).

[viii] Coppari R, Ichinose M, Lee C, e al. "The hypothalamic arcuate nucleus: A key site for mediating leptin's effects on glucose homeostasis and locomotor activity." *Cell Metabolism.*2009;1(1): 63- 72.

[ix] Hekerman P, Zeidler J, Korfmacher S, et al. "Leptin induces inflammation-related genes in RINm5F Insulinoma Cells." *BMC Molec Bio.* 2007; 41(8). http://www.biomedcentral.com/1471-2199/8/41 (Accessed July 26, 2009).

[x] Ibid.

[xi] Meigs JB, Jacques PF, Selhub J, Singer DE, et al. "Fasting plasma homocysteine levels in the insulin resistance syndrome: the Framingham offspring study." Diabetes Care. 2001 Aug;24(8):1403-10.

[xii] Meigs JB, Mittelmann MA, Nathan DM, et al. "Hyperinsulinemia, hyperglycemia, and impaired hemostasis. The Framingham Offspring Study." JAMA. 2000; 283:221-228.

[xiii] Chen, Shen-Song, Yiqun Zhang, and Tammy Santomango. "Glucagon chronically impairs hepatic and muscle glucose disposal." AJP - *Endocrinology and Metabolism.* 292 (3): E928 AJP - Endocrinology and Metabolism. http://ajpendo.physiology.org/cgi/content/full/292/3/E928 (Accessed July 26, 2009).

[xiv] Preedy VR, Garlick PJ. "The effect of glucagon administration on protein synthesis in skeletal muscles, heart and liver in vivo." *Biochem J.* 1985; June 15; 228(3): 575–581.

[xv] Anderson CCP, Flyvbjerg A, Buschard K, et al. "Periodontitis Is Associated with Aggravation of Prediabetes in Zucker Fatty Rats."*Journal of Perio.* 2007; 78, (3): 559-565.

[xvi] Engebretson SP, Hey-Hadavi J, Ehrhardt FJ, et al. "Gingival crevicular fluid levels of interleukin-1, and glycemic control in patients with chronic periodontitis and type 2 diabetes." *J Periodontal.* 2004; 75(9): 1203-1208.

[xvii] Salvi Ge, Yalda B, Collins JG, et al. "Inflammatory mediator response as a potential risk marker for periodontal disease in insulin-dependent diabetes mellitus patients." *J Periodontal.* 1997; 68(2): 127-135.

[xviii] Ibid.

[xix] Duarte PM, de Oliveira MCG, Tambeli CH, et al. "Overexpression of interleukin-1-beta and interleukin-6 may play an important role in periodontal breakdown in type 2 diabetic patients." *J Periodontal Res.* 2007; Aug42(4): 377-81.

[xx] Manouchehr-Pour M, Spagnuolo PJ, Rodman HM, et al. "Comparison of neutrophil chemotactic response in diabetic patients with mild and severe periodontal disease." *J Dent Res* 1981; 60(3):729-30.

[xxi] Mcmullen JA, Van Dyke TE, Horoszewicz HU, et al. "Neutrophil chemotaxis in individuals with advanced periodontal disease and a genetic predisposition to diabetes mellitus." *J Periodontal*, 1981; 52(4):167-173.

[xxii] Ficara AJ, Levin MP, Grower, MF, et al. "A comparison of the glucose and protein content of gingival fluid from diabetics and nondiabetics." *J Periodontal Res.* 1975: Jul10(3):171-175.

[xxiii] Nishimura F, Takahashi K, Kurihara M, et al. "Periodontal Disease as a Complication of Diabetes Mellitus." *Ann Periodontal.* 1998;3(1):20-29.

[xxiv] Liu R, Bal HS, Desta T, et al. "Diabetes Enhances Periodontal Bone Loss through Enhanced Resorption and Diminished Bone Formtion." *J Dent Res.* 2006: 85(6): 510-14.

[xxv] He H, Liu R, Desta T. et al. "Diabetes Casuses Decreased Osteoclastogenesis, Reduced Bone Formation, And Enhanced Apoptosis of Osteoblastic Cells in Bacteria Stimulated Bone Loss." *Endocrinology.* 2004: 145(1): 447-452.

[xxvi] Peppa M, Uribarri J, Vlassara H. "Glucose, Advanced Glycation End Products, and Diabetes Complications: What Is New and What Works." *Clinical Diabetes.* 2003: Oct 21(4): 186-187.

[xxvii] Ren X, Shao H, Wei Q, et al. "Advanced Glycation End-Products Enhance Calcification in Vascuar Smooth Muscle Cells." *The Journal of International Medical Research.*2009; 37:847-854. http://docserver.ingentaconnect.com/deliver/connect/field/03000605/v37n3/s29.pdf?expires=1250487834&id=51637127&titleid=75001442&accname=Guest+User&checksum=5A9AC72FAE8C22D7167129CCB67AF90B (Accessed August 16, 2009.)

[xxviii] Peppa M, Uribarri J, Vlassara H. "Glucose, Advanced Glycation End Products, and Diabetes Complications: What Is New and What Works." *Clinical Diabetes.* 2003: Oct 21(4): 186-187. .

[xxix] Vlassara H, Cai W, Crandall J, et al. *Proc Natl Acad Sci U.S.A.* 2003: Nov 26;99(24):15596-601.

[xxx] Viguet-Carrin S, Garner P, Delmas PD. "The role of collagen in bone strength." *Osteoporos Int.*2006;17(3):319-36.

[xxxi] Schmidt AM, Hori O, Brett J, et al. "Cellular receptors for advanced glycation end products. Implications for Induction of Oxidant Stress and Cellular Dysfunction in the Pathogenesis of Vascular Lesions." *Arterioscler Thromb.* 1994;Oct14(10): 1521-1528.

[xxxii] Schmidt AM, Hori O, Cao R, et al. "RAGE: A novel cellular receptor for advanced glycation end products." *Diabetes.* 1996; Jul45(supl 3): S77-80.

[xxiii] Vlassara H, Bucala R. "Recent progress in advanced glycation and diabetic vascular disease: role of advanced glycation end product receptors." *Diabetes.* 1996; 45(supl 3): S65-S66.

[xxxiv] Taylor GW, Burt BA, Becker MP, et al. "Severe periodontitis and risk for poor glycemic control in patients with non-insulin-dependent diabetes mellitus." *J Periodontol.* 1996; Oct67(10 suppl): 1085-1093.

[xxxv] Sammalkorpi K. "Glucose intolerance in acute infections." *J Intern Med.* 1989; 225(1): 15-19.

xxxvi Yki-Jarvinen H, Sammalkorpi K, Koivisto VA, et al. "Severity, duration, and mechanisms of insulin resistance during acute infections." *J Clin Endocrinol Metab.* 1989; Aug69(2): 317-323.

xxxvii Grossi SG, Skrepcinski FB, DeCaro T, et al. "Response to periodontal therapy in diabetics and smokers." *J Periodontal.* 1996; Oct67(10 suppl); 1094-1102.

xxxiii Grossi SG, Skrepcinski FB, DeCaro T, et al. "Treatment of periodontal disease in diabetics reduces glycated hemoglobin." *J Periodontal.* 1997; 68(8): 713-719.

xxxix Kiran M, Arpak N, Unsal E, et al. "The effect of improved periodontal health on metabolic control in type 2 diabetes mellitus." *J Clin Periotontol.* 2005; 32(3): 266-272.

xl Pontes Anderson CC, Flyvbjerg A, Buschard K, et al. "Periodontitis Is Associated With Aggravation of Prediabetes in Zucker Fatty Rats." *J Periodontal.* 2007; 78(3): 559-565. Pontes Anderson CC, Flyvbjerg A, Buschard K, and et al. "Lessons From Rodent Studies." *J Periodontal.* 2007; 78(7); 1264- 1275.

xli "Linus Pauling Institute at Oregon State University." Micronutrient Information Center. http://lpi.oregonstate.edu/infocenter/minerals/chromium/ (Accessed July 12, 2009).

xlii Ibid.

xliii Ibid.

xliv Prada PO, Hirabara SM, deSouza CT, et al. "L-glutamine supplementation induces insulin resistance in adipose tissue and improves insulin signaling in liver and muscle of rats with diet induced obesity."*Diabetologia.* 2007; 50(9): 1949-59.

xlv"Effects of Omega-3 Fatty Acids on Lipids and Glycemic Control in Type 2 diabetes and the Metabolic Syndrome and on Inflammatory Bowel Disease, Rheumatoid Arthritis, Renal Disease, Systemic Lupus Erythematosus, and Osteoporosis: Summary of Evidence Report." Agency for Health care Research and Quality (AHRQ) Home Page. http://www.ahrq.gov/clinic/epcsums/o3lipidsum.htm (accessed July 11, 2009)

xlvi Johnston CS, Kim CM, Buller AJ. "Vinegar Improves Insulin Sensitivity to a High-Carbohydrate Meal in Subjects With Insulin Resistance or Type 2 Diabetes." *Diabetes Care.* 2004; 27(1): 281-282.

xlvii Ogawa N, Satsu H, Watanabe H, et al. "Acetic acid suppresses the increase in disacchatidase activity that occurs during culture of Caco-2 cells." *J Nutr* 2000; 130(3): 507-513.

xlviii Fushimi T, Tayama K, Fukaya et al. "Acetic acid feeding enhances glycogen repletion in liver and skeletal muscle of rats." *J Nutr* 2001; 131(7): 1973-1977.

xlix Östman E, Granfeldt Y, Persson L, et al. "Vinegar supplementation lowers glucose and insulin responses and increases satiety after a bread meal in healthy subjects, by and colleagues." 2005; *Eur J Clin Nutr* 59(9):983–988, 2005.

l "Ayurvedic Interventions for Diabetes Mellitus: A Systematic Review: Summary of Evidence Report/Technology Assessment, No. 41." Agency for Health care Research and Quality (AHRQ) Home Page. http://www.ahrq.gov/clinic/epcsums/ayurvsum.htm (accessed July 11, 2009).

li Lee DH, Folsom AR, Harnack L, et al. "Does supplemental vitamin C increase cardiovascular disease risk in women with diabetes?" *American Journal of Clinical Nutrition,* 2004; Nov.80(5): 1194-1200.

lii Li S, Shin HJ, Ding, EL, et al. "Adiponectin Levels and Risk of Type 2 Diabetes." *JAMA.* 2009; 302(2): 179-188.

[liii] Geliebter A, Torbay N, Bracco EF. "Overfeeding with a diet of medium-chain triglycerides impedes accumulation of body fat."1980; *J Clinical Nutrition,* 33(4):921.

[liv] Geliebter A, Torbay N, Bracco EF, et al. "Overfeeding with medium-chain triglyceride diet results in diminished deposition of fat." *Am J Clin Nutr.*1983; Jan37(1):1-4.

## CHAPTER SIX
## WOMEN, SEX HORMONES, AND GUM DISEASE

[i] Machtei E, Mahler D, Sanduri H, et al. "The effect of Menstrual Cycle on Periodontal Health." *J Periodontol.* 2004; 75(3): Pages 408- 412.

[ii] Weinberg, MA, Maloney, WJ. "Periodontal Changes in Females." *US Pharm.* 2007; 32(9): 54-56.

[iii] Cavender JL, Murdoch WJ. "Morphological Studies of the Microcirculatory System of Periovulatory Ovine Follicles." *Biology of Reproduction,* 1988; 39: 989-997. http://www.biolreprod.org/cgi/reprint/39/4/989.pdf (Accessed May 10, 2007)

[iv] Ibid.

[v] Aiello, L, Avery RL, Arrigg PG, et al. "Vascular endothelial cell growth factor in ocular fluid of patients with diabetic retinopathy and other retinal disorders." *N. Engl. J. Med.* 1994; Dec331(22): 1480-1487.

[vi] Levin E, Rosen GF, Cassidenti D, et al. "Role of Vascular Endothelial Cell Growth Factor in Ovarian Hyperstimulation Syndrome." *J. Clin. Invest.* 1998; Dec102(11): 1978-1985.

[vii] Ashcroft GS, Dodsworth J, Boxtel, EV. et al. "Estrogen accelerates cutaneous wound healing associated with an increase in TGF-alpha- 1 levels." *Am J Pathol,* 1999; Oct155(4): 1137-1146.http://www.pubmedcentral.nih.gov/articlerender. fcgi?artid=1867002. (Accessed May 12, 2007)

[viii] Ibid.

[ix] Geurs NC, Lewis CE, Jeffcoat MK. "Osteoporosis and periodontal disease progression." *J Periodontol 2000.* 2003; 32:105-10.

[x] Ibid.

[xi] Levin E, Rosen GF, Cassidenti DL, et al. "Role of Vascular Endothelial Cell Growth Factor in Ovarian Hyperstimulation Syndrome." *J. Clin. Invest.* 1998; 102(11): 1978-1985.

[xii] Haytac C, Cetin T, Seydaoglu G. "The effects of ovulation induction during infertility treatment on gingival inflammation." *J Periodontol.* 2004; 75(6): 805-810.

[xiii] Offenbacher S, Katz Vern, Ferik G. "Periodontal infection as a possible risk factor I pre-term low birth weight." *J Periodontal* 1996; 67: 1103-3.

[xiv] Offenbacher S, Lieff S, Boggess KA, et al. "Maternal periodontitis and prematurity. Part I: Obstetric outcome of prematurity and growth restriction." *Ann Periodontol.* 2001; Dec6(1): 164-74.

[xv] Offenbacher S, Boggess KA, Murtha AP et al. "Progressive periodontal disease and risk of very pre-term delivery." Obstet Gynecol. 2006; 107(1): 29-36.

[xvi] Radnai M, Gorzo I, Urban E. et al. "Possible Association between mother's periodontal status and pre-term delivery." *J Clin Periodontal.* 2006; 33(11):791-6.

[xvii] Lopez NJ, Da Silva I, Ipinza et al. "Periodontal therapy reduces the rate of PT/LBW in women with pregnancy associated gingivitis." J.*N Engl J Med.* 2006 Nov 2;355(18):1885-94.

[xviii] Lin D, Moss K, Beck, JD et al. "Persistently High Levels of Periodontal Pathogens Associated With Pre-term Pregnancy Outcome" *J Periodontol.* 2007; 78(5): 833-841.

[xix] Hack M, Taylor, G, Drotar, D. et al. "Chronic Conditions, Functional Limitations, and Special Health Care Needs of Schoolaged Children Born With Extremely Low-Birth Weight in the 1990s." *JAMA.* 2005; Jul294(3)294:318-325.

[xx] Jeffcoat MK, Hauth JC, Geurs NC, et al. "Periodontal disease and pre-term birth: Results of a pilot intervention study." *J Periodontol.* 2003; 74(8): 1214–1218.

[xxi] López NJ, Patricio Smith PG, Gutierrez J. "Periodontal Therapy May Reduce the Risk of Pre-term Low Birth Weight in Women With Periodontal Disease: A Randomized Controlled Trial." *J Periodontol.* 2002; 73(8): 911-924.

[xxii] S. Offenbacher EL, Riché SP, Barros YA, et al. "Effects of Maternal Campylobacter rectus Infection on Murine Placenta, Fetal and Neonatal Survival, and Brain Development." *J Periodontol.* Nov2005, 76 (11-s): 2133-2143.

[xxiii] Barak S, Oettinger-Barak O, Machtei EE, et al. "Evidence of Periopathogenic Microorganisms in Placentas of Women With Preeclampsia" *J Periodontol.* 2007; 778(4): 670-676.

[xxiv] Bearfield C, Davenport ES, Sivapathasundaram V, et al. "Possible association between amniotic fluid micro-organism infection and microflora in the mouth." BJOG. 2002 May;109(5):527-33.

## CHAPTER SEVEN
## OSTEOPOROSIS: WOMEN – AND MATURE MEN – AT RISK!

[i] US Department of Health and Human Services; Office of the Surgeon General. "Bone Health and Osteoporosis: A Report of the Surgeon General." Rockville, MD: US Dept of Health and Human Sevices, Public Health Service, Office of he Surgeon General, 2004: Oct.

[ii] Randell A, Sambrook PN, Nguyen TV, et al. "Direct clinical and welfare costs of osteoporotic fractures in elderly men and women." *Osteoporos Int.* 1995; 5:427.

[iii] Kimmel, D. "Symposium on Bisphosphonate–Induced Bone Necrosis." *Journal of Oral and Maxillofacial Surgery.* Aug63(8 suppl 1): 16.

[iv] Ibid.

[v] Mendelsohn, ME, Karas, RH. "HRT and the Young At Heart." *N Engl J Med.* 2007; Jun356(25): 2639-2641.

[vi] Smith MR, "Selective Estrogen Receptor Modulators to Prevent Treatment-Related Osteoporosis." *Rev Urol.* 2005; 7(Suppl 3): S30– S35.

[vii] Chapin RE, Ku WW, McCoy H, et al. "The effects of dietary boron on bone strength in rats." *Fundam Appl Toxicol.*1997;Feb;35(2):205- 15.

[viii] Viguet-Carrin S, Garner P, Delmas PD. "The role of collagen in bone strength." *Osteoporos Int.*2006;17(3):319-36.

[ix] Jehle S, Zanetti A, Muser J, et al. "Partial neutralization of the acidogenic Western diet with potassium citrate increases bone mass in postmenopausal women with osteopenia." *J Am Soc Nephrol.* 2006; Nov17(11): 3213-3222.

[x] McLean RR, Jacques PF, Selhub, J, et al. "Homocysteine as a predictive factor for hip fracture in older persons." *New England Journal of Medicine* 2004; May13;350(20): 2042–2049.

[xi] van Meurs JB, Dhonukshe-Rutten R, Pluijm, S, et al. "Homocysteine Levels and the Risk of Osteoporotic Fracture." *New England Journal of Medicine.* 2004; May13;350(20): 2033-2041.

[xii] Lonn E, Yusuf S, Arnold MJ, et al. "Homocysteine Lowering with Folic Acid and B vitamins for Vascular Disease." *New England Journal of Medicine.* 2006; April13;354(15):1567-77

[xiii] "MedlinePlus ." National Library of Medicine - National Institutes of Health. http://www.nlm.nih.gov/medlineplus/ency/article/000318.htm (accessed June 1, 2007).

[xiv] Diem SJ, Blackwell TL, Stone KL, et all. "Use of Antidepressants and Rates of Hip Bone Loss in Older Women: The Study of Osteoporotic fractures." *Arch Intern Med* 2007;167(12):1240- 1245.

[xv] Busco M, Lie D. "SSRI Use in Older Women Linked to Accelerated Hip Bone Loss." *Arch Intern Med* 2007; 167(12)1240- 1245.

[xvi] Haney EM; Chan BKS, Diem SJ, et al. "Association of Low Bone Density with Selective Serotonin Reuptake Inhibitor Use by Older Men." 2007; *Arch Intern Med* 167(12):1246-1251.

[xvii] Yadav VK, Ryu JH, Suda N, et al. "Lrp5 Controls Bone formation by Inhibiting Serotonin Synthesis in the Duodenum." *Cell* 2008; 135(5): 8250837.

[xviii] Wactawski-Wende, J, Hausmann, Ernest, Hovey, K, et al. "The Association Between Osteoporosis and Alveolar Crestal Height in Postmenopausal Women." *J Periodontol.* 2005; 76(11-Suppl): 2116-2124.

[xix] Stepan, JJ, Alenfeld F, Boivin G, et al. "Mechanisms of Action of Antiresorptive Therapies of Postmenopausal Osteoporosis." *Endocr Regul.* 2003; 37, Dec37(4): 225-238.

[xx] Havemose-Poulson A, Wesergaard J, Stoltze K, et al. "Periodontal and Hematological Characteristics Associated With Aggressive Periodontitis, Juvenile Idiopathic Arthritis, and Rheumatoid Arthritis." *J Periodontal.* 2006; 77(2) 280-288.

[xxi] ADA Council on Scientific Affairs. "Dental Management of patients receiving oral bisphosphonate therapy. Expert panel recommendations." *JADA.* 2006; 137(8) 1144-1150.

[xxii] Anand G. "Jaw Ailment Shows Industry Moves Slowly on Drug Warnings." *Wall Street Journal.* December 8, 2004, B01 cxlvi Santini D, Caraglia M, Vincenzi B, et al. "Mechanisms of disease: Preclinical reports of antineoplastic synergistic action of bisphosphonates." *Nat Clin Pract Oncol.* 2006; 3(6): 325-38.

[xxiii] Santini D, Caraglia M, Vincenzi B, et al. "Mechanisms of disease: Preclinical reports of antineoplastic synergistic action of bisphosphonates." *Nat Clin Pract Oncol.* 2006; 3(6): 325-38.

[xxiv] Prasad, R. Ibanez, D, Gladman, D. "The role of non-corticosteroid related factors in osteonecrosis (ON) in systemic lupus erythematosus: a nested case-control study of inception patients." *Lupus.* 2007; 16(3): 157-162.

[xxv] Jin Q. Cirelli JA, Park CH, et al. "RANKL Inhibition Through Osteoprotegerin Blocks Bone Loss in Experimental Periodontitis." *J Periodontal.* 2007; 78(7): 1300-1308.

[xxvi] Meunier PJ, Roux C, Seeman E, et al. "The Effects of Strontium Ranelate on the Risk of Vertebral Fracture in women with Postmenopausal Osteoporosis." *NEJM.* 2004; Jan29; 350(5): 459-468.

[xxvii] Fogelman I, Blake GM. "Strontium Ranelate for the Treatment of Osteoporosis." *British Medical Journal.* 2005; June18;330:1400-1401.

[xxviii] O'Donnell S, Cranney A, Wells GA, et al. "Strontium Ranelate for Preventing and Treating Postmenopausal Osteoporosis." *Cochrane Database of Systematic Reviews* 2006;Issue 4. Art. No.: CD005326. DOI: 10.1002/14651858.CD005326.pub3. http://mrw.interscience.wiley.com/cochrane/clsysrev/articles/CD0053 26/frame.html. (Accessed July 5, 2009)

[xxix] Rodan GA, Martin TJ. "Therapeutic Approaches to Bone Diseases." *Science.* 2000; 289(5484): 1508-1514.

[xxx] Teronen O, Heikkila P, Konttinen YT, et al. "MMP inhibition and downregulation by bisphosphonates." *Ann NY Acad Sci.* 1999; 878(1): 453-465.

[xxxi] Sedghizadeh PP, Stanley K, Caligiuri, M, et al. "Oral bisphosphonate use and the prevalence of osteonecrosis of the jaw: an institutional inquiry." *J Am Dent Assoc.* 2009; 140(1): 61-66.

[xxxii] Ibid.

[xxxiii] Migliorati CA, Casiglia J, Epstein J, et al. "Managing the care of patients with bisphosphonate-associated osteonecrosis: An American Academy of Oral Medicine position paper." 2005; *J Am Dent Assoc* 136(12): 1658-1668.

[xxxiv] Marei MK, Saad, MM, El-Ashwah A, et al. "Experimental Formation of Periodontal Structure around Titanium Implants Utilizing Bone Marrow Mesenchymal Stem Cells: A Pilot Study." *J Oral Implantology.* 35(3): 106 – 129. http://www.allenpress.com/pdf/ORIM-35-3-106.pdf. (Accessed June 26, 2009)

[xxxv] Keller JC, Stewart M, Roehm M, et al. "Osteoporosis-like bone conditions affect osseointegration of implants." *Int J Oral Maxillofac Implants.* 2004; Sep-Oct19(5): 687-694.

[xxxvi] Basseri RJ, Basseri B, Chong K, Youdim A, Low K, Hwang LJ et al. "Intestinal methane production in obese humans is associated with higher body mass index." *Dig Dis Week* 2010; Abstr W1367.

[xxxvii] Larsen N, Vogensen FK, van den Berg FW, Nielsen DS, Andreasen AS, Pedersen BK et al. "Gut microbiota in human adults with type 2 diabetes differs from non-diabetic adults." *PLoS One* 2010; 5: e9085.

[xxxviii] Bell NH. "Renal and nonrenal 25-hydroxyvitamin D-1alpha-hydroxylases and their clinical significance." *J Bone Miner Res* 1998; 13: 350–353.

# CHAPTER EIGHT
## SMOKING INFLUENCES

[i] Tomar S, Asma S. "Smoking-Attributable Periodontitis in the United States: Findings from NHANESIII." *J Periodontol.* 2000; 71 (5): 743 – 751.

[ii] Johnson, GK, Hill, M. "Cigarette Smoking and the Periodontal Patient." *J Periodontol.* 2004; 75(2): 196-209.

[iii] Tomar S, Asma S. "Smoking-Attributable Periodontitis in the United States: Findings from NHANESIII." *J Periodontol.* 2000; 71(5): 743 – 751.

[iv] Kerdvongbundit V, Wikesjö U. "Prevalence and Severity of Periodontal Disease at Mandibular Molar Teeth in Smokers With Regular Oral Hygiene Habits." *J of Periodontol.* 2002; 73(7): 735- 740.

[v] McGuire MK, Nunn ME. "Prognosis versus actual outcome. III. "The effectiveness of clinical parameters in accurately predicting prognosis and tooth survival," *J Periodontol* 1996; 67(7):666-674.

[vi] Ibid.

[vii] Dietrich T, Bernimoulin Jean-Pierre, Glymn RJ. "The Effect of Cigareté Smoking on Gingival Bleeding." *J Periodontol.* 2004; 75(1) 16-22.

[viii] Meisel P, Schwahn C, Gesch D, et al. "Dose-Effect Relation of Smoking and the Interleukin-1 Gene Polymorphism in Periodontal Disease." *J Periodontal.* 2004;;75(2): 236-242.

[ix] Hanes PJ, Schuster GS, Lubas S. "Binding, Uptake, and Release of Nicotine by Human Gingival Fibroblasts." *J Periodontol.*1991; 62(2): 147-152.

[x] Tipton DA, Dabbous MK. "Effects of nicotine on proliferation and extracellular matrix production of human gingival fibroblasts in vitro." *J Periodontol* 1995; 66(12): 1056-1064.

[xi] James JA, Sayer, NM, Drucker DB. "Effects of Tobacco Products on the Attachment and Growth of Periodontal Ligament Fibroblasts." *J Periodontol.* 1999; 70(5): 518-525.

[xii] Guzzi G, Pigatto P, Ronchi A. "Periodontal Disease and Environmental Cadmium Exposure." *Environ Health Perspect.* 2009 December; 117(12): A535–A536.

[xiii] Position Paper: "Tobacco Use and the Periodontal Patient." *J Periodontal.* 1999; 70(11);1419-1427.

[xiv] Bostrom L, Linder LE, Bergstrom J. "Influence of smoking on the outcome of periodontal surgery. A 5-year follow-up." *J Clin Periodontol* 1998; 25(3):194-201. 75.

[xv] Erdemir EO, Nalcaci R, Caglayan O. "Evaluation of Systemic Markers Related to Anemia of Chronic Disease in the Peripheral Blood of Smokers and Non-Smokers with Chronic Periodontitis." *Eur J Dent.* 2008; 2: 102 – 109. http://www.pubmedcentral.nih.gov/articlerender.fcgi?artid=2633164 (accessed May 8, 2009)

[xvi] El-Ghorab N, Marzec N, Genco R, Dziak R. "Effect of nicotine and estrogen on IL-6 release from osteoblasts." *J Dent Res.* 1997; 76(Spec. Issue): 341.

[xvii] Pabst MJ, Pabst KM, Collier JA, et al. "Inhibition of neutrophil and monocyte defensive functions by nicotine." *J Periodontol.* 1995; 66(12):1047-1055.

[xviii] Payne JB, Johnson GK, Reinhardt RA, et al. "Nicotine effects on PGE2 and IL-1 Release by LPS-treated human monocytes." *J Periodont Res*1996; 31(2): 99-104.

[xix] Johnson GK, Organ CC. "Prostaglandin E2 and interleukin-1 levels in nicotine-exposed oral keratinocyte cultures." *J Periodont Res*1997; July32(5): 447-454.

[xx] Zambon JJ, Grossi SG, Machtei EE, et al. "Cigarette smoking increases the risk for subgingival infection with periodontal pathogens." *J Periodontol.*1996; 67(10-suppl):1050-1054.

[xxi] Zhang R, Brennan ML, Fu X, et al. "Association between myeloperoxidase levels and risk of coronary artery disease". *JAMA* 2001; 286(17): 2136–42. doi:10.1001/jama.286.17.2136. PMID 11694155.

xxii Nicholls SJ, Hazen SL. "Myeloperoxidase and cardiovascular disease". *Arterioscler. Thromb. Vasc. Biol.* 2005; 25(6):1102–11. doi:10.1161/01.ATV.0000163262.83456.6d. PMID 15790935.

## CHAPTER NINE
## ORAL CANCER

i Mager D, Haddad R, Wirth L, et al. "Oral Mucous Membrane Microbiota in Health and Oral Squamous Cell Carcinoma." *Grand Rounds in Oral-Systemic Medicine.*2007 2(3). http://www.dentaleconomics.com/display_article/296293/108/none/no ne/Oart/Oral Mucous Membrane Microbiota in Health and Oral Squamous Cell Carcinom?host=www.thesystemiclink.com. (Accessed August 6, 2009.)

ii Nosrat IV, Widenfalk J, Olson L. "Dental Pulp Cells Produce Neurotrophic Factors, Interact with Trigeminal Factors in Vitro, and Rescue Motoneurons after Spinal Cord Injury." *Dev Biol.* 2001; 238(1): 120-232.

iii Gandia C, Arminan, A., Garcia-Verdugo JM, et al. "Human Dental Pulp Stem Cells Improve Left Ventricular Function, Induce Angiogenesis, and Reduce Infarct Size in Rats with Acute Myocardial Infarction." *Stem Cells.* 2008; 26(3): 638645.

iv Mashberg A, Samit AM. "Early detection, diagnosis and management of oral and oropharyngeal cancer." *CA Cancer J Clin.* 1989; 39(2): 67-88.

v Shiboski CH, Shiboski SC, Silverman S. "Trends in oral cancer rates in the United States, 1973-1996."*Community Dent Oral Epidemiol.*2000;28(4):249-56.

vi Blot WJ, McLaughlin JK, Winn DM et al. "Smoking and Drinking in Relation to Oral and Pharyngeal Cancer." *Cancer Res.* 1988; June 1;48(11):3282-3287.

vii Rodriguez T, Altieri A, Chatenoud L, et al. "Risk factors for oral and pharyngeal cancer in young adults." *Oral Oncol,* 2004; 40(2): 207-13.

viii Blot WJ, McLaughlin JK, Winn DM et al. "Smoking and Drinking in Relation to Oral and Pharyngeal Cancer." *Cancer Res.* 1988; June 1;48(11): 3282-3287.

ix Castellsague X, Quintana MF, Martinez MC, et al. "The role of type of tobacco and type of alcoholic beverage in oral carcinogenesis."*Int J Cancer .*2004; 108(5): 741-749.

x "Smokeless Tobacco and Cancer: Q & A - National Cancer Institute." National Cancer Institute - Comprehensive Cancer Information. http://www.cancer.gov/cancertopics/ factsheet/Tobacco/smokeless (accessed June 17, 2007)

xi D'Souza, G, Kreimer, AR, Viscidi, R, et al. "Case-Control Study of Human Papillomavirus and Oropharyngeal Cancer." *N Engl J Med* 2007; May 10;356(19):1944-1956.

xii Perea-Milla Lopez E, Minarro-Del Moral RM, Martinez-Garcia C, et al. "Lifestyles, environmental and phenotypic factors associated with lip cancer: a case-control study in southern Spain." *Br J Cancer,* 2003; 88(11):1702-1707.

xiii Wirthlin R, Ahn BJ, Enriquez B, Hussain MZ. "Effects of stabilized chlorine dioxide and chlorhexidine mouthrinses in vitro cells involved in periodontal healing." *Periodontal Abstracts, The Journal of the Western Society of Periodontology.* 2006; 54(3).

xiiiKey TJ, Schatzkin A, Willet WC,et al. "Diet, nutrition and the prevention of cancer." *Public Health Nutr.* 2004; Feb7(1A): 187-200. cxci Ghadiran P. "Thermal irritation and esophageal cancer in northern Iran." *Cancer.*1987;60(8):1909-14.

[xiv] Ghadiran P. "Thermal irritation and esophageal cancer in northern Iran." Cancer.1987;60(8):1909-14.

[xv] Hitti, Miranda. "Study: Drinking Too-Hot Tea May Raise Esophageal Cancer Risk." WebMD - Better information. Better health. http://www.webmd.com/cancer/news/20090326/hot-tea-mayraise-esophageal-cancer-risk (accessed October 7, 2009).

[xvi] Wirthlin R, Ahn BJ, Enriquez B, et al. "Effects of stabilized chlorine dioxide and chlorhexidine mouthrinses in vitro cells involved in periodontal healing." *Periodontal Abstracts, The Journal of the Western Society of Periodontology.* 2006; 54(3).

[xvii] Mariotti AJ, Rumpf DA."Chlorhexidine-induced changes to human gingival fibroblast collagen and non-collagen protein production." *J Periodontol.* 1999 Dec;70(12):1443-8.

[xviii] Flemingson, Emmadi P, Ambalavanan N, et al."Effect of three commercial mouth rinses on cultured human gingival fibroblast: an in vitro study." *Indian J Dent Res.* 2008 Jan-Mar;19(1):29-35.

[xix] Murray AD; Kidby DK (Dept. of Microbiology, College of Biological Science, University of Guelph, Guelph, Ontario, Canada.); "Sub-cellular Location of Mercury in Yeast Grown in the Presence of Mercuric Chloride." *Journal of General Microbiology.* 1975; 86:66-74;

[xx] Tezal M, Sullivan, MA, Reid ME, et al. "Chronic Periodontitis and the Risk of Tongue Cancer." *Arch Otolaryngol Head Neck Surg.* 2007; 133: 450-454.

[xxi] Fox M, Trot B. "Gum disease may raise cancer risk" http://uk.reuters.com/article/id (Accessed October 13, 2009)

[xxii] Thomson CD, Chisholm A, McLachlan SK, et al. "Brazil Nuts: An Effective Way to Improve Selenium Status." *Am J Clin Nutr.* 2008; 87(2): 379-84.

[xxiii] Autier P, Gandini S. "Vitamin D Supplementation and TotalMortality." *Arch Intern Med.* 2007; 167(16): 1730-1737.

[xxiiv] "Mouthwash Cancer Test" Medport World Wide News. http://medport.jp/wwn.php?layout=topic_story&newsno=39599 (accessed June 11, 2007)

[xxv] Wang J, Henry S, Yu T, et al. "Salivary Oral Cancer Transcriptome Biomarkers (SOCTB) for Clinical Detection." In: *Proc Amer Assoc Cancer Res*; 2006 Mar 8-11; Orlando, FLA: AACR; 2006. Abstract Number: 4468.

## CHAPTER TEN
## KIDNEY TRANSPLANTS

[i] Fisher MA, Taylor GW. "A Prediction Model for Chronic Kidney Disease Includes Periodontal Disease." *J Periodontol.* 2009:80(1): 16-23. http://www.joponline.org/doi/pdf/10.1902/jop.2009.080226 (Accessed Septermber 26, 2009.)

[ii] Pontes Anderson CC, Holmstrup P, Buschard K, et al. "Renal Alterations in Prediabetic Rats wit Periodontitis." *J Periodontol.* 2008;79(4): 6840689.

[iii] Fisher MA, Taylor GW, Papapanou PN, et al. "Clinical and serologic markers of periodontal infection and chronic kidney disease." *J Periodontol*; 2008; Sep;79(9): 1617-9. http://www.ncbi.nlm.nih.gov/pubmed/18771368?ordinalpos=1&itool=EntrezSystem2.PEntrez.Pubmed.Pubmed_ResultsPanel.Pubmed_RV Abstract (Accessed September 25, 2009)

[iv] Borawski J, Wilczyska-Borawska M, Stokowska W, et al. "The periodontal status of pre-dialysis chronic kidney disease and maintenance dialysis patients." *Nephrol. Dial. Transplant.* Nov. 23, 2006. http://ndt.oxfordjournals.org/cgi/citmgr?gca=ndt;gfl676v1 (Accessed September 25, 2009.)

[v] Šedý J, Horká E, Foltán R , et al. "Mechanism of increased mortality in hemodialysed patients with periodontitis." *Medical Hypotheses.* 2009; June 24. http://uem.avcr.cz/miranda2/export/sitesavcr/data.avcr.cz/lifesci/uem/research/publications/neuroscience/files/sedy-2010-med-hypothese.pdf (Accessed September 25, 2009)

[vi] Szezech L, Lazar I. "Projecting the United States ESRDpopulation: issues regarding treatment of patients with ESRD." *Kidney Int Suppl.* Sept2004; 66 (Suppl 90)S3-S7. ccv

[vii] Shultis WA, Weil EF, Looker H, et al. "Effects of Periodontitis on Overt Nephropathy and End-State Renal Disease in Type 2 Diabetes." *Diabetes Care* 2007; 30(12): 306-311. ccvi Bansal R, Tiwari SC. "Back Pain in Chronic Renal Failure." *Nephrology Dialysis Transplantation.* 2006; 21(8):2331-2332.

[viii] Shultis WA, Weil EF, Looker H, et al. "Effects of Periodontitis on Overt Nephropathy and End-State Renal Disease in Type 2 Diabetes." *Diabetes Care.* 2007; 30(12): 306-311.

[ix] Bansal R, Tiwari SC. "Back Pain in Chronic Renal Failure." *Nephrology Dialysis Transplantation.* 2006; 21(8):2331-2332.

[x] Ayoob S, Gupta AK. "Fluoride in Drinking Water: A Review on the Status and Stress Effects." *Critical Reviews in Environmental Science and Technology* 2006; Dec36(6): 433-487.

[xii] National Research Council/National Academy of Sciences. "Fluoride in Drinking Water: A Scientific Review of EPA's Standards." *National Academies Press, Washington D.C.* 2006; 140.

[xiii] "Hyperkalemia." *eMedicine from WebMD* Garth, D. Updated Feb 20, 2007. http://www.emedicine.com/emerg/topic261.htm (Accessed Nov. 2, 2008)

[xiv] Ioannidou E, Kao D, Chang N, et al. "Elevated Serum Interleukin-6 (IL-6) in Solid-Organ Transplant Recipients is Positively Associated With Tissue Destruction and IL-6 Gene Expression in the Periodontium." *Journal of Perio.* 2006;77(11):1871-1878.

[xv] Fisher MA, Taylor GW, Shelton BJ, et al. "Periodontal Disease and Other Nontraditional Risk Factors for CKD." *Am J Kidney Dis.* 2008 Jan; 51(1):45-52.

## CHAPTER TWELVE
## THE SECRET: BEAUTY, BRAINS, AND BODY BALANCE

[i] McKeown, P. "Close Your Mouth; Buteyko Breathing Clinic Self Help Manual." Buteyko Books. 2004. page 30.

[ii] Timms DJ. "Rapid maxillary expansion in the treatment of nocturnal enuresis." *Angle Orthod.* 1990 Fall;60(3):229-33; discussion 234.

[iii] Samuels, C.A. & Elwy, R. "Aesthetic perception of faces during infancy". *British Journal of Psychology.* 1985; 3:221-228.

[iv] Bull, R. & Rumsey, N. "The social psychology of facial appearance." *Springer-Verlag,* New York. 1988.

[v] Cavior H , Hayes S, Cavior N. "Physical attractiveness of female offenders." *Criminal Justice and Behavior.* 1974; 1:321-331.

[vi] Lewison, E. "Twenty years of prison surgery: An evaluation." *Canadian Journal of Otolaryngology.* 1974; 3:42-50.

[vii] Ackerman, D. "A natural history of the senses." Cornell University. 1990. Knopf Doubleday Publishing. 1991.

[viii] Barsh, L. "The Origin of Pharyngeal Obstruction During Sleep." *Sleep and Breathing.* 1999; 3(1):17-21.

[ix] Myofunctional Research Co. "Soft Tissue Dysfunction Videos." Myofunctional Research Co.. N.p., n.d. Web. 25 Apr. 2011. <http://www.myoresearch.com/cms/index. php?id=153,215,0,0,1,0>.

[x] Jefferson, Y. "Mouth breathing: Adverse effects on facial growth, health, academics, and behavior." *Gen Dent.* 2010; 58(1):18-25.

[xi] Harvold, E, Chierici, G. and Vargervik, K. "Experiments on the development of dental malocclusion." *American Journal of Orthodontics.* 1972; 61:38-44.

[xii] Chervin, RD, et al. "Symptoms of sleep disorders, inattention, and hyperactivity in children." *Sleep.* 1997; 20(12):1185-1192.

[xiii] Ibid.

[xiv] Bat-Chen Friedman et al. "Adenotonsillectomy Improves Neurocognitive Function in Children with OSAS." *Sleep.* 2003; 26(8):999-1005.

[xv] Sun Z, Sun X, Wang W, et al. "Anti-Inflammatory effects of inhaled nitric oxide are optimized at lower oxygen concentration in experimental Klebsiella pneumoniae pneumonia." *Inflammation Research.* 2006. 55(10):430-440. DOI: 10.1007/s00011-006-6029-7

[xvi] Inoue M, Sate IF, Nishikawa M, et al. "Cross talk of nitric oxide, oxygen radicals, and superoxide dismutase regulates the energy metabolism and cell death and determines the fates of aerobic life." *Antioxid Redox Signal.* 2003 Aug;5(4):475-84.

[xvii] Ibid.

[xviii] McVeigh GE, Allen PB, Morgan DR, et al. "Nitric oxide modulation of blood vessel tone identified by arterial waveform analysis." *Clin. Science* (2001) 100, 387–393.

[xix] Farsi N, Salama F, Pedro C. "Sucking Habits in Saudi children: prevalence, contributing factors, and effects on the primary dentition." *Pediatr Dent* 1997;19(1):28-33.

[xx] Durmer, J et al. "Pediatric Sleep Medicine." *American Academy of Neurology Continuum.* 2007; 153-200. Cleveland Clinic Journal of Medicine. 2007 74:1.

[xxi] Hung, Whitford, Hillman, et al. "Association of sleep apnoea with myocardial infarction in men." *The Lancet.* 336, (8710):261-264. Jefferson, Y. "Mouth breathing: adverse effects on facial growth, health, academics, and behavior." *Gen Dent.* 2010; 58(1):18-25.

[xxii] Singh, GD, Keropian B., Pillar G. "Effects of the full breath solution appliance for the treatment of obstructive sleep apnea: a preliminary study." *Cranio.* 2009 Apr;27(2):109-17.

[xxiii] Puhan MA, Suarez A, LoCascio CL, et al. "Didgeridoo playing as alternative treatment for obstructive sleep apnoea syndrome: randomised controlled trial." BMJ. 2006;332:266.

## CHAPTER THIRTEEN:
## BEYOND THE DEATH SPIRAL: MODERN DENTISTRY 1908 – 1985

[i] Gutkowski S, DiGangi P, Harper M. "Economics of the Team Approach: How-to Guide for the Minimally Invasive Dental Practice." *Inside Dentistry*. 2009; 5(6).

[ii] No authors available. "The true cost of a cavity. When a little hole becomes a 2,000 dollar money pit." *Dent Today*. 2004; Oct 23(10):70.

[iii] Milicich G, Rainey JT. "Clinical Signs of Stress Distribution in Teeth and Significance in Operative Dentistry." *J Clin Pediatr Dent 1996;* 20(4):293-298.

[iv] Penning C, van Amerogen JP, et al. "Validity of probing, for fissure caries diagnosis." *Caries Res* 1993; 26(6):445-9.

[v] International Caries Detection and Assessment System Coordinating Committee. "Rationale and Evidence for the International Caries Detection and Assessment System (ICDAS III)." September 2005. Citing Ekstrand et al. 1987; Bergman and Linden, 1969.

[vi] Alsehaibany, White, and Rainey. "Caries Diagnosis and How to Use the Diagnodent". *J Clin Pediatr Dent* 1996; 20(4):293-298.

[vii] Ibid.

[viii] Ibid.

[ix] Ibid.

[x] 44 Magnum Caries by Tim Rainey, DDS

[xi] Futasuki M, Kubota K, et al. "Early loss of pit and fissure sealant: A clinical and SEM study." *J Clin Pediatr Dent* 1995; 19:99-104.

[xii] Simonsen RJ. 'Retention and effectiveness of dental sealant after 15 years." *JADA* 1991;122:34-42.

[xiii] Bravo M, Osorio E, Garcia-Anllo I, et al. "The Influence of dft Index on Sealant Success: A 48-month Survival Analysis." *J Dent Res 1996;* 75(2):768-774.

[xiv] Feigal RJ. "Sealants and preventive restorations: Review of effectiveness and clinical changes for improvement." *Pediatr Dent* 1998; 20:85-92.

[xv] Baysan, A., Whiley R. A., and Lynch E., 2000"Management of root caries using a novel ozone delivery system in vivo", submitted for publication)] Antimicrobial effect of a novel ozone- generating device on micro- organisms associated with primary root carious lesions in vitro, *Caries Res.* 34:498-501

[xvi] Holmes J. "Clinical reversal of root caries using ozone, double-blind, randomized, controlled 18-month trial." *Gerodontology* 2003; 20:106-114.

[xvii] Al Shamsi AH, Lynch E, Lamey PJ et al. "Influence of ozone on caries incidence around orthodontic brackets." *IADR Abstract 0604*, 2004.

[xviii] El Hadary A, Yassin H, Mekkhemer S, et al. "Evaluation of Ozonated Oils on Osseointegration of Dental Implants under the Influene of cyclosporinA: An In Vivo Study." *J Oral Implantol.* 2011; 37(2): 247-257.

[ixx] Ripamonti CI, Cislaghi C, Mariani L, et al. "Efficacy and safety of medical ozone (O3) delivered in oil suspension applications for the treatment of osteonecrosis of the jaw in patients with bone metastases treated with bisphosphonates: Preliminary results of a phase I–II study." *Oral Oncology* 2011; 47: 185-190.

[xx] Filippi A. "The influence of ozonated water on the epithelial wound healing process in the oral cavity." *Proceedings of the 15th Ozone World Congress,* Medical Therapy Conference (IOA 2001, Ed.), Speedprint MacMedia Ltd, Ealing, London, UK, 11th-15th Sept 2001;109-116.

[xxi] F. Foschi, J. Izard, H. Sasaki, et al. "Treponema denticola in Disseminating Endodontic Infections." *J Dent Res* 2006 85:761. DOI: 10.1177/154405910608500814 2006 85: 761.

[xxii] Roggenkamp, Clyde. "Dentinal Fluid Transport." Loma Linda , Calif., Loma Linda Univ. Press, 2004. Reviews work of Ralph R Steinman, Professor Emeritus at Loma Linda University/Founder of Loma Linda Dental School.

[xxiii] Mondelli, Steagall, Ishikiriama, et al. "Fracture Strength of Human Teeth With Cavity Preparations." *Journ Pros Dent 1980;* 43(4):419-422.

[xxiv] Wentworth P, McDunn JE, Wentworth AD, et al. "Evidence for antibody-catalyzed ozone formation in bacterial killing and inflammation." *Science (Journal)* 2002; 298 (5601): 2195-9.

[xxv] Babior BM, Takeuchi C, Ruedi J, Gutierrez A, et al. "Investigating antibody-catalyzed ozone generation by human neutrophils." *Proc. Natl. Acad. Sci. U.S.A.* 2003; 100 (6): 3031-4.

[xxvi] Zimran A, Wasser G, Forman L, et al. "Effect of ozone on red blood cell enzymes and intermediates." *Acta Haematol.* 102(3): 148-51. 2000. http://www.ncbi.nlm.nih.gov/pubmed/10692679

[xxvii] Wentworth P, Nieva J, Takeuchi C, et al. "Evidence for ozone formation in human atherosclerotic arteries." *Science (Journal)*2003; 302 (5647): 1053-6.

[xviii] Rothchild, JA, Mollica P, Harris R. "Current Concepts of Oxygen Ozone Therapy for Dentistry in the United States." *International Journal of Ozone Therapy 2010;* 9: 105-108.

## CHAPTER FOURTEEN
## FOOD AS MEDICINE

[i] Chilton, Floyd H. *Inflammation Nation: The First Clinically Proven Eating Plan to End Our Nation's Secret Epidemic.* New York: Fireside, 2005.

[ii] Lehrer, Jim. "Online News Hour: Oprah Winfrey Vs. The Beef People; January 20,1998." PBS. http://www.pbs.org/newshour/bb/law/jan-june98/fooddef_1-20.html (Accessed July 3, 2009).

[iii] Sutton, Tracy. "Md. Poultry Farmer's Struggle Featured in New Film | Lancaster Farming." Lancaster Farming: Ephrata, PA | Lancaster Farming. http://www.lancasterfarming.com/node/2030 (accessed July 3, 2009).

[iv] Bouchez, Colette. "Skin Nutrition: Vitamins and Minerals for Your Skin." WebMD - Better information. Better health. http://www.webmd.com/skin-problems-and-treatments/features/skinnutrition (accessed October 4, 2009).

[v] Prior IA, Davidson F, Salmond CE, et al. "Cholesterol, coconuts, and diet on Polynesian atolls: a natural experiment: the Pukapuka and Tokelau Island studies." *Amer J of Clin Nut.* 1981; 34:1552-1561.

[vi] Kaunitz H, Dayrit CS. "Coconut oil consumption and coronary heart disease." *Philippine Journal of Internal Medicine*.1992; 30:165-171.

[vii] Biasi F, Mascia C, Poli G. "The Contribution of animal fat oxidation products to colon carcinogenesis, through modulation of TGF-Beta1 Signaling." *Carcinogenesis*. 2008; 29(5):890-894.

[viii] Das, Undurti. "Can essential fatty acids reduce the burden of disease(s)?"*Lipids Health Dis.* 2008;7:19 Published online 2008 May 20. doi: 10.1186/1476-511X-7-19. http://www.pubmedcentral.nih.gov/articlerender.fcgi?artid=2276500 (Accessed October 9, 2009)

[ix] Nielsen FH."Dietary fat composition modifies the effect of boron on bone characteristics and plasma lipids in rats." *BioFactors*.2004;20.161-171.

[x] Ellis EF, Police RJ, Dodson LY, et al. "Effect of dietary n-3 fatty acids on cerebral microcirculation.."*AM J Physiol.* 1992; May262(5 Pt 2): H1379-H1386.

[xi] de Wilde MC, Farkas E, Gerritis M, et al. "The effect of n-3 polyunsaturated fatty acid-rich diets on cognitive and cerebrovascular parameters in chronic cerebral hypoperfusion." *Brain Res.* 2002; Aug947(2): 166-173.

[xii] Ziylan ZY, Bernard GC, LeFamconnier JM, et al. "Effect of dietary n-3 fatty acid deficiency on blood-to-brain transfer of sucrose, alpha-aminoisobutyrie acid and phenylalamine in the rat." *Neurosci Lett* 1992; 137: 9-13.

[xiii] Logan AC. "Neurobehavioral aspects of omega-3 fatty acids: possible mechanisms and therapeutic value in major depression." *Alt Med Rev.* 2003; Nov8(4):410-425.

[xiv] Ibid.

[xv] Adams PB, Lawson S, Sanigorski A, et al. "Arachidonic acid to eicosapentaenoic acid ratio in blood correlates positively with clinical symptoms of depression." *Lipids*. 1996; Mar31: Suppl: S157-S161.

[xvi] "USDA National Nutrient Database for Standard Reference." USDA; Agricultural Research Service; Nutrient Data Laboratory. www.nal.usda.gov/fnic/foodcomp/search/ (accessed July 3, 2009).

[xvii] Kaufman, Leslie. "Greening the Herds - Trying to Limit Cows' 'Emissions' - NYTimes.com." The New York Times - Breaking News, World News & Multimedia. http://www.nytimes.com/2009/06/05/us/05cows.html?_r=2 (accessed June 28, 2009).

[xviii] Pollan, Michael. *The Omnivore's Dilemma: A Natural History of Four Meals.* New York: Penguin, 2007.

[ix] Ibid.

[xx] Göritz C, Mauch DH, Nägler K, Pfrieger FW. "Role of glia-derived cholesterol in synaptogenesis: new revelations in the synapse–glia affair." *Journal of Physiology-Paris.* 2002;96(3-4):257-263.

[xxi] Okuyama H, et al. "Dietary Fatty Acids -- the N-6/N-3 Balance and Chronic Diseases. Excess Linoleic Acid and the Relative N-3 Deficiency Syndrome Seen in Japan." *Progress in Lipid Research*.1997; 35(4): 409-457.

[xxii] Innis SM, Dyer RA, "Dietary Canola Oil Alters Hematological Indices and Blood Lipids in Neonatal Piglets Fed Formula." *J Nutr*.1999;129:1261-1268.

[xxiii]Enig M, Fallon S. "Tripping Lightly Down the Prostaglandin Pathways."*Price-Pottenger Nutrition Foundation Health Journal*, Vol 20, No 3 (619) 574-7763. http://www.westonaprice.org/knowyourfats/tripping.html (Accessed October 10, 2009)

[xxiv] Wittenberg, Margaret M. *New Good Food, Essential Ingredients for Cooking and eating Well.* Berkely/Toronto: Ten Speed Press, 2007.

[xxv] Shimada K, Kawarabayashi T, Tanaka A, et al. "Oolong tea increases plasma adiponectin levels and low-density lipoprotein particle size in patients with coronary artery disease." *Diabetes Res Clin Pract.* 2004; Sept65(3):227-234.

[xxvi] Rude RD, Gruber HI, Wei, LY, et al. "Immunolocalization of RANKL is Increased and OPG Decreased During Dietary Magnesium Deficiency in the Rat." *Nutr Metab.*2005; Sept14;2(24).    http://www.pubmedcentral.nih.gov/articlerender.fcgi?artid=1266035. (Accessed July 9, 2009.)

[xxvii] "Indicators: Behind the Data." USDA Economic Research Service- Home Page. http://www.ers.usda.gov/Amberwaves/April03/Indicators/BehindData .htm (accessed June 9, 2007).

[xxviii] Lustig, M.D., Robert H. " UCTV; University of California Television – Sugar: The Bitter Truth ." First aired July 27, 2009. http://www.uctv.tv/search-details. aspx?showID=16717 (Accessed February 10, 2010.)

[xxxix] Avena NM, Rada P, Hoebel BG. "Sugar and Fat Bingeing Have Notable Differences in Addictive-Like Behavior." *J. Nutr.*2009;139(3):623-628.

[xxx] John Yudkin, M.D. *Sweet and Dangerous.* Peter H. Wyden, Inc.Publisher. 1972.

[xxxi] Amen, Daniel G. *Change Your Brain, Change Your Body: Use Your Brain to Get and Keep the Body You Have Always Wanted.* First ed. Harmony Books. February 2010.

[xxxii]Mercola, Dr. Joseph, and Dr. Kendra Degen Pearsall. *Sweet Deception: Why Splenda, NutraSweet, and the FDA May Be Hazardous to Your Health.* Nashville: Thomas Nelson, Inc., 2006

[xxxiii]Alaedini A, Green PH. "Narrative Review: Celiac Disease: Understanding a Complex Autoimmune Disorder." *Ann Int Med.* 2005; Feb 15;142(4):289-298.

[xxxiv] "Magnesium." National Institutes of Health/Office of Dietary Supplements - HOME. http://ods.od.nih.gov/factsheets/magnesium.asp (Accessed July 9, 2009).

[xxxv] Tebby, PW, Buttke TM. "Molecular basis for the immunosuppresive action of stearic acid on T cells." *Immunology.* 1990; March6;(70):379-384. http://www.ncbi. nlm.nih.gov/pmc/articles/PMC1384169/pdf/immunology00130-0101.pdf.(Accessed July 9, 2009).

[xxxvi] Vogiatzoglou A, Refsum H, Johnston C, et al. "Vitamin B12 status and rate of brain volume loss in community-dwelling elderly." *Neurology.* 2008; 71:826-832.

[xxxvii] Slavkin, H. "Health Promotion Made Easy-Give a Gift!" *J Am Dent Assoc.* 2000; 131(1): 87-91.

[xxxviii] Blount BC, Mack MM, Wehr CC, et al. "Folate deficiency causes uracil misincorporation into human DNA and chromosome breakage: Implications for cancer and neuronal damage." 1997; *Proc Natl Acad Sci* U.S.A. April 1(94(7): 3290-3295.

[xxxvix] Berlin. *A Personal Touch On... Celiac Disease (The #1 Misdiagnosed Intestinal Disorder).* San Diego: Personal Touch Publishing, Llc, 2004

## CHAPTER FIFTEEN
## IMMUNE SYSTEM SUPPORT

[i] "NOVA | scienceNOW | Epigenetics | PBS. http://www.pbs.org/wgbh/nova/sciencenow/video/3411/q02-220.html (Accessed September 24, 2009).

[ii] Wilson, Duff "Harvard Medical School in Ethics Quandary - NYTimes.com." The New York Times - Breaking News, World News & Multimedia. http://www.nytimes.com/2009/03/03/business/03medschool.html?_r=2 (accessed October 12, 2009).

[iii] Gardner JP, Shengxu L, Sathanur RS, et al. "Rise in Insulin Resistance Is Associated With Escalated Telomere Attrition." *Circulation.* 2005; May 5;111:2171-2177. http://circ.ahajournals.org/cgi/content/full/111/17/2171 (Accessed Sept. 23, 2009.)

[iv] Hugo FN, Hilgert JB, Bozzetti MC, et al. "Chronic Stress, Depression, and Cortisol Levels as Risk Indicators of Elevated Plaque and Gingivitis Levels in Individuals Aged 50 Years and Older." *J Periodontol.* 2006; 77(6)1008-1014.

[v] Shibata M, Yamakoshi T, Yamakoshi KI. "Physiological role of nitric oxide in oxygen consumption by anterior wall." Conference proceedings. Proc IEEE *Eng Med Biol Soc.* 2008;1:1389-1392.

[vi] Lundberg JO, Settergren G, Gelinder S, et al. "Inhalation of nasally derived nitric oxide modulates pulmonary function in humans." *Acta Physiol Scand.* 1996;158(4):343-347.

[vii] Cury PR, Araújo VC, Canavez F. et al. "Hydrocortisone Affects the Expression of Matrix Metalloproteinases (MMP-1, -2, -3, -7, and - 11) and Tissue Inhibitor of Matrix Metalloproteinases (TIMP-1) in Human Gingival Fibroblasts." *J Periodontol.* 2007; 78(7)1309-1315.

[viii] Peruzzo D, Bennatti B, Ambrosano G, et al. "A Systematic review of stress and Psychological factors as Possible Risk Facors for Periodontal disease." *J Periodontol..* 2007 (8):1491-1504.

[ix] American Academy of Periodontology. "Strong Connection Between Stress Periodontal Diseases." Gum Disease Information from the American Academy of Periodontology. http://www.perio.org/consumer/stress07.htm (accessed November 20, 2008)

[x] Kalemba D, Kunicka A. "Antimicrobial and antifungal properties of essential oils."*Curr Med Chem.*2003;.10(10):813-829.

[xi] Warnke PH, Becker ST, Posdchun R, et al. "The battle against multi-resistant strains: Renaissance of antimicrobial essential oils as a promising force to fight hospital-acquired infections."*J Craniomaxillofac Surg.*2009;37(7):392-7.

[xii] Cohen C, Doyle WJ, Alper CM, et al. "Sleep Habits and Susceptibility to the Common Cold." *Arch InternMed.* 2009;169(1):62- 67.

[xiii] Null, G. *Gary Null's Ultimate Anti-Aging Program.* 1999. New York: Kensington Publishing Corp., 1999.

[xiv] Berk LS, "The Laughter-Immune Connection: New Discoveries." *Humor & Health Journal.* 1996; Sept-Oct;5(5): 1-5.

[xv] Berenson, Alex. "Boom Times for Dentistry, But Not for Teeth." *New York Times,* October 11, 2007.

[xvi] Shareholder battle vs leading mfr of mercury fillings coming May 5. Consumers For Dental Choice. Mercury Fillings. http://www.toxicteeth.org/mercuryfillings_Danaher.cfm

[xvii] "Bank of America: Dental Products Manufacturer Update." Consumers for Dental Choice. October 16, 2007. http://www.toxicteeth.org/RB__565608.pdf (Accessed July 2, 2009.)

[xviii] FDA says dental amalgam safe. American Dental Association. http://www.ada.org/prof/resources/pubs/adanews/adanewsarticle.asp?articleid=3675 (Accessed September 25, 1009).

[xix] For a copy of this report see on the web: www.mercurypolicy.org or www.cleanwateraction.org/mercury.

[xx] "What Patients Don't Know; Dentists' Sweet Tooth for Mercury." *What Patients Don't Know; Dentists' Sweet Tooth for Mercury.* Mercury Policy Project;Consumers for Dental Choice; New England Zero Mercury Campaign;Sierra Club California; Clean Water Action California, 14 Feb. 2006. Web. http://mpp.cclearn.org/wpcontent/uploads/2008/08/whatpatientsdontknow.pdf (Accessed October 9, 2009)

[xxi] Jones, James Earl, Robert Kulacz, and Thomas E. Levy. The *Roots of Disease: Connecting Dentistry & Medicine.* New York: Xlibris Corporation, 2002.

[xxii] Mercury Study Report to Congress Volume IV: An Assessment of Exposure to Mercury in the United States. United States Environmental Protection Agency/Air. http://www.epa.gov/ttncaaa1/t3/reports/volume4.pdf(Accessed September 25, 2009).

[xxiii] Friberg, L. T., and G. N. Schrauzer). "Letter by Boyd Haley, PhD, is in response to an article on the ADA web site by the ADA President." WHALE. http://www.whale.to/m/haley.html (accessed October 12, 2009).

[xxiv] "A Study on the Release of Mercury From Dental Amalgams Made from Different Manufactured Materials and Produced by Nine Different Dentists" International Academy of Oral Medicine and Toxicology. May 3, 2007. http://www.iaomt.org/news/archive.asp?intReleaseID=240&month=7&year=2007 (Accessed August 3, 2007).

[xxv] "Federal Register Environmental Documents | USEPA. U.S. Environmental Protection Agency." Reference Dose for Methylmercury. http://www.epa.gov/fedrgstr/EPAMEETINGS/2000/October?Day-30/m27781.htm (Accessed June 2, 2007).

[xxvi] Leistevuo J, Leistvuo T, Helenium H, et al. "Dental amalgam fillings and the amount of organic mercury in human saliva." *Caries Res.* 2001; May-Jun;35(3):163-6.

[xxvii] Heintze U, Edwardsson S, Derand T, et al. "Methylation of mercury from dental amalgam and mercuric chloride by oral streptococci in vitro." *Scand J Dent Res.* 1983; Apr; 91(2): 150-152.

[xxviii] Rowland I, Davies M, Grasso P. "Biosynthesis of methylmercury compounds by the intestinal flora of the rat." *Arch Environ Health.* 1977 Jan-Feb; 32(1):24-8.

[xxix] Rowland IR, et al. "The methylation of mercuric chloride by human intestinal bacteria." *Experientia.* 1975 Sept 15; 31(9): 1064-1065.

[xxx] Department of Health and Human Services; Agency for Toxic Substances and Disease Registry. *2005 CERCLA Priority List of Hazardous Substances.* http://www.atsdr.cdc.gov/cercla/05list.html (Accessed August 4, 2007)

[xxi] Wiggers GA, Peçanha FM, Bariones AM, et al. "Low mercury concentrations cause oxidative stress and endothelial dysfunction in conductance and resistance arteries."

*Am J Physiol Heart Circ Physiol* 2008; 295: H1033-H1043.

xxxii Siblerud RJ. "The Relationship between Mercury from Dental Amalgam and the Cardiovascular System." *Sci Total Environ.* 1990; Dec 1;99(1-2): 22-35.

xxxiii American Heart Association (2002, April 29). Mercury Ups Heart Disease Risk. *ScienceDaily.* Retrieved July 3, 2009, from http://www.sciencedaily.com- / releases/2002/04/020429073754.htm

xxxivVia CS, Nguyen P, Niculescu,F, et al. "Low-dose exposure to inorganic mercury accelerates disease and mortality in acquired murine lupus." *Environ Health Perspect.* 2003; Aug111(10) 1273-1277.

xxv Silbergeld EK, /Silva IA, Nyland, JF. "Mercury and Autoimmunity: Implications for Occupational and Environmental Health." *Toxicol Appl Pharmacol.* 2005; Sep 1;207(2 Suppl):282-292.

xxxvi Ibid.

xxxvii Thompson AE, Pope JE. "Increased Prevalence of Scleroderma in Southwestern Ontario: A Cluster Analysis." *Journal of Rheumatology.* 2002; 29(9): 1867-1873.

xxxviii Dept of Health/Human Services; Agency for Toxic Substances and Disease Registry. CAS#: 7439-97-6 http://www.atsdr.cdc.gov/tfacts46.html (Accessed August 9, 2007)

xxxix Frustaci, Andrea."Marked elevation of myocardial trace elements in idiopathic dilated cardiomyopathy compared with secondary cardiac dysfunction." Journal of the American College of Cardiology. http://content.onlinejacc.org/cgi/content/full/33/6/ 1578?maxtoshow=&HITS=10&hits=10&RESULTFORMAT=&fulltext=Mercuryperc ent2F+IDCM&searchid=1&FIRSTINDEX=0&resourcetype=HWCIT (Accessed July 2, 2009).

xl Vimy MJ, Takahashi Y, Lorscheider FL. "Maternal-Fetal Distribution of Mercury (203(HG) Released From Dental Amalgam Fillings." *Amer J Physiol.*1990; 258(4):R939-R945.

xli Arenholt-Bindslev, D, Larsen, AH. "Mercury Levels and Discharge in Waste Water from Dental Clinics." *Water Air Soil Pollution.* 1996;86(1-4):93-9. http://www. springerlink.com/content/pp65v404t276p450/ accessed September 22,2007

xlii Rowe NH, Sidhu KS, Chadzynski L, et al. School of Dentistry, University of Michigan, Ann Arbor, USA. *J Mich Dent Assoc* 1996 Feb;78(2):32-6.

xliii Bagenstose LM, Salgame P, Monestier M, et al. "Murine mercury-induced autoimmunity: a model of chemically related autoimmunity in humans." *Immunol Res.* 1999; 20(1): 67-78.

xliv Bartova J, Prochazkova J, Kratka Z, et al. "Dental amalgam as one of the risk factors in autoimmune diseases." *Neuro Endocrinol Lett.* 2003; Feb-Apr; 24(1-2): 65-7.

xlvHultman P, Johansson SJ, Turley SJ, et al. "Adverse immunological effects and autoimmunity induced by dental amalgam and alloy in mice." *FASEB J.* 1994; Nov;8(14): 1183-90.

xlvi Gerhard I, et al. "Impact of heavy metals on hormonal and immunological factors in women with repeated miscarriages." *Hum Reprod Update.* 1998; May-Jun; 4(3): 301-9.

## CHAPTER SIXTEEN: RISK IS NOT DESTINY

[i] Oral Health Status of Georgia's Children, Facts at a Glance. http://health.state.ga.us/pdfs/familyhealth/oral/OralHealthStatusofGeorgia%27sChildren.pdf

[ii] Institute of Medicine of the National Academies. 2011. Advancing Oral Health in America. The National Academies Press. Prepublication. http://books.nap.edu/openbook.php?record_id=13086&page=35

[iii] Nidel C and Stockin DG. 2011. Fluoridegate and Fluoride Litigation: What Law Firms Need to Know About Fluoride Toxic Tort Actions. American Association for Justice Newsletter, Vol. 18, No. 2, Winter/Spring.
http://www.justice.org/cps/rde/xchg/justice/hs.xsl/14815_14817.htm

[iv] Letter from Rep. Frank Nicely, et al., to Commissioner Susan R. Cooper, Department of Health, Nashville, TN. February 7, 2011. http://fluoridealert.org/tn.letter.to.doh.2-7-11.pdf

[v] The New York City Council, A Local Law to amend the administrative code of the city of New York, in relation to the fluoridation of water, January 18, 2011. http://legistar.council.nyc.gov/LegislationDetail.aspx?ID=828442&GUID=B1B850E6-5BB5-4CC1-9492-6E1070A72B31&Options=&Search

[vi] Winter, Mark. "WebElements Periodic Table of the Elements | Fluorine | Essential information." WebElements Periodic Table ofthe Elements. http://www.webelements.com/fluorine/ (accessed September 12, 2009).

[vii] Helmenstine, Anne Marie, and Ph.D.. "Fluorine Facts - Periodic Table of the Elements." Chemistry - Periodic Table, Chemistry Projects, and Chemistry Homework Help. http://chemistry.about.com/od/elementfacts/a/fluorine.htm (accessed September 12, 2009).

[viii] Macpherson LM, Stephen KW. "The effect on human salivary fluoride concentration of consuming fluoridated salt-containing baked food items." Arch Oral Bio 2001; 46(10): 983-988.

[ix] Watson PS, Pontefract HA, Devine DA, et al. "Penetration of Fluoride into Natural Plaque Biofilms." J Dent Res 2005; 84(5): 451-455.

[x] Fagin, D. "Second Thoughts About Fluoride." Scientific American. 298(1) 74-81. Science News, Articles and Information | Scientific American. http://scientificamerican.com/article.cfm?id=second-thoughts-onfluoride (accessed July 9, 2009).

[xi] National Research Council. Fluoride in Drinking Water: A Scientific Review of EPA's Standards. Washington, D.C.: National Academies Press, 2006.

[xii] Ibid.

[xiii] Stannard, JG et al. "Fluoride levels and fluorides contamination of fruit juices." Journal of Clinical Pediatric Dentistry. 1991; 16(1): 38-40.

[xiv] Kiritsy MC, Levy SM, Warren JJ, et al. "Assessing Fluoride Concentrations of Juices and Juice-Flavored Drinks. J Am Dent Assoc, 1996; 127(7): 895-902.

[xv] Heilman JR, Kiritsy MC, Levy SM, et al. "Fluoride concentrations of infant foods." J A Dent Assoc. 1997; 128(7):857-863.

[xvi] Carton, RJ. Review of the 2006 United States National Research Council Report: Fluoride in Drinking Water. Guest editorial review. Fluoride. 2006; July-Sept;39(3):163-172.

[xvii] Bassin EB Wyppij D, Davis RB, et al. "Age-specific fluoride exposure in drinking water and osteosarcoma (United States)." *Cancer Causes and Control.* May 17(4):421-428. Published May 2006.

[xviii] Carton, RJ. Review of the 2006 United States National Research Council Report: Fluoride in Drinkng Water. Guest editorial review. Fluoride. 2006; July-Sept;39(3):163-172.

[xix] Limeback, H. "Should Juneau Fluoridate? A Risk and Benefit Analysis." Lecture presented in Juneau, Alaska Sept. 21, 2007.

[xx] E. Gazzano†, L. Bergandi†, C. Riganti, et al. "Fluoride Effects: the Two Faces of Janus." *Current Medicinal Chemistry.* 2010; 17( 21) 1-11.

[xxi] Fagin, D. "Second Thoughts About Fluoride." Scientific American. 298(1) 74-81. Science News, Articles and Information | Scientific American. http://scientificamerican. com/article.cfm?id=second-thoughts-onfluoride (accessed July 9, 2009).

[xxii] Burwell AK, Greenspan DC. "Potential for Dentifrice Protection Against Enamel Erosion in an In Vitro Model" *Caries Research.* 2007; June41(4): 309.

[xxiii] Featherstone JD, Rapozo-Hilo ML, Rechmann P, et al. "In Vitro Root Caries Inhibition by Phosphosilicate and Fluoride Dentifrices." IADE/AADR/CADR 85th General Session and Exhibition. New Orleans, La. March 22, 2007.Abstract #0501

[xxiv] Burt, BA. "The Use of Sorbitol-and Xylitol-Sweetened Chewing Gum in Caries Control." *J Am Dent Assoc.* 2006; 137(2): 190-196.

[xxv] Lynch H, Milgrom P. "Xylitol and Dental Caries: An Overview for Clinicians." *J Calif Dent Assoc.* 2003; 31(3): 205-9.

[xxvi] Peldyak J, Mäkinen KK. "Xylitol for Caries Prevention." *J Dent Hyg.* 2002 Fall76(4): 276-285.

[xxvii] Hayes C. "The Effect of Non-Cariogenic Sweeteners on the Prevention of Dental Caries: A Review of the Evidence." *J Dent Educ.* 2001; Oct65(10): 1106-1109.

[xxviii] Steinberg LM, Odusola F, Mandel ID. "Remineralizing Potential, Antiplaque and Antigingivitis Effects of Xylitol and Sorbitol Sweetened Chewing Gum." *Clin Prev. Dent.* 1992; Sept-Oct;14(5): 31-34.

[xxvi] Sengun A, sari Z, Ramoglu SI, et al. "Evaluation of the Dental Plaque pH Recovery Effect of a Xylitol Lozenge on Patients with Fixed Orthodontic Appliances." *Angle Orthod.* 2004; Apr74(2): 240-244.

[xxvii] California Dental Association. "Xylitol The Decay Preventive Sweetener." http:// www.cda.org/popup/xylitol. (accessed December 3, 2009).

[xxviii] Isokangas P. Soderling E, Pienihakkinen K,et al. "Occurrence of Dental Decay in Children after Maternal Consumption of Xylitol Chewing Gum, a Follow-up from 0 – 5 Years of Age." *J Dent Res.* 2000; 7911): 1885-1889.

[xxix] Uhari M, Tapiainen T, Kontiokari T. "Xylitol in preventing acute otitis media." *Vaccine.* 2000;19(sup-l): S144-S147.

[xxx] Mäkinen KK. "Long-term tolerance of healthy human subjects to high amounts of xylitol and fructose: general and biochemical findings." *Int Z Vitam Ernahrungsforsch Beih.* 1976;15: 92-104.

[xxxi] Paraskea,, S, Rosema, NAF, Versteeg, P, et al. "The Additional Effect of a Dentifrice on the Instant Efficacy of Toothbrushing: A Crossover Study." *J. Periodontal.* 2007; 78(6): 1011-1016.

xxxiiAmano K, Miyake K, Borke JL, et al. "Breaking Biological Barriers with a Toothbrush." *J Dent Res* 2007 86(8): 769-774.

xxxiii Asuarga, Juan Luis. Paleontology Professor. Reuters. 3:41PM CT Sept 11, 2007 as reported from newspaper El Pais. http://uk.reuters.com/article/idUKL1190325720070911

xxxivHague A., Carr MP. "Efficacy of an Automated Flossing Device in Different Regions of the Mouth." *J Periodontol.* 2007; 78(8): 1529-1537.

xxxv Featherstone, JDB. "The Science and Practice of Caries Prevention." *J Am Dent Assoc.* 2000; 131(7): 887-899.

xxxvi Pedrazzi V, Sato Maria S. "Tongue-Cleaning Methods: A Comparative Clinical Trial Employing a Toothbrush and a Tongue Scraper." *J Periodontal.* July 2004, Jul75(7):1009-1012.

## CHAPTER SEVENTEEN
## RESTRUCTURING TO MEET THE FUTURE!

i Nathe C. "Dental Hygiene's Historical Roots in Modern-Day Issues." *Contemp Dent Hyg.* 2003; 3: 24-5.

ii American Dental Hygienist's Association. How do You Know Dentistry is in Favor of On-The-Job Training? Copyright 2008, American Dental Hygienists Association. http://www.adha.org/profissues/preceptorship/paper.htm. Used with permission of the publisher. (accessed August 23, 2007)

iii Li Y, Denny P, Ho C-M, et al. "The Oral Fluid MEMS/NEMS Chip (OFMNC); Diagnostic and Translational Applications." *Adv Dent Res* 2005; Jun18(1):3-5.

## CHAPTER EIGHTEEN
## FINAL WORDS

i US Department of Health and Human Services. "Oral Health in America: A Report of the Surgeon General." Rockville, MD: US Department of Health and Human Services, National Institute of Dental and Craniofacial Research, National Institutes of Health, 2000.

ii Lipton JA, Ship JA, Larach-Robinson D. "Estimated Prevalence and Distribution of Reported Orofacial Pain in the United States." *J Am Dent Assoc.* 1993; 124(10): 115-21.

iii Cohen LA, Manski RJ, Magder LS, et al. "Dental Visits to Hospital Emergency Departments by Adults Receiving Medicaid: Assessing their use." *J Am Dent Assoc.* 2002;133(6):715-24.

iv Berenson, Alex. "Boom Times for Dentistry, But Not for Teeth." *New York Times,* October 11, 2007.[1]

# APPENDICES

## Appendix I. (Chapter Seven)
## A. Bone-Sparing Medications and Bisphosphonate Cancer Therapies

1. **FOSOMAX:** (Alenedronate nitrogen containing oral bisphosphonate.) Prescribed for osteoporosis in men and women and for Paget's Disease.
2. **ACTONEL:** (Resedronate nitrogen containing oral bisphosphonate.) Prescribed for osteoporosis in men and women and for Paget's Disease.
3. **BONIVA:** (Ibandronate nitrogen containing oral bisphosphonate.) Prescribed for osteoporosis in women. Approved to reduce spinal fractures. Also for Glucocorticoid-induced osteoporosis and Paget's Disease.
4. **DIDRONEL:** (Etidronate Disodium. Non-nitrogen containing oral bisphosphonate.) Prescribed for Paget's disease. Potency 10,000 times less than the weakest nitrogen containing bisphosphonates and not implicated in jaw osteonecrosis.
5. **SKELID:** (Tiludronate Disodium. Non-nitrogen containing oral bisphosphonate.) Prescribed for Paget's disease. Potency 10,000 times less than the weakest nitrogen containing bisphosphonates and not implicated in jaw osteonecrosis.
6. **AREDIA:** (Pamidronate Disodium.) Administered IV. Prescribed for bone cancers and moderate to severe Paget's disease.
7. **BONEFOS:**(Clondronate.) IV or oral tablets. Prescribed for excess calcium from malignant cells.
8. **ZOMETRA:** Zoledronic acid. IV. Prescribed for bone cancers and excess calcium from malignant cells.
9. **EVISTA:** Raloxifene. An orally administered modified estrogen (SERM or Selective estrogen receptor modulator). Evista is *not* a bisphosphonate, but one alternative to bisphosphonates.

## B. Expert Panel Clinical Recommendations For Managing
### Patients Receiving Oral Bisphosphonate Therapy*

### Recommendations:

"A comprehensive oral evaluation should be carried out on all patients about to begin therapy with oral bisphosphonates (or as soon as possible after beginning therapy). The dentist should inform the patient taking oral bisphosphonates that:

1.  There is a very low risk (estimated at 0.7 cases per 100,000 person-years' exposure) of developing BON (Bisphosphonate-induced osteonecrosis of the jaw);
2.  There are ways to minimize the risk, but not to eliminate the already low risk;
3.  The consensus is that good oral hygiene along with regular dental care is the best way to lower risk;
4.  There are no diagnostic techniques to identify those at increased risk of developing BON.

The patient also should be informed of the dental treatment needed, alternative treatments, how any treatment relates to the risk of BON, other risks associated with various treatment options, and the risk of foregoing treatment, even temporarily. The patient should be encouraged to consult with his or her treating physician about any health risks. BON can occur spontaneously, owing to dental disease or secondary to dental therapy. Therefore, patients taking oral bisphosphonates should be instructed to contact their dentist if any problem develops in the oral cavity. Routine dental treatment generally should not be modified solely on the basis of oral bisphosphonate therapy. However, patients with possible risk factors for BON may benefit from assessment by an expert in metabolic bone diseases. These risk factors may include concomitant use of estrogen or glucocorticoids, older age (over 65 years) and prolonged use of bisphosphonates. For more information, readers may consult the National Osteoporosis Foundation ("www.nof.org") or the American Society for Bone and Mineral Research ("www.asbmr.org")."

See Chapter Thirteen: ozone therapy, if you are unfortunate enough to suffer from osteonecrosis of the jaw due to bisphosphonates.

* From: "Dental management of patients receiving oral bisphosphonate therapy." *ADA*, Vol. 137 http://jada.ada.org August 2006 p.1147

## Appendix II. (Chapter Eight)
## Tobacco Quitlines

About seventy percent of smokers report a desire to quit. When smoking cessation includes clinicians, the number of people who quit smoking doubles, so many medical and dental offices incorporate private smoking cessation programs. Some offices refer clients to statewide tobacco "Quitlines."

These Quitlines are now available in every state to all individuals over age 18 by calling 1–800 QUITNOW. (1–800–784–8669 or TTY 1–800–332–8615). Canada, Mexico, and the EU also have Quitlines.

If you google "quitline," many websites appear. This web site: http://www.aafp.org/online/en/home/clinical/publichealth/tobacco/quitlines.html, from the American Academy of Family Physicians, provides numerous links that inform you of ways to access individual state Quitline telephone numbers, language availability information, program explanation, self-help materials, and availability of smoking cessation medication. The American Cancer Society, American Lung Association, and American Legacy Foundation's Great Start (for pregnant smokers) also offer help. Instant messaging is available via a National Cancer Institute smoking cessation counselor. (English only, specified hours.)

These Quitlines offer multiple free professional counseling sessions by phone. Most provide special services for specialized populations such as pregnant smokers and spit tobacco users. Clients appreciate the convenience and anonymity. Because they operate on a state-by-state basis, they can be sensitive to ethnic and geographic disparities. Self-help materials are mailed or available online. Discounted or free cessation medications are also offered, depending on the state. These usually fall into the category of nicotine replacement therapies. Arizona, Wyoming, and Nevada, at the time of this writing, also offer limited access for the prescription Bupropion Sustained Release (Zyban), thought to work by reducing the neurotransmitters dopamine and norepinephrine in the brain.

Abstinence rates correlate with the number of counseling sessions completed.

Some clients have suggested books by Allen Carr such as *Easy Ways to Quit Smoking* were useful. (http://www.theeasywaytostopsmoking.com)

Quitnet (www.quitnet.com) hosts a "thriving, supportive online community of current and ex-tobacco users," according to their web site. Many clients find the chat forums, help lines, and other support invaluable.

## Appendix III. (Chapter Ten)
## Kidney Transplants

**Blood Tests for Kidney Function:**

Serum Creatinine – Serum creatinine is a waste product that comes from normal wear and tear on body muscles. Creatinine levels >1.2 for females and >1.4 for men may be an early sign that the kidneys are not working properly.

Glomerulation Filtration Rate (GFR) – This test is a measure of how well the kidneys are removing wastes and excess fluid from the blood. A GFR below 60 is a sign that the kidneys are not working properly. A GFR below 15 indicates that a treatment for kidney failure, such as dialysis or a kidney transplant, will be needed.

Blood Urea Nitrogen (BUN) – Urea nitrogen comes from the breakdown of protein in the foods you eat. A normal BUN level is between 7 and 20.

Symptoms of Chronic Kidney Disease:

- Low energy
- Poor appetite
- Difficulty sleeping
- Difficulty concentrating
- Gum disease because the body does not absorb calcium properly. Osteoporosis generalizes to the bones that support the teeth.
- Breath smells like ammonia because the kidneys do not remove urea from the blood. The urea breaks down into ammonia.
- Swollen feet and ankles and morning puffiness around eyes
- Itchy, dry skin
- Need to urinate often, especially at night

## Appendix IV. (Chapter Twelve)
## Reflux and a Restricted Tongue (Tongue-Tied)

Dr. Palmer researched how frenums impact airway development. A person with a tied tongue creates a vacuum/negative pressure as he or she swallows. This can collapse the airway, alter the proper development of the epiglottis (which develops between four and six months) and potentially stretches/elongates the soft palate, reducing the airway further. It exacerbates the initial problem, and increases the risk of apnea and other respiratory issues. It can also create a 'sucking' effect on stomach acids – causing reflux!

He likens the reflux problem a small airway generates to a perfume atomizer, using two principles:

- **Venturi Principle** – Moving the same amount of air, the smaller the tube/airway, the faster the air must move.
- **Bernoulli Principle** – The faster the flow of air, the greater the inward vacuum and inward collapse of the walls of the tube.

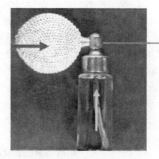

He gives an example of a patient, age 40, who suffered significant gastric distress, bloating and gas build up and who was significantly tongue tied. After the simple surgery that freed her tongue, she successfully stopped all the medications she had been taking all her life for gastric distress. Why? She can now chew better and does not swallow air as she used to.[1]

Ironically, the Proton Pump Inhibitors often prescribed for reflux, have been shown to cause small intestinal bacterial overgrowth in half of users – resulting in diarrhea, related infections, potential food intolerance – and reflux.[2]

Recent ultrasound images have shown tongue tied infants do not use a typical tongue action. Instead, they use two distinct sucking patterns that either resolved entirely or lessened after frenulotomy.

---

1 Frenulotomy for Breastfeeding Infants With Ankyloglossia: Effect on Milk Removal and Sucking Mechanism as Imaged by Ultrasound, doi:10.1542/peds.2007-2553
2 Increased incidence of small intenstinal bacterial overgrowth during proton pump inhibitor therapy. Clinical Gastroenterology and Hepatology - June 2010 8(6)504-508.

## Appendix V (Chapter Thirteen)
## Beyond the Death Spiral: Modern Dentistry

### A. Advancing Modern Dentistry

In our market-driven economy, I do believe we receive what we ask for. In the 1980s and 1990s, Americans clambered for picture-perfect smiles. Big Case marketers emerged, offering $60,000.00 seminars to teach dentists how to present and execute these large aesthetic cases.

If we in turn, value whole body health, we will vote to go to dental professionals who have invested in learning about and offering oral/systemic health counseling and therapies that includes appropriate, early diagnosis and intervention.

Developing this more robust second edition, I was fortunate to meet with leaders in the profession who have worked tirelessly for decades to develop methodologies and procedures that benefit people for a lifetime. They are the natural partners for those already practicing oral/systemic medicine. Out of need, we are forming the Academy of Biomimetic Dentistry (AMD: http://www.academyofbiomimeticdent.org/), offering a network of accredited dentists and hygienists to the public, courses, and an informational library. Se also: www.mouthmattersbook.org.

### B. The Potential for "Brain Dysfunction"
### Enough is Enough: No More Routinely Putting Kids to Sleep:
### An Opinion on Time for Change
### J Tim Rainey, DDS
### Scientific Research in Operative Dentistry

Over the years we have been instrumental in forcing change in dentistry for the patient's benefit. After moments of monumental resistance, my colleagues have been swift to adapt to the new technology once somebody points out a way to make money. One of those changes was in the area of "Soft Tissue Management", or providing a higher level of gum care for patients. Twenty-five years after we helped introduce this life saving technology to dentistry, it is considered a standard of care.

Organized dentistry has conveniently ignored other life saving technology we have helped introduce over the years. It is time to put a stop to unnecessary dentistry. Several things that have been in our cross hairs over the years are amalgam fillings, stainless steel crowns accompanied by the unnecessary placing of kids under general anesthesia, placing unnecessary tubes in kids' ears, and one of the biggest financial scams and frauds in history, placing sealants on kids' teeth.

Recently, there have been several ground-shaking articles outlining the desperate need for change in a profession still stuck on 19th century dental technology. Considering recently released data and peer reviewed articles, it is time for major changes in dentistry. With the past a good predictor of the future, in my opinion nothing will change unless YOU, the consumer, demand immediate change and put a stop to the carnage, starting with "sealants", "amalgam" and simple "bonding" technology. Placing sealants, amalgam or improperly done bondings in teeth virtually assures future dentistry, resulting in an estimated lifetime cost to the patient in excess of $2000. PER TOOTH.

In one of the most stunning developments, the U.S. government has recently reversed its stand on mercury amalgam fillings and has called for a phase out of this devastating, 19th century technology that is incompatible with tooth structure. To read more on this issue go to: www. toxicteeth.org. The technology we developed twenty-five years ago to eliminate sealants and amalgam technology can carry a lifetime warranty. (Go to www.jtimrainey. com. Click on "Articles, "Dead Elephant".)

**Background:** When I was in dental school, I recognized that high speed drills shatter healthy tooth structure and that amalgam "filling" technology, as still taught nearly worldwide, causes future breakdown of teeth. I set out on a life's mission to find a better way to stop the decay process. This odyssey resulted in our introduction twenty-five years ago for a method of "sealing" teeth that actually worked. This potentially lifesaving technology has been continently ignored by organized dentistry and the dental universities. To see what the American Dental Association doesn't want you to know about sealants, go to www.jtimrainey.com, Click on "Articles", "JADA cover story on Sealants 2009".

Recent research and the science are also pointing in the direction of questioning the wisdom of routinely putting kids to sleep. (Bob Rappaport, M.D., R. Daniel Mellon, Ph.D., Arthur Simone, M.D., Ph.D., and Janet Woodcock, M.D. March 9, 2011 (10.1056/NEJMp1102155). Meanwhile, we have treated thousands of teeth and hundreds of kids who would routinely have been put to sleep for simple dental procedures. The research is leaning towards findings of significant changes resulting in "brain dysfunction" associated with multiple episodes of general anesthesia.

Bottom line, when technology has been developed to circumvent the need for general anesthesia, why are dental professionals, in particular, pediatric dentists, insisting on using technology more than a half century old when proven alternatives exist? To see just one of the many kids we have rescued from general anesthesia and unnecessary stainless steel crowns, go to http://www.jtimrainey.com/Videos.aspx.)

It is important to note this child was referred by his pediatric physician to a pediatric dentist for unnecessary dentistry and general anesthesia.

**Note:** National Public Radio just ran a story, *A Curious Case of Foreign Accent Syndrome.* "When Karen Butler went in for dental surgery, she left with more than numb gums: She also picked up a pronounced foreign accent. It wasn't a fluke, or a joke — she'd developed a rare condition called foreign accent syndrome that's usually caused by an injury to the part of the brain that controls speech.... "(The unusual problem) is usually the result of a brain injury," Lowenkopf says, "which can come from stroke...") It was surmised she had a small stroke due to the anesthesia used for her dental work. In this case, the patient considered it an amusing, small brain injury. Most brain injuries are not so benign. The use of anesthesia is always a serious decision.[1]

## C. Ozone

Doctors Mollica and Harris teach ozone therapies from a medical perspective. A few of their insights into how beneficial ozone can be:

* **Ozone significantly raises Interferon levels.** Interferons are globular proteins that orchestrate every aspect of the immune system. Cells infected by viruses produce certain interferons. These interferons warn adjacent, healthy cells of the likelihood of infection; in turn, they are rendered nonpermissive host cells. They inhibit viral replication. Other interferons are produced in muscle, connective tissue, and by white blood cells. Ozone can raise gamma interferon levels 400-900 percent. Gamma interferon helps control phagocytic cells that engulf and kill pathogens and abnormal cells. Synthetic interferons are FDA approved for the treatment of chronic hepatitis B and C, genital warts (caused by the papilloma virus), hairy-cell leukemia, Kaposi's sarcoma, relapsing-remitting multiple sclerosis and chronic granulomatous disease. Interferons are currently in clinical trials for throat warts caused by the papilloma virus, HIV infection, chronic myelogenous leukemia, non-Hodgkins lymphoma, colon tumors, kidney tumors, bladder cancer, malignant melanoma, and basal cell carcinoma. While levels induced by ozone remain safe, interferon levels that are FDA-approved (and in clinical trials) are extremely toxic.
* **Ozone stimulates the production of Tumor Necrosis Factor.** TNF is produced by the body when a tumor is growing. The greater the mass of the tumor, up to a point, the more the body produces tumor

---

1 Greenhalgh, Jane. "NPR.org » A Curious Case Of Foreign Accent Syndrome." NPR. org. N.p., 1 June 2011. Web. 1 June 2011. <http://m.npr.org/news/Health

necrosis factor. When a tumor metastasizes, it means cancer cells break off from the original tumor and are carried away by the blood and lymph. This allows the tumor to take up residence elsewhere in the body. These lone cancer cells have little chance of growing when sufficient TNF is produced to inhibit the original tumor. If a tumor is removed surgically, TNF levels drop dramatically. New tumors emerge from seemingly healthy tissue.

- **Ozone stimulates the secretion of Interleukin-2 (IL-2).** IL-2, secreted by T-helper cells, is a cornerstone of the immune system. In this autostimulation process, the IL-2 then binds to a receptor on the T-helper, which causes it to produce more IL-2. Its main duty is to induce lymphocytes to differentiate and proliferate, yielding more T-helpers, T-suppressors, cytotoxic T's, T-delayeds and T-memory cells.

- **Ozone kills most bacteria at low concentrations.** Most bacteria's metabolism is about one-seventeenth as efficient as our own, therefore they cannot afford to produce disposable anti-oxidant enzymes such as catalase. Very few types of bacteria can live in an environment composed of more than two percent ozone.

- **Ozone is effective against all types of fungi.** This includes systemic Candida albicans (a fungal yeast), athlete's foot, molds, mildews, and other yeasts.

- **Ozone is the best virucide.** As discussed above, ozone goes after viral particles directly. The part of the virus most sensitive to oxidation is its reproductive structure. This is how the virions enter cells. When this structure is inactivated, the virus is essentially "dead". Infected cells already have a natural weakness to ozone. Because infections cause a metabolic burden on cells, they can no longer produce the protective enzymes necessary to deal with the ozone or repair themselves.

- **Ozone oxidizes arterial plaque.** It breaks down the plaque involved in both arteriosclerosis and atherosclerosis. This means ozone has a tendency to clear blockages of small and even large vessels. This allows for better tissue oxygenation in deficient organs.

- **Ozone increases red blood cell flexibility and elasticity.** Red blood cell are disc-shaped. In lung capillaries, where they pick-up oxygen, and in tissue capillaries where they release oxygen, these discs stretch into an oval or umbrella shape, so they can more easily pass through tiny capillaries and efficiently exchange gases. [Remember AGE products work against this?] The increased red blood cell flexibility allows elevated oxygen levels for days, or even weeks after ozone treatment.

- **Ozone significantly accelerates the Citric Acid Cycle** (also known as the Kreb's Cycle or TCA Cycle), an important step in carbohydrate metabolism that takes place in the cellular mitochondria. Most energy stored in glucose (sugar) is converted in this pathway. Ozone makes the anti-oxidant enzyme system more efficient. Cells respond to the beneficial oxidative stress by increasing their production of protective enzymes.
- **Ozone breaks down petrochemicals.** This is why many people "gas" their produce, since many pesticides are petrochemically-based. These chemicals place a great burden on the immune system. They also worsen and even cause allergies and are detrimental to your long-term health. And of course ozone is a better way to preserve your produce anyway.
- Ozone helps red blood cells carry more oxygen.

If you or a loved one has HIV/AIDS and found this list of ozone's benefits enlightening, you may appreciate this small study that took place in Uganda. Since Africa's HIV/AIDS challenge and accompanying costs are overwhelming, an inexpensive alternative therapy was tried. Patients were given a rectal suppository of ozonated hemp oil three times a day. After thirty days, HIV viral loading was reduced and 'T' Cell counts increased. All patients expressed energy and wanted to return to active employment.

People often ask me what kind of ozonated oil is best. They are right to ask. Some oils have much higher concentrations of ozonoids than others, given the same ozone concentration/time/bubble size times. Ozonoids are formed when ozone attacks an oil's double bonds. The higher the omega 3s, 6s, or 9 content, the higher their ability to form ozonoids. For example linseed oil is twice as concentrated as olive oil. Linseed is inexpensive. The following chart shows the potential of other oils.

| Plant Oil | % Omega 3s | %Omega 6s | %Omega 9s | Ozonoid-forming potential |
|-----------|-----------|-----------|-----------|----------------------------|
| Hemp | 20 | 60 | 12 | 192 |
| Sunflower | 0 | 65 | 23 | 153 |
| Canola | 7 | 30 | 54 | 135 |
| Olive | 0 | 8 | 76 | 92 |
| Avocado | 0 | 10 | 70 | 90 |

**Note: Avoid ozonated oils incorporating essential oils or scents.**

Though Europe has used ozone in medicine for decades, we are all in a discovery zone as we learn of its healing benefits. Almost daily I receive e-mails detailing some new use. Here is one edited example:

- "Patient: a sixty-some semi-controlled diabetic came in with a very sore tongue down the sides and ventral surface. (It looked very much like hairy leukoplakia, but that is generally not painful. There were fibrous bands of white, keratinized tissue running anteroposteriorly.)
- We did a split mouth approach. On the right side, we used the diode laser (specifics omitted).
- On the left side we simply used the ozone handpiece at the maximum concentration of 115 micrograms/ml at a 1/32 LPM flow rate. The tip is around 3/4 inch, so with a sixty second exposure per site, it took around five minutes to step down the extent of the lesion.
- Comments from the patient next day: 'Get me back and use ozone on my right side. It still hurts. The left side is almost better."
- On return the next day, most of the leukoplakia was gone, revealing what appeared to be fairly classic looking roundish ulcerations of various sizes down the right side of the tongue. Suspect it was viral in nature.
- The left side looked somewhat similar, but was much less inflamed and was essentially pain free.
- We ozoned the right side, and our conversation in the evening indicated it was then feeling considerably better, but not 100%.
- We had her back the next day and ozoned just the right side one more time. By evening she said she was feeling 100% and is now able to eat.

### D. Burning Tongue

Many people complain of a burning mouth, especially the tongue. This accompanies gum disease and cavities as a symptom of an unbalanced oral flora. Microorganisms are extremely sensitive to the acid-base balance (pH) in the mouth/body. Mineral balance and hydration are central to oral health. Poor mineral balance also alters the voltage of everything in the body. Though I have not touched on this important emerging medical field, do not overlook the overriding fact that our bodies run on electricity. We need minerals and hydration for optimal health.

My personal batteries were severely depleted towards the end of writing this book. I could feel how the exhaustion and lack of balance in my life were affecting my health. Among other symptoms, my tongue felt as though it was mildly burning all the time. My challenge pH was around 6. I added kale, sometimes chard to my morning vegetable mix and immediately my burning tongue abated; my challenge pH reverted to where it should be – around pH 6.8.[2]

Typically, a burning tongue indicates a dietary deficiency. Calcium, phosphate, magnesium, and iron minerals play an important role in reversing burning mouth syndrome. One must also erase $B_{12}$ and $B_9$ deficiencies and of course, improve hydration.

Sometimes health is so challenged that one's body hosts systemic yeast infections. Yeast is often subclinically present in the mouth, where it causes burning. The key is to change systemic pH through diet, but this can take awhile. In the meantime local therapy helps. Rinse with Caphasol or its generic (prescription) several times a day. Brush with CariFree[3] toothpaste (nonprescription) or MI paste (prescription) in the morning and straight baking soda out of the box (pH 10!) in the evening. Work the baking soda in between the teeth with a interdental brush if you like for added benefit. If baking soda is initially intolerable due to a deep-seated yeast infection, a kick start of ozone therapy is helpful.

An alternative to the baking soda routine is the alkaline rinse "CariFree Treatment Rinse" (www.carifree.com). The same caveats apply as with baking soda, that is, it can burn until the yeast comes under control. Before ozone came into use, many doctors prescribed the anti-fungal Nystatin rinse prescription. The rinse contains intolerably high levels of sugar, which yeast bugs love. At most, use it twice a day for two weeks. By then, you should be able to use the baking soda or Carifree rinse pain-free.

Add Evora, an oral probiotic, to help repopulate the mouth.

These therapies incidentally help with tooth sensitivity, a red, smooth tongue, and what is called geographic tongue. If you rinse with Caphasol and swallow, it may incidentally eliminate any reflux problems you may have. Be sure B-complex intake and absorption is excellent.

If you have an intense localized burning or other problem around a crown, it could be from an economically-made crown. Many people have high sensitivity to the beryllium used in economical crowns. At the very least, have your dentist smooth the margins.

---

2 The most accurate pH saliva testing strips: pHion Diagnostic Test Strips. Find them and more resources at: http://www.phionbalance.com/.

3 CariFree CTx3 contains 20nm particles of HAP. See Chapter 16.

### Appendix VI. (Chapter Fifteen)
### Root of the Matter: Immune System Support

Additional anti-amalgam websites:

1.  http://www.flcv.com/indexa.html
2.  http://www.flcv.com/amalg6.html **Mercury Exposure Levels from Amalgam Dental Fillings; Documentation of Mechanisms by Which Mercury Causes over 30 Chronic Health Conditions**; Bernard Windham, Editor – Chemical Engineer
3.  http://www.mercurypoisoned.com/new/mercury_connection_ and_seizures.html **Dental Amalgam Mercury Syndrome** B. Windham (Ed.) includes further links.
4.  http://www.fda.gov/cdrh/meetings/090606-summary.html US/FDA Center for Devices and Radiological Health: **Joint Meeting of the Dental Products Panel (CDRH) and the Peripheral and Central Nervous System Drug's Advisory Committee (CDER)–September 6-7, 2006 (Summary).** Text downloaded at: http://www.fda.gov/AdvisoryCommittees/ CommitteesMeetingMaterials/MedicalDevices/ MedicalDevicesAdvisoryCommittee/DentalProductsPanel/ ucm125150.htm
5.  www.toxicteeth.org. Consumers For Dental Choice, a consortium of consumer advocates from all walks of life whose goal is education and effective government oversight on mercury use in dentistry.
6.  http://articles.mercola.com/sites/articles/archive/2009/08/22/

Once people learn more about the concerns of many regarding dental amalgams: their continuous vapor emissions, their constant galvanic electrical currents, and their occasional contra indicated position next to another metal, they often immediately want their amalgams replaced. This sounds reasonable until one realizes removal presents several problems. First it releases a tremendous burden of vaporized mercury. Remember the vaporization measured in Dr. Boyd Haley's study was emitted from one exposed surface. In drilling for removal, the surface area is exponentially increased. Don't overlook that fillings are removed by grinding away material with a drill. This exposes vastly more surface area than the original amalgam presented. Also, the drill produces friction expressed as heat! Heat significantly vaporizes mercury.

If you make a personal decision to replace your amalgam fillings, the International Academy of Oral Medicine and Toxicology offers guidelines for amalgam removal. Many doctors prepare their patients for the procedure by boosting their immune systems in various ways, making sure they digestive tracts are working optimally, then using the following the protocol as a minimum starting point:

**Suggestions from the International Academy of Oral Medicine and Toxicology (www.iaomt.org) over the years for safe mercury filling removal that protects both staff and client.**

During chewing the patient is exposed to intraoral levels, which are several times the EPA allowable air concentration. Once the drill touches the filling, temperature increases immediately vaporize the mercury component of the alloy. Jerome mercury vapor analyzers used by industry have measured upwards of 1000 mc/l concentrations of mercury arising from drilling to remove these fillings.

**Eight steps greatly reducing everyone's exposure.**

1.  **Keep the fillings cool**
    All removal must be done under cold-water spray with copious amounts of water. Once the removal has begun, the mercury vapor will continuously release from the tooth.

2.  **Use a high volume evacuator**
    Keep a high volume evacuator tip near the tooth (1/2 inch) at all times to evacuate this vapor from the area of the patient. If using a rubber dam, use high speed suction under the dam, too. Polishing amalgam creates very dangerous levels of mercury and should be avoided especially for the mercury toxic patient.

3.  **Provide an alternative air source**
    All patients having amalgam removed or placed should be provided with an alternative air source (oxygen mask) and instructed to not breathe through their mouth during treatment. If just air is used it should be clean and free of mercury vapor preferably from outside the dental office.

4.  **Immediately dispose of the mercury alloy**
    Wash and vacuum particles of mercury alloy as soon as they are generated. The filling should be sectioned and removed in large pieces to reduce exposure.

At present the International Academy of Oral Medicine and Toxicology (IAOMT) has approved removal both with and without the use of a rubber dam. Some evidence exists to support both views since high levels of mercury and amalgam particles can be found under the dam. All members are agreed that whether or not a rubber dam is used the patient should be instructed to not breathe through their mouth or swallow the particles. Some experts feel that it is better to remove the amalgam first and then apply the dam if needed for restorative procedures.

5.  **Lavage, and change gloves**
    After the fillings have been removed, take off the rubber dam if one was used and lavage the patient's mouth for at least 30 seconds with cold water and vacuum. Remove your gloves and replace them with a new pair. If a restorative procedure is next then reapply a new dam and proceed.

6.  **Immediately clean patient**
    Immediately change patient's protective wear and clean their face, including their protective face cover.

7.  **Consider nutritional support**
    Consider appropriate nutritional support before, during and after removal. Before beginning, be certain the patient is eliminating regularly so released mercury is not reabsorbed.

8.  **Keep room air pure**
    Install room air purifiers or ionizers and fans for everyone's well being.

**Staff Protection:**

OSHA requires employees be given written informed consent before the use of any toxic chemicals of which mercury is one. Elemental mercury vapor is one of the most toxic forms of mercury and should not breathed. Women of childbearing age should be exposed to no more than 10 percent of the OSHA MAC. Women who are pregnant should be exposed to no mercury. If you use mercury or remove mercury in any form the National Institute of Occupational Safety and Health (NIOSH) has recommended that your employees be medically monitored annually.

**Any mercury exposure requires that the employee wear an approved mercury filter mask!**

An approved mask is appropriate for wearing during all dental procedures, which will expose you or your staff to mercury.

The manner in which dentists operate their equipment dramatically affects the amount of mercury released. Never drill on mercury high dry. It is hazardous to you, your staff, and your patient. Levels as high as 4000 m g/M3 have been measured 18" from the drill when used high dry. Levels over 1,000 m g/M3 are measurable upon opening an amalgam-mixing capsule.

1. IAOMT Standards of Care Preferred Procedure Approved 9/27/92. [These are minimal guidelines. The IOAMT constantly upgrades suggestions as research illustrates better precautions.

2 EPA United States Environmental Protection Agency Office of Health and Environment Assessment Mercury health effects update Final Report EPA–600/8–84–019F 1971 EPA

3. Cooley RL, Barkmeier WW: Mercury vapor emitted during ultra speed cutting of amalgam. J Indiana Dent Assoc 57:28–31, 1978

4. OSHA Job Health Series: Mercury.(2234)8/1975

5. Hazard Communication Program Federal Register/ Vol. 52. No. 163 / Monday, August 24, 1987

6. OSHA MAC is Threshold Limit Value of 100 micrograms/ cubic meter or 100 PPM This is a never to be exceeded standard.

7. Koos BJ and Lango LD, "Mercury Toxicity in the pregnant woman, fetus, and newborn infant: A review." *Am J Obstetrics and Gynecology* 1976;126(3):390–409.

8. Mine Safety Association high levels and 3M mercury dust mask lower levels.

## Appendix VII. (Chapter 16)
## A. In Between Clean!
## Flossing

Fewer and fewer people choose to floss manually. That is, most clients now use the various flossers now available. The Johnson and Johnson Reach flosser is popular because of its size and design.

Many still want to use their fingers, yet remain awkward because they are self-taught. Their main obstacle is how to anchor the floss and to know which fingers do what. The most common difficulty arises when one anchors the floss using the most dexterous and independent fingers – the index fingers. The lassoed index fingers are then used to awkwardly manipulate the floss around the teeth.

Or more awkwardly, the middle fingers manipulate the floss while the index fingers – get in the way. Not only are most people's middle fingers inept at maneuvering floss in the back of the throat, but also all the other fingers create an artificial "stop." It becomes difficult to reach the back teeth or manipulate the floss adequately.

I ought to know. I stubbornly followed this technique during my first year in hygiene school. When I finally tried the following technique, flossing was far simpler!

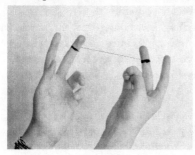

Anchor about 18" of floss by lightly wrapping it around the first knuckle of the middle fingers. Leave about 5 inches of floss in between the fingers.

Move your middle fingers out of the way to allow the index fingers to floss your lower teeth.

- For best control your fingertips should be only slightly further apart than the width of your teeth.
- Gently tease the floss through tight tooth contacts with a light sawing or rocking motion. If necessary, go through a tight contact with the floss at a slant.
- Once through the contact, as you reach the gum line, curve the floss into a "C" shape against one of the teeth.

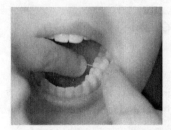

• Gently scrape **vertically** up and down each tooth, including behind the back tooth. Unwind new floss as necessary, though it is not critical to use a new portion of floss each time. You are simply breaking the bonds of the sticky plaque from your tooth. Your gums produce a fluid that constantly clears the "collar"; your saliva then clears it from your mouth. I suggest burnishing the surface with about 5 vertical repetitions or until "squeaky-clean."

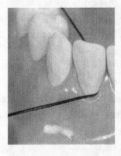
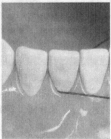

• Reverse the "C" shape to floss the opposite tooth. Avoid cutting across the base of the triangular-shaped tissue that fills the space between the teeth. You will eventually obliterate it!
• **Do not feel you must push hard against your gums. Once you reach the bottom, if the floss is curved, only go as far as the gums allow you to. If you force it, you can create permanent tears (floss clefts) in your gums.**

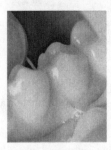

**Left: The floss does not curve around the tooth enough. The tissue is blanched from inappropriate pressure and could tear permanently if hard downward pressure is repeated over time.**

Remember, your gums may bleed for the first few days, indicating your gums are infected. As your gums heal, the bleeding stops.

Those with dental bridges, multiple fused implants, and orthodontic arch wires and brackets might consider using Oral B® Superfloss with a stiffened tip that threads under dental work. These are often easier than using loop threaders. Floss Fish and Platypus flossers also simplify flossing around orthodontic appliances.

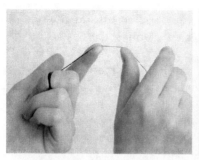 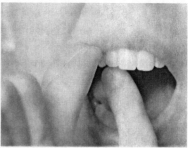

Floss the top teeth using a thumb and an index finger; again fingers are closely spaced on the floss. Reach your thumb under your cheek to reach your back teeth. This means if you are flossing your left side, your left thumb and right forefinger are used. On the right side, use your right thumb and left forefinger.

Many dental care specialists suggest various mechanical flossers. The Sonicare AirFloss has helped many of my clients, who could or would not otherwise clean between their teeth. Many other interdental cleaners are available to try. Anything that can be reliably and gently slipped under the gums on **both** sides of each space without damaging teeth or gums is useful.

When gum disease is present, it is crucial to seek advice from a professional, as specialized techniques may be necessary.

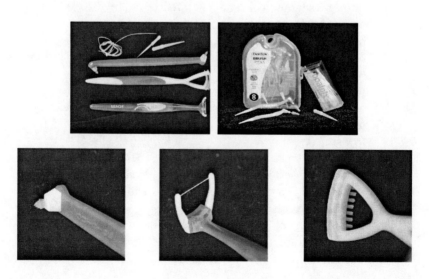

## B. What Water Fluoridation Opponents Say
### more online links and information:

- Link to an interview with Dr. Hardy Limeback, Bsc, PhD, DDS, Associate Professor and Head of Preventive Dentistry, University of Toronto and President of the Canadian Association of Dental Research, Dr. Limeback was originally Canada's primary proponent of fluoride, but now feels strongly against its use in public water systems. See: http://video.google.com/videoplay?docid=-3153312008186362773

- http://www.youtube.com/watch?v=aK9LfSqoHAk relates an interview with Dr. Hardy Limeback about his recent change of heart on fluoridation.

- http://www.zerowasteamerica.org/ADA,Fluoride,&Liability.htm highlights practical viewpoints about why water should not be fluoridated – in line with what dentistry has said about overexposure. Fluoride seems to have the same "whoops factor" mercury fillings have. Concerns about environmental dissemination that leads to unacceptable biological concentrations might just be what makes us all finally reevaluate the science and reasoning behind past common practice and thought.

- http://www.youtube.com/watch?v=SoJ0EQE4KEo

- http://articles.mercola.com/sites/articles/archive/2010/07/01/paul-connett-interview.aspx

- http://www.zerowasteamerica.org/Fluoride.htm

- http://www.zerowasteamerica.org/CaseAgainstFluoridation.htm

- www.nofluoride.com

- www.fluoridealert.org (Note this is: ".org." " .com" will lead you to an ADA sponsored web site, which you should also feel free to visit.)

- http://www.youtube.com/playlist?list=PL616C72C204DF8901. A historical view is introduced in this video link that chronicles a renowned investigative journalist, Christopher Bryson, as he spends ten years investigating fluoride. It discusses why and how the "science" of fluoridation became so accepted.

- One may want to read *Fluoride, the Aging Factor* by John Yiamouyiannis, PhD in which he explains:

1. "Hydrofluoric acid is used to refine high octane gasoline, to make fluorocarbons and chlorofluorocarbons for freezers and air conditioners, and to manufacture computer screens, fluorescent light bulbs, semiconductors, plastics, herbicides, and toothpaste.
2. Once in the body, fluoride is a destroyer of human enzymes. It does this by changing their shapes. In human biochemistry, thousands of enzymes are necessary for various essential cell reactions that take place every second we're alive. Without enzymes, we'd die instantaneously.
3. Since enzymes are proteins, once they've been changed, they're now foreign-looking. The body now treats them as invaders, even though they're part of that body. This is known as an autoimmune situation – the body attacks itself.
4. Another way to look at it: enzymes are long-chain proteins held in certain shapes. Hydrogen bonds are the Velcro strips that hold the enzyme in a certain shape. Fluoride comes along and hydrolyzes the enzyme: cuts the Velcro strips away. The shape collapses. It is no longer an enzyme; now (it's) just a foreign protein."

Many people attempt to avoid fluoride through filtration or by buying non-fluoridated bottled water. They need to check carefully because most bottled water contains fluoride. Ozarka and Mountain Valley water do not. Additionally, Mountain Valley water uses glass bottles that do not leach bisphenols. Some people use reverse osmosis to filter the tiny fluoride element and other contaminants. It does work, but be aware it leaches out all minerals. Since most of us are mineral deficient, it is imperative to replace the minerals.

Other ways to avoid fluoride exposure: avoid processed and restaurant foods and beverages as much as possible. Stick to organic foods and wash them well, since they can be sprayed with cryolite. Avoid non-stick cookware. The fluorine atoms in nonstick coatings are not as biologically inert as we were assured. Toxic fluorine gases emitted while cooking are called perfluorochemicals (PFCs). They have come under serious scrutiny as a major toxin. See: http://www.ewg.org/search/site/perfluorochemical%20other.

"Mineral Waters of the World" (http://www.mineralwaters.org/) is creating a database that lists the contents of bottled waters all over the world. It is far from complete, but for the United States, one can click on www.waters.com to find a company that has fluoridated and non-fluoridated water available in at least 40 states.

*Note for those undergoing orthodontics: about fifteen percent of people undergoing orthodontics manifest a nickel allergic reaction to their appliances. The gums appear infected. Fluoride mouthrinses (especially stannous fluoride compounds) corrode the common metallic brackets and wires, exacerbating this allergy.

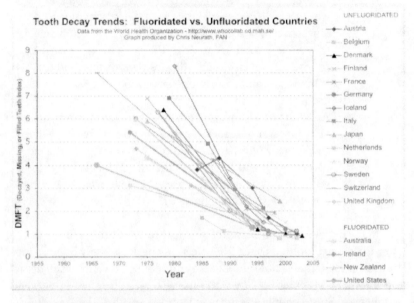

Tooth Decay Trends: Fluoridated vs. Unfluoridated Countries
Data from the World Health Organization - http://www.whocollab.od.mah.se/
Graph produced by Chris Neurath, FAN

**Decay rates around the world have decreased about at the same rate, whether one lives in a fluoridated or non-fluoridated area. Factors outside of enforced water fluoridation must be at work. Chart courtesy of Dr. Paul Connett, Professor of Chemistry at St. Lawrence University, and founder of Fluoride Action Alert.**

## Appendix VIII.
## X-Ray Guidelines

Many clients take a cautious approach towards x-rays and appropriately ask if there are official guidelines for frequency. I encourage them to discuss their particular concerns with their dentist. Official guidance comes from the American Dental Association, the U.S. Department of Health and Human Services, and the FDA. The guidelines call for reorganizing the practice format of dentists to bring them into line with the ALARA Principle (As Low As Reasonably Achievable). The principle states:

"Radiographic screening for the purpose of detecting disease before clinical examination should not be performed. A thorough clinical examination, consideration of the patient's history, review of any prior radiographs, carries (decay) risk assessment, and consideration of both the dental and general health needs of the patient should precede radiographic examination." Clients deserve a clear, communicated need for x-rays based on individual risk.

A critical, but often overlooked good practice guideline requires using a leaded collar over the neck to protect the radiation-susceptible thyroid gland. This collar is sometimes integrated into the required apron, but is sometimes separate.

The website: http://www.ada.org/sections/professionalResources/pdfs/Dental_Radiographic_Examinations_2012.pdf documents these guidelines as well as those governing frequency. Insurance codes are beginning to reflect more conservative benefit schedules to reflect these guidelines.

Dental offices that use medical practice formats and follow their state Dental Practice Acts (in states where hygienists do not have independent practice) practice as follows:

– Conduct a thorough clinical exam

– Order appropriate x-rays. Refer to specialists for therapy as necessary. This includes specific recommendations for hygiene therapy.

– Conduct a pretreatment conference with a written estimate, the opportunity to discuss treatment options, and documented informed consent.

Those that follow this protocol find it simplifies trust, time, and fee issues between clients and their doctors.

Note: As you have read, x-rays are evidence of damage long past. X-rays begin to show loss only when bone mass reaches sixty percent, decay when it has progressed about two to three millimeters into the sub-enamel layer. Minimally Invasive Dentists rely on earlier and more accurate detection in conjunction with x-rays.

## Appendix IX
## Resources

**Academy of Biomimetic Dentistry**. An organization of professionals dedicated to conservative dental techniques that improve the typical quality of dental care through early diagnosis & intervention, minimally invasive procedures for oral hard and soft tissues, adhesive bonding techniques, and innovative biomaterials. These techniques reduce the need for tooth preparation, strengthen the remaining tooth, and help prevent the repair-replacement-repair cycle currently utilized in traditional dentistry. About eighty percent of a traditional dental practice is currently focused on replacement of previous restorations. **They also encourage dental sleep medicine training.** (www.AcademyofBiomimeticDent.org.)

**American College of Integrative Medicine and Dentistry** (ACIMD). http://www.ozonefordentistry.com The medical community determines the standard of care for ozone, its purity, and its uses. Frank Shallenberger, MD, the president of the American Academy of Ozonetherapy (AAOT), is also a founding member of the International Scientific Committee on Ozonotherapy (ISCO3), whose purpose was to standardize scientifically acceptable ozone practice. The resulting "Madrid Protocol." was signed by the AAOT, and European, and Latin American ozone societies. A key point of the protocol is that ozone generators meet EU standards to assure the public the ozone product is pure/medical grade. The Longevity ozone generator (www.ozonegenerator.com) complies with the Madrid Protocols. The AAOT can guide you to protocol-compliant educational groups, of which the American College of Integrative Medicine and Dentistry (ACIMD) is one. These practitioners are noted on my database. Be sure to contact me if you are ACIMD-trained and want to be included! The public is searching for you!

**The North American Association of Facial Orthotropics (NAAFO):** An organization of doctors, myofunctional therapists, and other associated professionals who implement techniques that bring good facial balance through proper oral posture. Not only does this help children remain attractive throughout life, but appropriate therapy can open their airways up to 31%. This should keep many young patients from snoring and/or having obstructive sleep apnea in adulthood. Parents will find their website invaluable: www.orthotropics-na.org

**Advanced "Plug and go" clean air/clean water system for dentists available soon.** I will post it on my website when it is available.

**Gut/Brain Connection:** Cyrex labs offers tests that "evaluate complex thyroid, gluten, and gut-associated disorders and its related neurodysregulation." Repeated exposure to inflammatory messengers from constant gut inflammation and leakiness can disrupt the blood brain barrier, eventually leading to neurodegenerative disorders. Their tests assist health care practitioners to sort out leaky gut syndrome problems like gluten allergies. To help patients reestablish gut barrier function, they test for predictive antibodies that identify dietary and environmental triggers. (www.cyrexlabs.com)

**pHion Diagnostic Test Strips:** The most accurate pH saliva testing strips. Strips and resources for building alkaline reserves at: http://www.phionbalance.com/.

**Tom's of Maine and The Natural Dentist:** Gluten-free oral hygiene products.

**Respected Supplement Companies – there are many other good neutraceutical companies available now.**

**Exceptional Nutritionals:** Supplements and protocols designed to help support various health concerns. They will soon offer educational courses by DVD. (ExceptionalNutritionals.com)

**Glutathione:** Protandim® can boost levels. So can liposomal gluathione. (RediSorb by Complementary Prescriptions) The fatty exterior of liposomal GSH is made from the same material as cell membranes , which allows it to bypass the digestive tract to enter the blood stream. The lipid exterior also protects the water-soluble interior that keeps glutathione in its active state. Again, maintain good digestive tract flora and a high fiber diet when detoxing or chelating with glutathione or any other agent to prevent toxin reabsorption.

**ProBiora3™ oral probiotic (Evora):** Contains three bacterial strains (*Streptococcus oralis, Streptococcus uberis,* and *Streptococcus rattus)* isolated from orally healthy humans. These strains normally colonize the mouth and have well documented oral health benefits. The first two (*S. oralis* and *S. uberis*) inhibit gum disease-causing pathogens by producing hydrogen peroxide. As an added benefit, hydrogen peroxide helps whiten teeth and oxidize the volatile sulfur compounds (VSC) responsible for bad breath. *S. rattus* is a very close relative of a bacteria hghly implicated in decay called *S. mutans.* However *S. rattus* is unable to make the acidic metabolic waste product of sugar metabolism its cousin uses to cause tooth decay. It helps crowd out its decay-causing cousin in the mouth. Though we all can benefit, especially consider it for those who are disabled, institutionalized, have a dry mouth whether from pharmaceuticals or from other reasons, the aging, and for those undergoing orthodontic care. Find it at: Walgreens, Target, CVS Pharmacies.

**Standard Process:** Whole Food Supplements and purifying programs marketed through professionals.

**Xymogen:** Partners with some of the most respected international manufacturers, universities and researchers to offer its proprietary formulas. Many of them are based upon exclusive licenses from partners such as Johns Hopkins University. They have found a place in many functional medicine practices. I particularly recommend their products designed to boost energy production (ALAmax and Resveratin and their CoQ10 supplement: CoQ Max CF. See Menu items #4 and #6.)

## Thyroid issues

**Iodine loading test:** ZRT's Comprehensive Iodine Thyroid Test in Dried Urine and Blood Spot: While measurement of urinary iodine levels may provide useful information on one's iodine nutritional status, sufficient levels does not always guarantee that adequate amounts of thyroid hormones will be synthesized by the thyroid gland. ZRT combines the technology of measuring iodine in dried urine (DU) with thyroid hormone measurements in finger prick dried blood spots (DBS) to create what is called the Comprehensive Iodine Thyroid Test. The Iodine-Thyroid Profile is designed to evaluate not only iodine availability, but also its capacity to be utilized for thyroid hormone synthesis. The thyroid gland's capacity to utilize iodine for thyroid hormone synthesis is determined by measuring thyroglobulin, TSH, total T4, free T4, free T3, and TPO antibodies in finger-prick whole blood dried on filter paper. (http://www.zrtlab.com/patients/iodine)

**Lugol's solution:** A highly recommended form of iodine supplementation, but regulations make its availability difficult. Over-the-counter solutions are often diluted. Many states now require a prescription for regular Lugol's solution (10% total iodine from 10% potassium iodide and 5% iodine in water). Currently, Ioderal tablets may be the easiest way to supplement. Enhance iodine uptake with riboflavin and niacin; these help incorporate iodine into hormones and cells.

**OralDNA® Labs** (a subsidiary of Quest Diagnostics® Incorporated (www.oraldna. com): Provides diagnostic tests based on DNA testing of saliva. Currently, OralDNA® Labs offers:

- MyPerioPath® - Salivary DNA test that determines the cause of periodontal infections
- MyPerioID® PST® - Salivary DNA test that determines increased risk for severe periodontal infections
- OraRisk® HPV - Salivary DNA test that determines who is at increased risk for HPV-related oral cancers

**Dental DNA:** Polymerase chain reaction DNA testing for 147 pathogens frequently found in root canals and cavitations. The report states areas of the body commonly affected by these anaerobes. They also offer tests for gluten intolerance and genetic susceptibility for Alzheimer's Disease. (5082 List Drive; Colorado Springs, Colorado 80919; 719-219-2826; RWheeler@DentalDNA.us)

## Appendix X
### Menu For Immune System Support
### Synopsis from Text

Synopsis of many of the immune boosting suggestions recommended in *Mouth Matters*:

**1. Address grief and anger.** These emotions block or limit nutrient transport into and toxin transport out of cells. High magnification of cell membranes show these transport systems shut down when angry, are active when happy, and even more active when meditating/praying. These transport systems operate at full speed when laughing.

**2. So laugh often!**

**3. Learn to manage stress.** Through the adrenal hormones cortisol and DHEA, the precursor to human sex hormones, the adrenal glands influence most body functions. Poorly functioning adrenals leave a person exhausted and hormone depleted. The destruction of the adrenal glands may be the most significant challenge a person faces as they try to overcome health problems. Cortisol, an adrenal hormone, works with insulin to maintain healthy levels of circulating glucose (blood sugar) and to regulate the flow of glucose (the chief source of cellular energy) into cells for energy production. (There is a pithy saying, "Sugars feed cancers.") To generate energy for your response to the stressor, the adrenal glands produce more cortisol. This helps raise blood sugar levels so cells can accept more glucose. Elevated blood sugar, in turn, requires higher levels of insulin to get the glucose from the blood into the cells. When this cycle repeats frequently, cells fatigue.

**4. Alpha Lipoic Acid (ALA).** The more energy generators (mitochondria) you have within each cell and the more ALA available, the more body fat you will burn. ALA increases the number of mitochondria within each cell and is also a critical coenzyme that helps the mitochondria generate energy. This antioxidant also recycles other antioxidants – vitamins C and E. ALA is known to lower blood sugar levels. Diabetics use it to treat nerve damage. ALA also elevates glutathione levels! (See #5 below)

Since ALA is both water and fat soluble, it can move into all parts of a cell to neutralize free radicals. Vitamin C, on the other hand, is limited to the watery parts of cells because it is soluble only in water, while vitamin E is only fat soluble. ALA is particularly good at crossing the blood-brain barrier to reduce oxidative stress in the brain.

ALA further regulates immune cells, called T-cells and provides protection against the toxins arsenic, cadmium, and mercury. I recommend those with pink-colored dental appliances take it due to the released cadmium. It may bind to other metals like iron, copper and zinc. It may be beneficial to include a B-complex supplement in a regimen containing alpha lipoic acid. The preferred form is R-alpha lipoic acid in conjunction with methylated resveratrol and quercetin, which extends the life of resveratrol.  Example: Xymogen's:  ALAmax CR Take two tablets 30 minutes before breakfast and 1 tablet 30 minutes before dinner. You may take this with Xymogen's Resveratin. Take one 2 X per day. Many people take ALA in conjunction with Acetyl L-Carnitine. Together they are known to boost the immune system even in HIV patients.

**5. Glutathione.** Glutathione levels are deficient in many inflammatory disease states. Glutathione (GSH) is so protective of our well being that every human cell can synthesize it from three amino acids (L-cysteine, L-glutamic acid and glycine). GSH's most important functions are commonly remembered with the acronym "AIDE": Anti-oxidant, Inflammation reducer, Detoxifier, Energizer.

**6. CoQ10.** CoQ10 has been shown to significantly enhance immune cells' ability to kill bacteria and elevate the immune system's antibody response, especially in those with cancers and degenerative diseases like diabetes and heart disease. It seems to decrease tumor numbers in those exposed to carcinogens. For those that do develop tumors, it seems to increase survivor rates.

Further, CoQ10 helps drive mitochondrial energy production in each cell and helps fight the oxidation that happens as that energy is produced. The heart is the body's hardest working organ. Beating incessantly, its cells require more oxidation protection than any other organ. CoQ10 minimizes oxidation partly because it recycles antioxidant vitamins C and E. Antioxidants reduce damage to DNA, especially mitochondrial DNA. Most of the damage the heavy metals mercury, plutonium, and lead produce, stems from the proliferation of the free radicals they cause and the resultant decrease in cellular energy production (ATP). If you suspect you have heavy metal toxicity from any source, including "silver fillings", it is important to supplement with CoQ10. CoQ10 will help maintain an efficient heart, normalize blood pressure, and lower cholesterol and blood sugar levels. Aging, infections, and statin drugs like Lipitor and Crestor lower naturally occurring CoQ10 levels. (Xymogen's CoQ Max CF is an example of one supplement with superior absorption.)

**7. Limit or curtail simple carbohydrates** in your diet, including refined flours, sugars, and alcohol. Among many other things, sugars feed cancers, decrease white blood cells' ability to fight bacterial invaders, and cause glycation of red blood cells. These glycated hemoglobins are large, sticky and sharp. They can severely damage blood vessel walls, especially in fragile tissues like those of the eyes and kidneys. Sugars also raise insulin levels. Insulin in low levels promotes healing; at consistently high levels, health deteriorates.

**8. Limit fruit juice and fructose-laden beverages.** The liver metabolizes the fructose into the worst kind of LDLs, called VLDLs. These are the "bad cholesterols" that indicate blood vessel damage. Drink water; eat whole foods. Whole foods are perfect little nutrition and fiber packets. Doctors often encourage people with high levels of VLDL cholesterol to consume more green vegetables, fresh fruits and whole grains. This increases dietary fiber, which regulates the speed of sugar entrance into the bloodstream and also helps lower cholesterol levels.

**9. Limit caffeine and chocolate.** Both raise blood glucose, cholesterol, and uric acid. They decrease levels of chromium, magnesium, and zinc. They also help create leaky gut syndrome. See Cyrex Lab video.

**10. Limit alcohol consumption,** which, like other sugars, also raises levels of blood glucose, cholesterol, and depletes magnesium, manganese, potassium, and folic acid.

**11.** Low **DHEA** levels encourage diabetes through several pathways, including increased inflammation, decreased insulin sensitivity, and control of fat to muscle ratios. Several forms of dementia are increasingly associated with diabetes and low DHEA levels. Supplements are available.

**12. Biotin.** (Egg yolks, milk, poultry, broccoli, and fish) or supplement. They are rich in biotin, an important B vitamin. Biotin is involved in many steps of energy metabolism.

**13. Vanadyl sulfate,** sometimes prescribed for diabetics, Vanadyl sulfate and insulin each move glucose out of the bloodstream. Because they use different pathways, vanadyl supplements may help lower insulin levels. They may also help protect pancreatic beta cells that produce insulin.

**14. Chromium.** Found in whole grains, nuts, and particularly broccoli, chromium works with insulin to utilize glucose. It activates insulin and changes cell membranes to allow sugars to exit the bloodstream to enter cells. Chromium, though stripped from sugars and grains during the refining process, is nonetheless essential for their metabolism. Worse, diets rich in sugars accelerate chromium excretion. This means that chromium stores are depleted rather than augmented every time one eats refined carbohydrates. Chromium insufficiency has been hypothesized to be a contributing factor to the development of Type 2 diabetes.

**15. Zinc.** Excessive sugar consumption also depletes zinc. Zinc is a component of the insulin molecule that moves sugar out of the blood stream. Zinc combats cold and flu viruses. It also aids wound healing and supports the immune and reproductive systems, especially the prostate. Zinc also supports healthy liver function.

**16. Probiotics.** Liberally enjoy unpasteurized fermented foods like natto, miso, kefir, and sauerkraut to help repopulate your gut with good bacteria, destroyed by antacids, sugars, and other processed foods. While fermented foods deliver many times the beneficial bacteria of supplements at a fraction of the cost, probiotic supplements can help, especially after taking antibiotics or straying from a healthy diet. Take quality supplements with fiber so they last long enough to survive  until they get to the intestines. Prebiotic, high fiber foods like bananas, whole grains, greens, tomatoes, onions, legumes, and garlic are important because they help probiotic bacteria survive long enough to gain a foothold in your gut. Yogurt has many beneficial bacteria, but if you are using it to replace good bacteria destroyed by refined carbohydrates, it makes no sense to add sugar. Unpasteurized kefir contains friendly bacterial strains as well as beneficial yeasts. These yeasts likewise maintain balance. They control and eliminate pathogenic yeasts because these small molecules can penetrate the intestinal lining where unhealthy bacteria and yeasts reside. Kefir also helps digest the food you eat. Beyond improved food digestion and assimilation, probiotics influence genes' disease-fighting capabilities. They may even help lower blood pressure!
Note: Fermented soy increase isoflavone availability, and decreases the negative effects of phytic acid found in nonfermented soy products such as tofu, soy milk, nuts, baby formula, and other processed foods. Phytic acid binds to nutrients and thus, hinders their absorption. Nattokinase, found in natto, has an enzyme produced in the fermentation process that has a powerful ability to dissolve blood clots and seems to dissolve the amyloid plaques in the brain associated with Alzheimer's. (Fibrin is a key indicator of whole-body inflammation.)

**17. Drink pure, filtered water.** Realize whatever is flushed into the city water supply is in your water – hormones, heavy metals, cleaners, solvents, medical wastes, and prescription drugs. Chlorine reacts with organic materials in water to form trihalomethanes and other compounds far more toxic than chlorine itself. Reverse osmosis (RO) filtration is an option, if wasteful. Some specialized filters that remove fluorine as well as chlorine, both of which displace iodine in your thyroid. The removed minerals can then be added back in several ways such as Himalayan or Celtic salts and other mineral mixtures designed to adjust water. Try to avoid bromine, such as in brominated flour and processed foods that contain bromine, which also displaces iodine in the thyroid.

**18. Avoid or limit processed foods.**

**19. Exercise.** Exercise improves your blood chemistry. Doctors can look at your red blood cells and easily tell if you do. It increases the number of energy generators in each cell (mitochondria), which profoundly influences how you process energy. Remember, Lance Armstrong's muscle fibers had about 23,000 mitochondria/cell at one time. Since diabetics have trouble in all ways with energy use This affects how energetic you feel. It changes hormone balance, stabilizes insulin levels, and improves digestion, circulation, mental and physical agility, blood pressure, oxygen transport, liver function, metabolism, sleep patterns, reaction time, mood, and sexuality. Exercise reduces stress, depression, breast cancer risk, heart attack, and osteoporosis. Exercise curbs emotional eating. When you exercise, muscular contractions pump lymph throughout your body. The lymphatic system is integral to immune system function. Unlike the heart that pumps blood through the circulatory system, the immune system has no pump. It depends on muscular contractions to pump lymph. A regular exercise routine creates improved discipline and self-esteem. Finally, exercise sculpts your body. You may not lose a lot of weight, but fat pounds convert to muscle. Exercise until you feel energized, but not exhausted. Enjoying a massage after exercising is a pleasurable way to augment lymph movement.

**20. Get eight hours of sleep every night.** Work with your circadian rhythms, largely defined by your body's natural rhythm of cortisol. Go to bed and rise with the sun. Sleep in a completely dark room. Even the lights of an alarm clock can rocket cortisol levels and interfere with restful sleep.

**21. Know the smoking points of your cooking oils.** Don't ever let them smoke. Smoking is the sign that oils are deforming and oxidizing, otherwise known as going rancid. Smoking point depends on purity, acidity, and the age of the oil, as well as how it is manufactured. Roughly here are the smoking points of a few oils:

| | | | |
|---|---|---|---|
| "Off the shelf" butter | 250° | Almond oil | 420° |
| Clarified butter | 300° | Palm oil | 455° |
| Ghee | 485° | Avocado oil, refined | 520° |
| Unrefined coconut oil | 350° | Olive oil, extra virgin | 320°+ |
| Refined coconut oil | 450° | Olive oil, virgin | 391° |

Avoid "heart healthy" canola oil. See Chapter Fourteen.

**22. Selenium** assists the body to make glutathione peroxidase, an important antioxidant enzyme. Glutathione peroxidase reduces inflammatory mediators. Deficiencies are seen in conditions oxidative stress such as some cancers, cataracts, asthma, Parkinson's, and Alzheimer's disease.

The inorganic form, selenite, is often offered in supplements because it is cheaper. This form is somewhat toxic however, and it reacts with vitamin C to form elemental selenium that humans cannot absorb. In studies, scientists use L-selenomethionine, the organic, bioavailable form. Plants that provide us with cereal grains and nuts convert inorganic selenite to L-selenomethionine. Two Brazil nuts equal 100 micrograms of L-selenomethionine supplementation. Mushrooms and sunflower seeds are also excellent sources if grown in non-depleted soils. Animal proteins and eggs also provide this source. Plants in the onion/garlic and broccoli families might provide the most important cancer-protective and bioavailable form of selenium, L-Se-methylselenocysteine. These also activate tumor-suppressor genes that fight cancers.

**23. If you are going to eat meat, eat only pasture-raised meat and eggs, butter, and cheese from animals that are truly pasture-raised.** The typical American diet drips with the omega-six fatty acids that accelerate inflammation and that derive from corn-fed animals. These feedlot agribusiness-raised animals cause most of us to have a dietary fatty acid ratio of about 25/1 (omega-6/omega-3) instead of the healthier goal of 1/1. Pasture-raised animals and their products bring a diet much closer to the ideal: about 4/1.

**24. Supplement with high quality, carefully-handled omega 3 oils** or eat cold-water seas fish often. Eat only wild salmon, not farm-raised. Omega-3 oils are generally anti-inflammatory. I like krill oil because it is harvested from cold-water seas and, if kept cool during processing and transportation, it has not oxidized into a damaging compound. Krill is so low on the food chain it is not a source of additional mercury.

**25. Supplement with potassium citrate** while you adjust to eating mainly foods that alkalize the body. Enzymes work in a very narrow pH range. If your diet is mainly highly processed foods, your body will always be trying to neutralize the acidity, to the detriment of your health.

**26. Vitamin D** is actually a steroid hormone with far-ranging influences on health through its interactions with thousands of genes. Beyond cancer protection (vitamin D kills cancer cells), vitamin D is the body's main calcium regulator. It maximizes calcium absorption, which encourages strong bones. Just as importantly, when blood does not maintain proper calcium levels, the parathyroid hormone signals bones to release calcium, which exacerbates osteoporosis. Anything that causes bone loss is generalized to the jawbone, causing gum disease to accelerate.

Vitamin D may help prevent falls by making muscles stronger and by improving coordination. Preliminary evidence suggests vitamin D may fight inflammation, which in turn helps control gum disease. The Public Health Agency of Canada is investigating whether optimal vitamin D levels diminish flu severity. Vitamin D can also protect against respiratory infections and stroke.

As with so many things, the dose makes the poison. Vitamin D is fat soluble, therefore it is stored in fat tissues. Toxic doses can accumulate, so check blood levels before you supplement. DiaSorin, Inc. has recently developed an automated immunoassay called Liaison, which provides clinically accurate results. If necessary, I suggest liquid vitamin D$_3$ drops to be used under the tongue.

Before choosing to take Vitamin D, however, be sure you evaluate "Vitamin D as a Paradox" in the osteoporosis chapter.

**27. Curcumin (found in the spice, turmeric)** inhibits the transformation of cells into tumor cells and inhibits tumor cell proliferation. It helps the body destroy cancer cells so they can't metastasize and helps blunt blood supply formation in tumors so they can't grow. Turmeric also decreases inflammation. Use it in cooking, as heat releases its powers.

**28. Magnesium** – to balance calcium. Magnesium relaxes blood vessel walls, helps maintain normal muscle and nerve function, keeps heart rhythm steady, supports a healthy immune system, and keeps bones strong. Magnesium also helps regulate blood sugar levels, promotes normal blood pressure, and is involved in energy metabolism and protein synthesis. There is increasing interest in magnesium's role in preventing and managing disorders such as high blood pressure, cardiovascular disease, and diabetes. Magnesium can help slow noise-related hearing loss and can reduce ringing and buzzing in the ears. Since an excessive influx of calcium ions can cause nerve death, a balanced calcium/magnesium intake ratio can provide protection.

In the pre-agrarian days when humans evolved, calcium to magnesium intake was about 1:1. Diets today usually reflect a skewed ratio. In dairy products it is often about 12:1. As magnesium and calcium compete for absorption in the gut, modern diets are often deficient in magnesium. High sugar intake depletes magnesium for instance. Low magnesium levels impair absorption of vitamin D, calcium, and phosphorus. If you supplement with these vitamins, be sure you also supplement with magnesium.

Try to avoid magnesium stearate. Magnesium stearate is an excipient with no nutritive value. It is a filler, carrier, and adds anti-caking properties. Stearates are most commonly produced by hydrogenating cottonseed oil. They are pre-oxidized and contain heavy pesticide residues. Those made with organic palm oils would be a better choice. Stearates can coat every particle in a supplement, which may lead to compromised nutrient absorption. Magnesium may suppress the immune system's T-cells. A rule of thumb when buying vitamins in general is to buy only veggie caps. Magnesium stearate is a particular hallmark of shellacked, hard-shelled vitamins, which often exit the digestive tract completely intact. Preferred forms: magnesium citrate, picolate, or magnesium L-lactate dihydrate. Telling you to avoid magnesium stearate is easy. Doing it is difficult because most vitamins include it. The best advice is to avoid vitamins with a hard, shellacked outer coating. Choose gel-caps when possible. Best to enjoy green leafy veggies in abundance!

**29. Vitamin $K_1$** is necessary for clot or scab formation. Without it, hemorrhaging risks increase. People with stroke risk should be aware of this since careful control of blood viscosity is a preventive goal for their condition. Vitamin $K_1$ also plays a role in normal bone growth and development.

$K_2$ plays a vital role in orchestrating where and how calcium in the body will be utilized. It deposits calcium in the right places like bone and blood and keeps it from being deposited in the wrong places, like arterial plaques where it stiffens blood vessels, or into oral plaque which create hardened deposits.

**30. Test for iodine.** If after an iodine loading test you are found to be deficient, supplement with Ioderol or Lugal's solution. Iodine is essential for preventing breast and prostate cancers and for proper thyroid function. Its natural place in the human body is often supplanted by excess sources of the other halide elements, especially fluoride and bromide. See resources section.

**31. Remove sources of heavy metal toxicity and think carefully about your position on the wisdom of root canals.**

**32. Trocotrienols (known together as "Vitamin E")** are some of the most important phytonutrients in edible oils. Beyond their well-known antioxidant powers, various forms can help reduce cholesterol, reverse atherosclerosis in the carotid artery, protect the heart from oxidative stress, inhibit clotting, and can inhibit some kinds of tumor growth, especially of breast and prostate.

There are eight naturally occurring forms – four tocopherols and four tocotrienols. Plant-based edible oils are rich source for tocotrienols. Crude palm oil extracted from the fruits of oil palm are particularly high in tocotrienols. Palm, rice, wheat barley, rye, oats and raw almonds are good sources. Tocomin® is a good supplement source.

**33. If you smoke, stop.**

**34. Always breathe with your diaphragm.** Practice several meditative breathing periods during each day.

**35. Control your body's acid-alkaline balance.**

**36. Coconut oil.** Great for diabetics because it provides instant energy without blood sugar spikes. It also stabilizes weight gain and is easily digestible, needing no special enzymes to be easily utilized. It speeds up metabolism! (By trying to fatten up their livestock with inexpensive coconut oil, farmers found out in the 40s that it had the opposite effect. Their livestock because lean and active. Many animal and human research studies have demonstrated that replacing long chain fatty acids like vegetable fats with medium chain fatty acids like coconut oil results in both decreased body weight and reduced fat deposition.) Coconut oil also increases thyroid activity. A sluggish thyroid is one reason why some people can't lose weight, no matter what they do. It is also anti-microbial and a good oil for the brain and for cell membranes.

Degenerative diseases circle around three primary concerns: what kinds of oils you choose to incorporate into your diet; how they are manufactured and used (including omega-3/omega-6 fatty acid ratios), glycation from simple carbohydrate intake and other sources, and free radical damage (oxidation).

**37. Keep it clean! (Your mouth, that is.)**

**38. Eat foods high in anti-oxidants. (See chart in book.)**

## Tests to consider:

- Vitamin D test: Through a compounding pharmacy or Diasorin Lab
- hsCRP test: Tests for total inflammatory load. Available at compounding pharmacies or visit www.mouthmattersbook.com for links to two options
- Iodine Loading Test: See Resources section.
- A1C test that measures blood sugar control over about a three-month period. At compounding pharmacies, online, or visit www.mouthmattersbook.com for links to two options
- IL-1 levels (PST test – Oral DNA Labs) a test for genetic predisposition. Especially helpful for smokers.
- Thermography imaging: to test for inflammatory "hot spots". (about $300.00 and up)
- Darkfield microscope to examine blood quality – can visualize fibrinogen and red blood cell clumping, indicating inflammatory mediators are high.
- Many dental offices offer hs-C-Reactive Protein tests as an adjunct to treating gum disease and its risks. Administered in-office or in the home, one source for these tests is Healthy Life Labs (www.healthy-lifelabs.com). Another company, Direct Labs (https://www.direct-labs.com/Home/tabid/36/language/en-US/Default.aspx), offers the same tests, but also measures VLDLs in their lipid panel. Anyone can order a test from Direct Labs, but they must visit a LabCorp lab (3000 locations nationwide) for the test and access results with any mobile device or a computer.
- PLAC Test, measuring LP-PLA$_2$ levels. Approved for assessing stroke risk. Those with gum disease are at 1.8 times the risk of significantly elevated levels.

## Appendix XI
### RDA Toothpaste Abrasivity Index

The RDA Index here is a toothpaste abrasivity index. The higher the value, the more abrasive it is. Loss of tooth structure is based on abrasivity, frequency of use, type of toothbrush, and brushing technique. If you do not know the RDA of your toothpaste, call the consumer contact information on the package.

04 Toothbrush with plain water
07 **Plain baking soda**
15 Waleda Salt Toothpaste
19 CariFree CTX Gel
30 Waleda Plant Tooth Gel
35 Arm & Hammer Dental Care
40 Waleda Children's Tooth Gel
45 Walenda Calendula Toothpaste
45 Oxyfresh
49 Tom's of Main Sensitive
52 Arm & Hammer Peroxicare Regular
53 Rembrandt Original
53 Closys
57 Tom's of Main Children's
63 Rembrandt Mint
68 Colgate Regular
70 Colgate Total
70 Arm & Hammer Advance White Sensitive
78 Biotene
79 Sensodyne
80 Close-up
83 Colgate Sensitive Max Strength
87 Nature's Gate
94 Rembrandt Plus
95 Oxyfresh with Fluoride

95 Crest Regular
103 Arm & Hammer Sensitive
104 Sensodyne Extra Whitening
106 Colgate Platinum
117 Arm & Hammer Advanced White Gel
107 Crest Sensitive Protection
120 Closeup with Baking Soda
124 Colgate Whitening
130 Crest Extra Whitening
144 Crest Multicare Whitening
145 Ultra Brite Advanced Whitening
150 Pepsodent Tartar Control
165 Colgate Tartar Control
176 Nature's gate Paste
200 Colgate 2-in-1

200 **FDA Recommended upper limit**

250 **ADA Recommended upper limit**

Some companies like Natural Dentist consider RDA values to be proprietary information. Other companies like Young Living, Jason, and Peelu are unavailable because these companies do not test abrasivity.

## Appendix XII
### Is There Really Such a Thing as "Metal-Free Dentistry"?
Posted by Gary M. Verigin, DDS, CTN at drvee.wordpress.com

As more people become aware of the health risks of mercury amalgam fillings, you see more dental practices marketing themselves as "metal-free." Sounds great, no? It's also inaccurate – and not just because these dentists often do place metal restorations such as gold crowns. As dental materials expert Jess Clifford has noted, "There is no such creation as a metal-free restorative" – not even tooth-colored restorations. All modern composites, glass ionomers (dental cements), porcelain and ceramics contain some metal. It's not that "metal-free" dental offices are trying to mislead you. They just seem to be using it as shorthand for "mercury-free dentistry." But it's still inaccurate.

And it makes it very easy to think of just about any non-precious metal as dangerous. Consider, for instance, this excerpt from an article on the website of Dr. Hal Huggins, a pioneer in the fight against dental mercury:

> I became curious about the composition of porcelain crowns and called one of the manufacturers. I was told their porcelain was pure ceramic. Thanks. I called another and asked what their ceramic was made out of. Porcelain I was told. I called another and asked what their porcelain ceramic was made out of. Natural products. Knowing that mercury was "natural" I went to scientists other than manufacturers. Natural porcelain ceramic is made from clay B kaolin specifically B which is 45 percent aluminum oxide. Oh! So porcelain crowns are really aluminum. The aluminum does come out of the crown and I have personally seen some tragic cases of poisoning from dental porcelain ceramic aluminum crowns. Obviously not everyone has violent reactions, but when they occur, it is not a happy site [sic].

Scary, no? Makes you want to avoid porcelain all together, doesn't it? There's just one problem: aluminum oxide is a benign form of the element. As Clifford explains while aluminum in its "fully reduced (shiny metal) form…will react with a vast number of chemical constituents," some of which are highly toxic,

> "not all forms of aluminum are readily reactive, nor do they have appreciable toxicity concerns. In order to be a toxic problem, aluminum must be ionizable or dissociable or otherwise available to bind chemically with tissue constituents. **If the aluminum does not have opportunity to chemically separate and bind, toxic constituents are simply not formed.** [emphasis added]

In short, it's not the metal itself but the kind of metal that matters. According to Clifford, "benign" forms of aluminum include alumina and aluminosilicate, in addition to aluminum oxide.

*In such fully oxidized forms, the aluminum is either completely bound, or is part of a chemical matrix in crystalline lattice form, or both. Some common occurrences of these forms of aluminum are quartz, mica, feldspar, opal, glass and basic sand. While it is technically possible to force aluminum to chemically separate from any of these materials, it would require extreme furnace heat or high irradiation energy. These conditions are not commensurate with life and tissue survival.*

\*\*\*

*Dental products are not the only ones where we find the benign forms of aluminum. The glass jars which contain our foods and beverages on the grocer's shelf are basically barium-boro-aluminosilicates. Sand on the seashore is a rich mix of aluminum oxide and various aluminosilicates. Glass utensils, dishes and vessels in the kitchen (ie., Pyrex, Kimax, Corningware, Stoneware, Anchor-Hocking) are similar aluminosilicates and aluminum oxides. In our bodies, by nature, the bones are comprised of 2.0% – 2.5% aluminosilicate, aluminum oxide or alumina. If the patient can safely have food or beverage stored in glass, or can safely eat food prepared in a Pyrex pan or bowl, or can safely walk on sand, then it becomes immediately obvious that these forms of aluminum are not a threat to good health. The aluminunosilicate/ aluminum oxide content of the bones is supplied and replenished daily from the fruits, grains and vegetables of the diet. The aluminosilicate content of lettuces and other vegetables in a single fresh garden salad serving will easily exceed the total quantity of aluminum released in ionized form from a mouthful of porcelain or ceramic crowns over a period of years.*

*He adds that only time when even benign forms of aluminum are contraindicated is when an individual tests sensitive to both aluminum and silicates.*

You can read his complete paper – "Should I Be Worried About Aluminum in Fillings and Crowns?" at http://biologicaldentalhealth.com/Data/cliff_al.pdf.

Where sensitivity or reactivity is a concern, we always recommend testing to be absolutely sure we choose restorative materials that the client will be able to tolerate. This includes both energetic and blood serum compatibility evaluations. Energetic testing is done via EAV and matrix imaging. For blood serum analysis, we rely on the Clifford Materials Reactivity Test, which reports on 94 chemical groups and families in more than 11,000 trade name dental products. For assessing material quality, it's the method of choice for conscientious holistic and biological practitioners. Energetic testing, on the other hand, gives us insight to the quantitative scenario, as well – how much of any given material may be safely used.

You may also want to consult http://drvee.wordpress.com/?s=implants

# Index

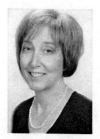

Carol Vander Stoep brings a combination of experience, research, and passion to this book. Over her thirty-year career in dental hygiene she has looked into the mouths of thousands of people and observed the startling range of what can result from poor lifestyle choices and the neglect of oral care.

She has observed that problems are not confined to the poor or uneducated – behind those winning smiles of the rich and famous can lie inflamed sores and degenerative bone disease. Too few realize the consequences of neglect go beyond teeth and gums, sweet breath or captivating smiles; the mouth is the most exposed gateway into our bodies and what goes on within it or passes through it has profound implications elsewhere in our bodies, undermining overall health.

While acquiring extensive clinical experience, Carol came to realize that the place of oral hygiene within dentistry and the place of dentistry within preventive medicine hinders public and professional awareness of the role oral care should play in our daily lives and how medical providers approach patient care. A Bachelor of Science degree from Baylor University provided the foundation of knowledge, enhanced by extensive research and study with leaders in a wide variety of fields in the professional medical community. Applying science in her clinical practice helps refine simple techniques that work for her clients and help her hone her verbal motivational skills.

As Carol's concerns grew, her awareness of the system and respect for the importance of professional discipline convinced her to carry her message beyond the confines of her place in a dental office. That realization led her to bring together the perspectives, the stories, and the knowledge she has acquired to prepare this book.

Carol is active in the Academy of Biomimetic Dentistry and is a founding member of The American Academy of Oral Systemic Medicine (AAOSH). She finds time to kayak and travel while continuing her professional work as a hygienist, consultant, orofacial myofunctional therapist, and speaker to professional audiences and the general public.

~ ~ ~

*It's not that some people have willpower and some don't. It's that some people are ready to change and others are not.*

**James Gordon, M.D**

CPSIA information can be obtained at www.ICGtesting.com
Printed in the USA
LVOW06s0809240713

344286LV00004B/7/P